THE MEDICAL SERVICES HANDBOOK FUNDAMENTALS AND BEYOND

Second Edition

Cindy A. Gassiot, CPMSM, CPCS
Program Coordinator, Medical Staff Services Degree Program
El Centro College
San Antonio, Texas

Vicki L. Searcy, CPMSM
Vice President, Consulting Services
Morrisey Associates, Inc.
Temecula, California

Christina W. Giles, CPMSM, MS
President
Medical Staff Solutions
Nashua, New Hampshire

With Foreword by Hugh Greeley
HG Healthcare Consultants, LLC

JONES AND BARTLETT PUBLISHERS
Sudbury, Massachusetts
BOSTON   TORONTO   LONDON   SINGAPORE

World Headquarters
Jones and Bartlett Publishers
40 Tall Pine Drive
Sudbury, MA 01776
978-443-5000
info@jbpub.com
www.jbpub.com

Jones and Bartlett Publishers
Canada
6339 Ormindale Way
Mississauga, Ontario L5V 1J2
Canada

Jones and Bartlett Publishers
International
Barb House, Barb Mews
London W6 7PA
United Kingdom

Jones and Bartlett's books and products are available through most bookstores and online booksellers. To contact Jones and Bartlett Publishers directly, call 800-832-0034, fax 978-443-8000, or visit our website, www.jbpub.com.

Substantial discounts on bulk quantities of Jones and Bartlett's publications are available to corporations, professional associations, and other qualified organizations. For details and specific discount information, contact the special sales department at Jones and Bartlett via the above contact information or send an email to specialsales@jbpub.com.

Copyright © 2011 by Jones and Bartlett Publishers, LLC

All rights reserved. No part of the material protected by this copyright may be reproduced or utilized in any form, electronic or mechanical, including photocopying, recording, or by any information storage and retrieval system, without written permission from the copyright owner.

This publication is designed to provide accurate and authoritative information in regard to the subject matter covered. It is sold with the understanding that the publisher is not engaged in rendering legal, accounting, or other professional service. If legal advice or other expert assistance is required, the service of a competent professional person should be sought.

Production Credits
Publisher: David Cella
Associate Editor: Maro Gartside
Editorial Assistant: Catie Heverling
Senior Production Editor: Renée Sekerak
Marketing Manager: Grace Richards
Manufacturing and Inventory Control
 Supervisor: Amy Bacus
Composition: Toppan Best-set Premedia Limited
Cover Design: Nancy Deutsch and Kristin E. Parker
Cover Image: © Bocos Benedict/ShutterStock, Inc.
Printing and Binding: Malloy, Inc.
Cover Printing: Malloy, Inc.

Library of Congress Cataloging-in-Publication Data
Gassiot, Cindy A.
 The medical staff services handbook : fundamentals and beyond / Cindy A. Gassiot, Vicki L. Searcy, Christina W. Giles ; with foreword by Hugh Greeley.—2nd ed.
  p. ; cm.
 Rev. ed. of: The medical staff services handbook / [edited by] Cindy A. Gassiot, Vicki L. Searcy, Christina W. Giles. c2007.
 Includes bibliographical references and index.
 ISBN 978-0-7637-8441-6
 1. Hospitals—Personnel management—Handbooks, manuals, etc. I. Searcy, Vicki L. II. Giles, Christina W. III. Medical staff services handbook. IV. Title.
 [DNLM: 1. Medical Staff, Hospital—organization & administration. 2. Credentialing. 3. Managed Care Programs. 4. Quality of Health Care. WX 203 G253m 2010]
 RA971.35.H366 2010
 362.11068'3—dc22
                                                                              2009053268
6048

Printed in the United States of America
14 13 12   10 9 8 7 6 5 4 3 2

Dedication

This book is dedicated...

To John, my best friend and soul mate; to my wonderful friends and colleagues in medical staff services, some of whom I have known for 35 years; and to my students.
    C.A.G.

To all the people who have supported me throughout my years in working in health care. That includes my three children, who were always supportive of everything that I wanted to try. And now my grandchildren—Summer, John Thomas, Samantha, Sabrina, Xander, and Cathryn—who help keep me grounded into what is really important: love, laughter, and time spent with people who you love and who love you back unconditionally.
    V.L.S.

To all newcomers to the field and those who continue to strive to better themselves and their organizations; to my children, Brett and Amy, and my grandchildren, Elle, Evelyn, Cade, and Angel—the hope for the future!
    C.W.G.

Contents

Foreword	xv
Preface	xvii
Acknowledgments	xix
About the Editors	xxi
Contributors	xxiii
Reference Materials Provided on Accompanying CD	xxv

CHAPTER 1 ■ Introduction to Medical Staff Services — 1

Jodi Schirling, CPMSM

The National Association Medical Staff Services	1
Certification Programs	1
Formal Education Programs	2
The Medical Staff Services Professional	2
The Medical Staff Services Department	18
Performance Improvement in the MSSD	31
Expanded Roles	33
Conclusion	38
Notes	38

CHAPTER 2 ■ Healthcare Organization Accreditation 39

Cindy A. Gassiot, CPMSM, CPCS
Mary A. Baker, CPMSM, CPCS, DHA

Introduction	39
Hospital Accreditation	39
International Healthcare Accreditation	49
Long-Term Care Accreditation	51
Managed Care Organization Accreditation	52
Ambulatory Care Accreditation	54
Rehabilitation Facility Accreditation	56
Commission on Accreditation of Rehabilitation Facilities	57
Centers for Medicare and Medicaid Services	57
International Organization for Standardization	59
Reviewing Credentials Files in an Accreditation Survey	60
Notes	61

CHAPTER 3 ■ The Medical Staff Organization 63

Cindy A. Gassiot, CPMSM, CPCS
Vicki L. Searcy, CPMSM

Introduction	63
The Medical Staff Organization	64
Accountability	65
The Traditional Model Medical Staff Organization	66
Developing Medical Staff Leaders	72
Medical Staff Bylaws	72
Relevance of the Medical Staff Organization	73
Barriers to Success with the Traditional Medical Staff Organization	73
Alternatives to the Traditional Medical Staff Organization	74
Notes	77

CHAPTER 4 ■ Medical Staff Bylaws and Related Documents — 79

Christina W. Giles, CPMSM, MS

Definitions	79
Medical Staff Bylaws and Related Manuals	80
Medical Staff Bylaws and Related Manuals Revision Project	83
Reviewing the Amendment Process	86
Major Considerations for a Medical Staff Bylaws Revision Project	87
Distribution of New Documents	92
Conclusion	92
Notes	93

CHAPTER 5 ■ Physician Executives — 95

Vicki L. Searcy, CPMSM

Historical Perspective	95
Hospital Trustee Accountability	95
Hospital Reimbursement	96
Problems of Traditional Hospital Medical Staff Leadership	97
The Physician Executive	98
Notes	102

CHAPTER 6 ■ The Hospital Credentials Process — 103

Vicki L. Searcy, CPMSM

Why Credential? What Are Credentials?	103
Key Terms	105
Key Players and Their Roles	106
Applicable Standards	110
Credentialing Documents	110
The Pre-application Process	113
Application for Membership and Privileges	116
Processing the Application	120
Red Flags	134

Evaluation and Decision-Making Process	142
Staff Reappointment	143
Conclusion	149
Notes	150

CHAPTER 7 ■ Hospital Privileging — 151

Christina W. Giles, CPMSM, MS

Delineation of Privileges	151
The Joint Commission Requirements	157
Centers for Medicare and Medicaid Services Requirements	158
Developing and Revising Privileges	159
Implementation of New Forms	160
Criteria for Granting Privileges	162
Process for Adding New Privileges	166
Focused Professional Practice Evaluation	167
Proctoring	174
Ongoing Professional Practice Evaluation	176
Temporary Privileges	182
Locum Tenens Privileges	183
Disaster Privileges	185
Telemedicine Privileges	186
Privileges That Cross Specialty Lines	188
Turf Battles	189
Documentation of Privileges	189
House Staff, Medical Students, and Other Trainees	190
Practitioners with Low Volume of Activity	192
Reprivileging and Profiling	192
Clinical Activity Requirements Related to Competency	197
Privileging Questions	198
An Innovative and Creative Solution	199
Acknowledgment	200
Notes	200

CHAPTER 8 ■ Credentialing Allied Health Professionals — 213

Cindy A. Gassiot, CPMSM, CPCS

What Is an Allied Health Professional?	213
Historical Perspective	213
The Current Picture	214
Who Must Be Credentialed and Privileged	216
Multidisciplinary AHP Committees	216
AHP Policy	217
The Application Form	217
Delineation of Privileges	219
Scope of Practice	219
Processing the Application	219
Reappointment of AHPs	220
Competency Assessment	221
Maintaining Expirables	221
Due Process for AHPs	222
Conclusion	222
Web Sites	223
Notes	223

CHAPTER 9 ■ The Managed Care Credentials Process — 225

Christina W. Giles, CPMSM, MS

Background on the Managed Care Credentials Process	225
Types of Managed Care Organizations	226
The NCQA Accreditation Process	227
Practitioner Credentialing	228
Contracting Versus Credentialing	233
Managing Credentialing Operations	234
Automation	235
Organization of the Credentialing Department	238
State and Federal Requirements	239
Notes	239

CHAPTER 10 ■ Health System Credentialing and Credentials Verification Organizations 241

Margaret Palmer, MSA, CPMSM, CPCS

Credentialing in a Healthcare System	241
Credentials Verification Organizations	249
To Outsource or Not to Outsource to a CVO	252
NCQA CVO Certification Standards	253
URAC CVO Certification Standards	257
The Joint Commission CVO Guidelines	257
CVO Operating Models	258
CVO Computer Operations	259
Security of Practitioner Data	260
Conclusion	260
Notes	261

CHAPTER 11 ■ The Role of the Medical Staff in Quality Improvement 263

Curtis Pulllman, MHA

Introduction	263
The Transparent Environment of Health Care	263
Historical Overview: Form Versus Function	265
Quality Functions That Involve the Medical Staff	267
The Role of the Medical Staff in Quality Improvement	268
Patient Safety	278
Reporting Quality Functions	281
Case Review	287
Notes	292

CHAPTER 12 ■ Program-Specific Accreditation 293

Cindy A. Gassiot, CPMSM, CPCS

Institutional Review Boards	293
Approved Cancer Programs	297
Approved Trauma Centers	301

Continuing Medical Education Programs	303
Graduate Medical Education	306
Notes	308

CHAPTER 13 ■ Physician Health and Behavior Issues — 311

Cindy A. Gassiot, CPMSM, CPCS

The Impaired Practitioner	311
Causes of Practitioner Impairment	312
Hospital-Based Programs	312
A Contract with an Impaired Practitioner	317
Monitoring Recovery	319
The Americans with Disabilities Act	319
The Aging Physician	320
The Disruptive Practitioner	321
Assistance in Dealing with Practitioner Behavior and Health Problems	323
Assistance for Other Professionals	324
Notes	324

CHAPTER 14 ■ Effective Meeting Management — 325

Jodi Schirling, CPMSM

When to Establish Committees	325
Understanding the Role of the Committee	326
Effective Meetings	327
Preparation Phase	328
Conducting Phase	334
Purpose of Meeting Minutes	338
Recording and Documenting Meeting Minutes	339
Minutes Formats	344
Legal Aspects of Minutes Documentation	345
Follow-up Phase	346
Virtual and Paperless Meetings	347

Tools for Effective Meetings	348
Conclusion	352
Notes	352
Bibliography	353

CHAPTER 15 ■ Introduction to the Law — 355

Carla DiMenna Thompson, JD

The Legal System	355
The Courts	356
What Happens in a Civil Lawsuit?	358
Statutes, Laws, and Regulations	360
Tort Law	362
Restraint of Trade	366
Notes	367

CHAPTER 16 ■ Medical Staff Law and Important Legal Cases — 369

Joanne P. Hopkins, JD, BSN, MSN

The Medical Staff	369
Medical Staff Liability Issues	372
Appointment and Clinical Privileges	374
Quality Improvement and Corrective Action	386
Procedural Rights of Review	391
Legal Issues in Corrective Action and Hearings	394
Peer Review Privileges of Confidentiality and Immunity	401
Credentialing in the Managed Care Setting	406
Conclusion	410
Notes	410
Appendix A: Significant Case Law Summary	413
Appendix B: The Practitioner's Hearing Rights Under the Health Care Quality Improvement Act	422
Appendix C: Recommended References on Legal Issues	423

CHAPTER 17 ■ Supporting Corrective Action and Fair Hearing Procedures — 425

Cindy A. Gassiot, CPMSM, CPCS

Role of the Medical Staff Services Professional	425
Corrective Action	425
Steps in the Corrective Action Process	426
Planning for a Hearing	426
Correspondence	427
Orientation of the Hearing Panel	428
Evidence Notebook	428
Arranging the Hearing Room	428
The Hearing	429
Follow-up	430
Examples of Language to Insert in Notice Letter	430

Instructions for Completion of the Continuing Education Quizzes — 434

Index — 435

Chapter Quizzes — 453

Foreword

When asked to write the foreword for this important new addition to credentialing literature, I felt honored. After reviewing the excellent chapters I am hopeful that many others will feel the same. The authors have accomplished a marvelous objective by synthesizing an enormous amount of critical material in a very readable format. Medical staff service professionals, credentials coordinators, managed care associates, and physician leaders will undoubtedly find this book to be a valuable and continuing resource as they constantly improve their own individual credentialing programs and enhance their knowledge of this important patient safety program.

The process of "credentialing" exists for three vital purposes. The first is to protect the patient, who has very little ability to question or determine the qualifications and competence of any particular physician; the second is to facilitate clinical practice because no physician may legally practice in a hospital without a grant of clinical privileges; and the last is to protect the organization from legal, regulatory, societal, and accreditation embarrassments.

One wonders what would have been the fate of Darling, Johnson, and Elam had the hospital's credentialing programs been administered by well-read and highly skilled credentialing professionals? Might Michael Swango have been prevented from injuring patients throughout the United States if the credentialing process had followed the advice of dedicated credentialing experts? Is it likely that Mr. Themoglie would not have been allowed to provide clinical service to hundreds of managed care patients if a simple licensure check had been performed by a certified credentialing coordinator? Would "Doc Barns" have been allowed to conduct physical exams on FBI agents if his credentials had been verified by a certified MSSP instead of an HR specialist?

A few readers of this excellent new book may not be familiar with the names in the foregoing paragraph; however, once you have had an opportunity to study the following chapters you will be well versed in concepts behind these and many other poignant examples of credentialing failures. You will better understand how to assist in preventing such catastrophes in the future. As you peruse this book you will also gain valuable insight concerning various accreditation options, the need for adequate form to follow function and substance, physician leadership development, and much, much more.

Congratulations to Cindy, Vicki, Chris, Jodi, Margaret, Curtis, Carla, and Joanne.

Hugh Greeley
Managing Director
HG Healthcare Consultants, LLC

Preface

The *Second Edition* of *The Medical Staff Services Handbook: Fundamentals and Beyond* has been revised and updated to reflect changes in hospital accreditation standards and practices relating to credentials verification and support for the organized medical staff in healthcare organizations. The intended audience for this book includes students in medical staff services academic programs, medical staff and credentialing service professionals, those individuals who are studying for the certification exams provided by the National Association Medical Staff Services, students in other allied health programs, professionals working in the quality and risk management departments in hospitals, paid and voluntary medical staff leaders, and those who have an interest in the organized medical staff and its functions.

Competent professionals working in medical staff service departments in hospitals and other healthcare delivery organizations, as well as managed care organization credentialing departments and credentials verification organizations, are key to successful administration of the organized medical staff or a panel of providers in a managed care organization. This book presents how-to information on state-of-the-art processes that are crucial to the functions performed by those departments.

Patient safety begins with the credentialing and privileging of all licensed independent practitioners and the identification of the level of competency of each practitioner. All of those activities are the primary functions carried out by the medical staff services or credentialing professional. In this *Second Edition*, both chapters on credentialing and privileging have been revised and updated. There still remains a great deal of confusion about what is best practice for credentialing and privileging allied health professionals. These professionals are playing an increasingly important role in healthcare delivery and, therefore, are becoming much more common in the hospital and ambulatory care arenas. The difficulty and confusion about their credentialing and privileging persist because of the variations in state laws and regulations governing allied health professionals; this book outlines a basic approach and discusses the various issues that should be considered as part of these processes. All other chapters in the text have been likewise revised and updated.

Whether the reader is a seasoned veteran of medical staff services or a student just learning the ins and outs of the field, this book offers solutions to the dilemmas most commonly encountered by the medical staff services professional. The CD that accompanies the book contains all exhibits from the text as downloadable and printable PDF files as well as many other helpful forms, policies, and samples, some of which are only included on the CD.

In addition to the useful CD, at the end of this book there is a series of quizzes that readers can complete for as many as 16 National Association Medical Staff Services–endorsed CEUs.

We hope that our readers will gain valuable information and timely answers and will grow professionally by reading about the experiences and knowledge of the many successful and experienced medical staff service professional contributors.

Acknowledgments

The editors are grateful once again to the contributors for their work. These very busy people time and again have dropped what they were doing to update and add to their previous work so that we may impart the latest information on state-of-the-art processes in medical staff services for our readers and students in the field. We also acknowledge two new authors, Curt Pullman and Maggie Palmer. We thank Maro Gartside, Associate Editor, and David Cella, Publisher, at Jones and Bartlett Publishers.

About the Editors

Cindy A. Gassiot, CPMSM, CPCS, began her career in medical staff services in 1970 and has held the position of director of medical staff services in several hospitals in Texas and Florida. She is currently the coordinator for the Associate of Science in Medical Staff Services degree program for El Centro College, Dallas.

Ms. Gassiot is past president of the National Association Medical Staff Services (NAMSS) as well as cofounder and charter president of the Texas Society for Medical Staff Services. She served on the NAMSS Board of Directors for six years and was a member of both the Certification and Education Councils. She wrote a column for the NAMSS publication, *OverView* (now called *Synergy*), for several years. Cindy was the driving force behind the certification program of NAMSS and chaired the first Certification Committee, which administered the first certification examinations. She was the first recipient of the Golden Key Award by NAMSS for contributions made to the certification program. The Texas Society for Medical Staff Services also honored her by establishing the Cindy Gassiot Scholarship Award.

Ms. Gassiot is a full-time faculty member at El Centro College, Dallas, and instructs distance education courses for the online medical staff services degree program, for which she wrote the curriculum and syllabus. She is coauthor and coeditor of *Medical Staff Services Manual* published by Center for Health Education (1981), *Principles of Medical Staff Services Science* published by NAMSS (1987), and the previous editions of *Handbook of Medical and Professional Staff Management*, published by Aspen Publications and the Texas Society for Medical Staff Services (1990, 1998, and 2002) as well as the *First Edition of Medical Staff Services Handbook: Fundamentals and Beyond* (published in 2006). She is also coauthor of *AHP Competencies: A Method for Effective Assessment* published by HcPro in 2005.

Ms. Gassiot lives in San Antonio, Texas, with her husband John. The Web site for the medical staff services degree program is http://www.elcentrocollege.edu/Program/Health/_docs/packet/MSST%2009.pdf.

Vicki L. Searcy, CPMSM, is Vice President, Consulting Services for Morrisey Associates (www.morriseyonline.com). Vicki has also been the Practice Director,

Credentialing and Privileging, for the Greeley Company as well as President of the Searcy Resource Group. She was also a partner with BDO Seidman, LLP, a leading accounting, tax, and consulting firm, heading up its national healthcare accreditation and compliance consulting practice.

Vicki is a popular speaker at conferences, seminars, and medical staff and board retreats, speaking on a variety of topics such as credentialing, privileging, peer review, and competency management.

She is recognized as a leading innovator in medical staff services. For example, she has assisted organizations across the United States to achieve operational excellence and has been a successful implementer of the "paperless" medical staff office.

In addition, Vicki has been a pioneer in the field of designing systems related to physician competency, development of privilege delineation systems, and physician profiling. In her position with Morrisey Associates, she has been responsible for the development of the Privileging Content and Criteria Builder, a Web-based system that allows organizations to develop their own privilege forms from Morrisey-provided content.

Vicki was the founding editor for *Health Care Competency & Credentialing Report*. She is a coauthor of *Professional Excellence = Professional Advancement: 101 Smart Things Every Medical Staff Services Professionals Should Do* (published by Searcy Resource Group, September 2005, and available from the National Association Medical Staff Services). Vicki has written numerous articles related to issues in medical staff organization management and quality management, which have been published in a variety of newsletters and magazines.

Vicki lives in Temecula, California.

Christina W. Giles, CPMSM, MS, is President of Medical Staff Solutions, a healthcare consulting company specializing in medical staff administrative issues. Chris has been in the field of medical staff services since 1981, and has served as President of the Massachusetts Association of Medical Staff Services, Northeast Regional representative on the board of directors of the National Association of Medical Staff Services (NAMSS), as a member of the Education Council, and as a NAMSS faculty member since 1989. She has created and presented national seminars on various medical staff administrative and management topics since 1989. She is a founding member of Edge-U-Cate, a speakers' bureau providing seminars, webinars, and training on current healthcare topics.

Ms. Giles is a member of the advisory board for many of the HcPro newsletters. She is a contributing author to *The Credentialing Handbook* (Aspen Publishers), contributing author to *A Guide to AHP Credentialing* (HcPro), and coauthor of *Health Care Credentialing: A Guide to Practical Innovations*.

Ms. Giles lives in Nashua, New Hampshire. The Web site for her consulting firm is www.medicalstaffsolutions.net.

Contributors

Dr. Mary A. Baker, CPMSM, CPCS, DHA
Contract Consultant, Medical Administration
Sidra Medical & Research Center
Doha, Qatar

Cindy A. Gassiot, CPMSM, CPCS
Program Coordinator, Medical Staff Services Degree Program
El Centro College
1719 Red Leaf Drive
San Antonio, TX 78232
PH: 210-494-2847

Christina W. Giles, CPMSM, MS
President, Medical Staff Solutions
Partner, Edge-U-Cate, LLC
32 Wood Street
Nashua, NH 03064
PH: 603-886-0444

Joanne P. Hopkins, JD, BSN, MSN
Attorney at Law
P.O. Box 162834
Austin, TX 78716-2834
PH: 512-327-4647

Margaret Palmer, MSA, CPMSM, CPCS
Director, Credentialing Consulting
Scripps Healthcare System
500 Washington Street, Suite 705
San Diego, CA 92103
PH: 619-260-7294

Curtis Pullman, MHA
Director of Medical Staff/Credentialing Services
University of Texas Southwestern Medical Center
Dallas, TX
PH: 817-313-0265

Jodi Schirling, CPMSM
Manager, Corporate Credentialing
Nemours Foundation
1600 Rockland Road
Wilmington, DE 19899
PH: 302-651-5938

Vicki L. Searcy, CPMSM
Vice President, Consulting Services
Morrisey Associates, Inc.
222 S. Riverside Plaza
Chicago, IL 60606
PH: 312-784-5579

Carla DiMenna Thompson, JD
Attorney
Reed Opera House
260 Lafelle St. 5
Salem, OR 97302
PH: 503-588-2440

Reference Materials Provided on Accompanying CD

EXHIBIT 1-1	Sample Job Descriptions
TABLE 1-1	Competency Checklist
TABLE 1-2	Competency Checklist for Department Using More Electronics
TABLE 1-3	Example of Staffing Analysis for One Committee
EXHIBIT 1-2	Sample Performance Improvement Plan–Medical Staff Services Department
EXHIBIT 1-3	Perfomance Improvement Report–Medical Staff Services Department
EXHIBIT 3-1	Sample Job Description for a Medical Staff Leader
TABLE 4-1	Comparison of 2009–2010 Joint Commission and CMS Bylaws Requirements and NCQA's Policies and Procedure Requirements
TABLE 4-2	Sample Format for Distributing Proposed Bylaws Revisions
EXHIBIT 6-1	Verification Requirements and Methods Document
EXHIBIT 6-2	Sample Initial Application Cover Letter
EXHIBIT 6-3	Sample Initial Application Follow-up Letter
EXHIBIT 6-4	Sample Letter Returning Incomplete Initial Application
EXHIBIT 6-5	Sample Letter Requesting Additional Information for Initial Application
EXHIBIT 6-6	Sample Letter Notifying Applicant of Status of Initial Application
EXHIBIT 6-7	Sample Letter for Voluntary Withdrawal of Initial Application
EXHIBIT 6-8	Sample Policy and Procedure on Credentials Files
EXHIBIT 6-9	Sample Peer Reference Letter and Questionnaire
EXHIBIT 7-1	New Privilege/Service/Treatment Criteria Development and Authorization Form
EXHIBIT 7-2	Sample Proctoring Policy and Procedure and Attachments
EXHIBIT 7-3	Sample Application for Temporary Privileges
EXHIBIT 7-4	Sample Policy and Procedure for Privileges That Cross Specialty Lines
EXHIBIT 8-1	AHP Credentialing Policy and Procedure
EXHIBIT 8-2	AHP Delineation of Privileges
EXHIBIT 8-3	Sample Scope of Practice

EXHIBIT 8-4   Screening Tool for Nurse-Midwife
EXHIBIT 8-5   Screening Tool for CRNA
EXHIBIT 9-1   Job Description for Credentialing Manager
EXHIBIT 9-2   Job Description for Credentialing Specialist
EXHIBIT 10-1   Sample Policies for Shared Credentialing Service
EXHIBIT 13-1   Sample Policy on Physician Health
EXHIBIT 13-2   Responding to Inappropriate Physician Conduct
FIGURE 14-1   Clinical Department Meeting Agenda
FIGURE 14-2   A Guideline to the Basics of Parliamentary Procedure
EXHIBIT 14-1   Meeting Checklist
FIGURE 14-3   Reporting Calendar
FIGURE 14-4   Pending Log
EXHIBIT 17-1   Notice of Hearing
EXHIBIT 17-2   Hearing Committee Recommendations
EXHIBIT 17-3   Notice of Final Decision by Governing Body

Introduction to Medical Staff Services

Jodi Schirling, CPMSM

If you have chosen medical staff services as your career path, you have chosen a challenging, exciting, sometimes frustrating, but ultimately very satisfying career. Many of the veteran medical staff services professionals (MSSPs) are passionate about what they do, and they can't imagine working in any other field. Although most days in a medical staff services department are a whirlwind of meetings, telephone calls, conferring with physicians, and many interruptions, the work is consummately interesting, challenging, and fulfilling. Working with a group of highly educated individuals who always strive for perfection and admire competence (physicians) is gratifying.

■ The National Association Medical Staff Services

The medical staff services profession has evolved over the past 40 years from a strictly clerical position to one that requires a specific knowledge base. This evolution has been greatly assisted by the professional association, National Association Medical Staff Services (NAMSS). Charlotte Cochrane and Joan Covell Carpenter of California established a medical staff services association in southern California in 1971, which evolved into a national organization in 1976. NAMSS offers education and many other resources to its members. Affiliated organizations can be found in all states, and many local chapters exist throughout the country. Information about NAMSS and membership can be found at www.namss.org.

■ Certification Programs

Recognizing that specific knowledge was required to perform the medical staff services and credentialing functions effectively, NAMSS developed a certification program within the first five years of its existence as a national organization. The Certified Medical Staff Coordinator (CMSC) examination was established by a committee led by Cindy Gassiot and was first offered in 1981. It has since evolved into today's Certified Professional Medical Services Management (CPMSM) credential. The CPMSM exam focuses on the management functions in a medical staff services or provider credentialing organization. In 1995, a second certification program was developed by NAMSS for those who specialize in practitioner credentialing, including the managed care arena, known as the Certified Provider Credentialing Specialist (CPCS) examination. The CPCS exam focuses on the functions of provider credentialing. At the time of this writing, in the United States there are currently 1767 CPMSMs, 2557 CPCSs, and 903 individuals who hold dual certification, for a total of 4324 certified persons.

■ Formal Education Programs

Formal education programs in medical staff services have also evolved over the years. The first program was established in Orange County, California, at Cypress College in the mid-1980s, and currently offers an associate degree in medical staff services science. The program consists of 60 semester units and is part of the college's health information technology program. Courses cover medical staff services science, medical quality management, healthcare law, information technology, medical terminology, anatomy and physiology, and supervision and management, among others.

Beginning in 2000, El Centro College in Dallas, Texas, began offering the first distance education associate degree program. An associate of applied science in medical staff services degree is offered with most of the courses presented online. The 64-credit-hour curriculum includes general education courses as well as courses that address credentialing, privileging, healthcare accreditation, organization of the medical staff services department, medical staff law, performance improvement, medical terminology, anatomy and physiology, pathophysiology, and supervisory management courses, among others. During the final semester, students serve an internship in a medical staff services department.

In 2006, the National American University started an online degree program in medical staff services management. The associate of applied science degree focuses on medical staff services administration, accreditation and regulatory compliance, management of credentialing processes, privileging, risk management, medical staff law, medical terminology, peer review, and information management.

NAMSS also offers noncredit online courses on various medical staff services and credentialing topics.

■ The Medical Staff Services Professional

The evolution of the medical staff services profession can be traced back to the development of the medical staff organization. As hospitals began to be held liable for the negligent acts of their medical staff members, and as accrediting organizations strengthened their standards for verifying physician credentials and peer review activities, hospitals began to take a hard look at support for the organized medical staff. In the 1970s, the titles of veteran medical staff secretaries changed to *medical staff coordinators*. Hospital leaders relied more and more on the coordinator to provide guidance and administrative support for regulatory and accreditation requirements for the medical staff organization. Over the years the position expanded and experience gained by the medical staff coordinator was amplified by more formal education provided both by NAMSS and college degree programs. Currently, leaders in the medical staff services department (MSSD) hold titles such as manager, director, and even vice president.

Today, the MSSP plays a vital role in the various healthcare delivery systems. Whether in a hospital, ambulatory care center, credentials verification organization, or managed care setting, the MSSP brings a range of knowledge and skills essential for each type of organization. This chapter focuses on the role of the MSSP and MSSD in the hospital setting.

The MSSP provides coordination for the day-to-day activities of the organized medical (professional) staff. Whether in a multifacility organization, an integrated healthcare delivery system, or a small rural hospital, the MSSP acts as the link between the medical staff, the administration, and the board. This link is facilitated by the access the MSSP has to both the medical staff and the members of the administrative team.

In most cases, the MSSP will be one of the first contacts a physician has with the organization. Through the initial credentials verification process and orientation to the organization, the MSSP and MSSD establish a unique relationship with the practitioner. Medical staff members look to the department for interpretation of bylaws, information on hospital policies and procedures, advice on maneuvering through the sometimes complex administrative structures, and support for the activities of the organized medical staff.

The MSSP also provides a unique service to the hospital administration. Due to the relationships that develop between the department staff members and physicians, MSSPs are sometimes first to know of an underlying issue within the medical staff organization. The issues can be as minor as changes in the physician parking lot or as major as a controversy over new hospital ventures. This information can then be transmitted to the appropriate administrative staff member for attention or resolution.

The MSSP's role is one that engenders trust—from both the medical staff and the hospital administration. Medical staff members need to trust that the MSSP and MSSD maintain confidential information, provide accurate and timely information, and respect the confidences of the physicians. The administration needs to trust that the MSSP and the MSSD will maintain accurate records, follow established procedures and practices in all activities, maintain activities that meet accreditation standards, alert the administration when accreditation standards are out of compliance, and apprise the administration of major issues within the medical staff organization.

Knowledge

To be effective, the MSSP must have a wide breadth of knowledge and the ability to apply that knowledge in several key areas. The U.S. healthcare delivery system is extremely complex. Emphasis on health care in both the political and legal arenas results in an ever-changing system. Both the medical staff and the hospital must deal with the complexity of the various payment systems daily. The MSSP should understand the various components of the delivery system, including how they operate in an integrated fashion. An understanding of the legal system and how the law shapes the delivery system is helpful. There is also a need to understand how the political system impacts the healthcare environment. Healthcare reform has been a hot political topic since the early 1990s, when the Clinton administration first broached the subject.[1] As of this writing, the U.S. government, under the leadership of the Obama administration, is again embroiled in a debate on the need to overhaul the healthcare delivery system. Past attempts at government healthcare reform have resulted in the healthcare industry and private sector reacting and responding to the governmental proposals.

Past issues affecting health care included the implementation of the regulations under the Health Insurance Portability and Accountability Act of 1996 (HIPAA), including the creation of the Health Care Integrity and Protection Data Bank to provide a resource to organizations to help fight healthcare fraud and abuse. More recently, sweeping Medicare reform and Centers for Medicare and Medicaid Services (CMS) compliance guidances have had profound effects on hospital operations. There has been increased Office of Inspector General enforcement within the healthcare industry regarding compliance with such laws as the Emergency Medical Treatment and Active Labor Act (EMTALA), the False Claims Act, and all other aspects of federally funded healthcare programs. Successful MSSPs pay attention to current political agendas that have the potential to affect health care.

Healthcare Financing

An appreciation of the financial components of the healthcare system is required of all MSSPs. At a minimum, a basic understanding of utilization management is essential. The MSSP should be familiar with basic terms used in managed care. The difference between a health maintenance organization, preferred provider organization, or independent practice association should be understood.

In addition, the role of the CMS should be appreciated. In recent years, there has been an increased scrutiny of hospital reimbursement and quality-of-care concerns by CMS. The CMS Quality Improvement Roadmap has as one of its five strategies to pay for health care "in a way that expresses our commitment to supporting providers and practitioners for doing the right thing—improving quality and avoiding unnecessary costs—rather than directing more resources to less effective care."[2] This practice, which is referred to as "pay for performance," has clear import for both hospitals and physicians. In the past, hospitals and physicians have experienced difficulty in getting reimbursed for improving quality and reducing costs because resources have been directed toward providing more care. In 2009, however, CMS adopted a process for denying payment of any patient care services related to a preventable medical error. These events, which include things such as wrong-site surgery, are referred to as "never events." Medical staff services professionals should be aware of the CMS program.

Likewise, the MSSP must be familiar with the various reimbursement systems, with a special focus on how the physician is affected by their rules. One of the many criteria that may be used during the reappraisal and reappointment period is utilization information. Efficiency of physician practice is becoming increasingly more important to hospitals. The MSSP must assure that appropriate information is provided while maintaining a balance between clinical and economic criteria for reappointment.

Medical Staff Organization

The MSSP also needs to understand the basic concepts of medical staff organization—for example, whether the medical staff organization accomplishes its functions in a departmentalized or nondepartmentalized structure. The medical staff organizational structure is defined in the organization's bylaws or other governance documents.

Accreditation Knowledge

Perhaps the most important aspect of the knowledge that an MSSP brings to the hospital is that of accreditation standards. As mentioned in Chapter 2, there are many accrediting agencies with which the MSSP should be familiar, including the Joint Commission, National Committee for Quality Assurance (NCQA), Utilization Review Accreditation Commission (URAC), Centers for Medicare and Medicaid Services (CMS), and Commission on Accreditation of Rehabilitation Facilities (CARF). Additional accrediting bodies include the American College of Surgeons' Commission on Cancer and Committee on Trauma certification programs, the Food and Drug Administration's (FDA's) institutional review boards, and continuing medical education (see Chapter 12). The MSSP must maintain current knowledge of the accreditation standards applicable to his or her facility.

Understanding the standards is not enough, however. The MSSP must also be able to interpret the standards and implement systems to comply with them. For example, the MSSP may need to assist the medical staff in policy development or expansion of their quality improvement process as the standards change. The MSSP must be familiar with *all* of the Joint Commission's standards—not just the section containing medical staff standards. Currently, many standards that affect the medical staff are noted throughout the Joint Commission's manual. In larger facilities, the Joint Commission network standards or the ambulatory care standards may also apply, and the MSSP needs to have a working knowledge of those standards as well.

The Law

Knowledge and understanding of state and federal laws related to licensure and peer review is required for all MSSPs. Because the MSSP may serve as a resource for physicians applying for a state medical license, he or she must understand the requirements for licensure. The MSSP should also know the differences between the various medical training programs—for example, is an MD equivalent to a DO?

In addition to laws and statutes that regulate the practice of medicine, the MSSP must be aware of state laws that have an effect on the medical staff or hospital. Examples of such laws would be those related to organ donation or use of advance directives.

The MSSP also needs to have knowledge of medical staff laws, particularly those relating to medical staff issues such as credentialing, privilege restriction, medical staff membership, restraint of trade, and peer review. Knowledge of the various laws and legal precedents will help the MSSP understand what has to be done and why. The MSSP can then communicate information about the legal implications of peer review to the medical staff. Although the MSSP is not a substitute for legal counsel, he or she can be instrumental in advising the staff when legal counsel should be sought.

The Credentials Process

The MSSP must have a complete understanding of the credentialing process—from initial appointment to privilege delineation to focused and ongoing monitoring to reappointment. This knowledge must encompass not just what to do, but why it is important, and how to establish systems for assuring that the processes are carried out efficiently and correctly.

Technology

The MSSP must have an understanding of current technology. It is up to the MSSP to determine which information is available through computerized or electronic sources. The MSSP must also determine which of the many electronic sources is the most accurate and reliable for the purpose of primary source verification in the credentials process. The acceptable sources should be documented in MSSD policies and procedures. In addition to understanding which sources are available through the Internet or other electronic media, the MSSP must have a good understanding of computers and databases. This professional may find himself or herself in the position to evaluate and select credentialing software, for example. The MSSP must be able to identify the desired features of the software, evaluate and compare products, and then select the product that best meets the needs and the budget of the organization.

The MSSP must also be able to adapt processes and the work flow to maximize efficiencies found through automation. For example, using a software program to send notices to the medical staff members' e-mail addresses or office fax machine can save the MSSD countless person-hours that would otherwise be spent copying, stuffing envelopes, and mailing the same notice. Through this use of technology, staff efficiency would increase while supply costs would decrease.

The technology related to electronic content management has improved significantly in recent years and is widely available. The MSSP must be aware of this type of technology. Using electronic content management systems will facilitate the medical staff services department in limiting or eliminating paper-driven processes. With this kind of system, important documents such as bylaws, policies, procedures, and forms may be scanned and stored electronically. The electronic content management can save costs related to paper, supplies, and storage. Using electronic content management with companion electronic work flows can reduce process time and increase staff efficiencies. The initial investment is well worth the efficiencies gained by adopting this technology.

Information Management

As accreditation organizations such as the Joint Commission and professional certification boards under the auspices of the American Board of Medical Specialties strive to implement processes that focus on competency assessment and evidence-based privilege delineation, the role of the MSSP has evolved to one that includes information management. The MSSP of today must be able to understand how medical staff data interfaces with other databases. He or she must also be aware of the types of databases that exist in the hospital or ambulatory setting and the information contained in each. Such databases may include those holding billing information, clinical informatics (electronic health records), and performance improvement/quality outcome data. The information that comes from the various databases is important for competency management and privileging decisions.

The MSSP serves as a resource to the medical staff in the development of reports that reflect practitioner-specific data. Such practitioner-specific data should focus on providing evidence of competency in clinical care to the medical staff leaders charged with making privileging decisions.

Ethical Issues

Understanding ethical issues surrounding medical staff activities is another important part of the body of knowledge an MSSP brings to the job. Professional ethics, such as codes of ethics related to maintaining professional relationships and confidentiality, must be practiced by the MSSP. The MSSD may be instrumental in assisting the medical staff in establishing an ethics committee. For this reason, the MSSP must understand medical ethics such as patients' rights and responsibilities as well as requests for treatment withdrawal.

Quality and Resource Management

The MSSP should understand the basics of utilization management, quality improvement, risk management, and continuous quality improvement. This understanding can be obtained by working collaboratively with the hospital departments devoted to quality, risk, and utilization management. MSSPs should take advantage of continuing education programs on these topics. Another way to obtain information on these subjects is to keep abreast of current literature. As previously noted, the MSSP should be knowledgeable in database management, which is a key aspect of these disciplines.

Management

The MSSP must be a competent manager. Regardless of the size of the facility or the medical staff organization, the MSSP acts as a manager for many functions and may also manage staff. Knowledge of basic management theory and the ability to apply management skills are essential to the MSSP who wants to advance in the profession.

The MSSP must be involved in planning. Planning focuses on what needs to happen, how it should happen, and which resources are required to make something happen. The annual budgeting process is a good example of planning. A successful MSSP also conducts future planning. What will the department look like in 5 years? In 10 years? This future thinking gives the MSSP the opportunity to incorporate long-range plans in the budgeting process.

Finally, the MSSP needs to be versed in strategy management. Each organization has an overall strategy developed by its leadership, which defines the mission, vision, and goals that need to be accomplished to turn the vision into reality. The MSSP must be aware of the organization's strategy so that any planning and future thinking will support the overall goals of the organization.

Understanding Processes

Many functions are the responsibility of the MSSD. The MSSP must understand and be able to break down a process into distinct tasks and develop procedures for the staff to follow. This type of "assembly-line thinking" is a critical skill for the MSSP who is serving at the coordinator or director level. Multiple staff members must perform a specific function in a consistent manner. In developing systems that are efficient and effective, the MSSP must embrace the available technology and remain open to automating processes. A basic principle underlying continuous quality improvement is the need to understand causes of variation in a process. Embracing technology and automating processes, along with having clearly defined procedures to follow, helps to reduce the variation. Understanding a process makes it easier to develop the necessary procedures.

Budgeting and Finance

The MSSP working in a single-person office or in the role of supervisor or director must have a basic understanding of the budgeting process as well as financial management. He or she must be able to calculate staffing needs and forecast expenses for the department. Most medical staff departments do not produce revenue (an exception might be application fees and/or medical staff dues that are deposited into the organization's general funds). Therefore, the MSSP needs to manage resources prudently. During the fiscal year, this professional must be able to review monthly financial reports to determine any areas that are out of line with the budget. The MSSP should develop strategies for managing the department's resources, such as having the hospital library purchase key journals rather than purchasing them with department funds. Other strategies might include placing controls on ordering office supplies, sharing high-cost resources (such as fax machines) with other departments, or providing staff with the opportunity to participate in continuing education through audio conferences or webinars rather than incurring higher-cost travel to seminars.

Medical Terminology

MSSPs use knowledge of medical terminology in many ways—most specifically in developing systems for the delineation of clinical privileges. Additionally, a good understanding of basic terminology is required for those in the department who support specific committees. Although the MSSP may never be asked to identify the root of a specific medical term, knowledge and correct use of medical terminology enable the professional to communicate more effectively with the medical staff.

Skills

In addition to the requisite knowledge outlined previously, the MSSP must possess the work skills that will enable him or her to run an efficient MSSD. He or she must establish policies and procedures; define processes for work completion; write job descriptions; interview, hire, discipline, and terminate staff; facilitate meetings; manage multiple projects; and implement quality control mechanisms.

Supervision of Staff

The MSSP must be able to perform all the functions and skills necessary to recruit, train, and maintain staff. Whether the department is a small one with one MSSP and a volunteer, or a large one with a director and ten support staff, personnel management is a necessary skill for this position. The MSSP must be able to create criteria-based job descriptions and conduct interviews that gather information to assess how well the candidate meets the criteria for the position.

Once a hire is made, the MSSP must be able to orient the new person to the department. This departmental orientation complements the organization orientation offered to all staff. Topics covered during a departmental orientation may include the hours of operation, the manner in which breaks and lunch are handled, the process for requesting time off, review of policies and procedures, fire drills, and so on. The department orientation should also include a review of the tasks the new employee will be performing. Along with the review of tasks, the new employee should be informed of any intradepartmental standards for the task. For example, the employee responsible for responding to requests for applications needs to know that the departmental standard is that application forms must be mailed within 48 hours of the request.

Establishing Staff Competency Requirements

For each task that must be carried out, the MSSD director needs to identify the steps and the skill or competency required to complete the task. Once the tasks and competencies are identified, the various tasks can be assigned to specific individuals who possess the required skills. Alternatively, job descriptions can be created that require varying degrees of skills based on the tasks assigned to that particular position within the MSSD. A sample skills (competency) list and a competency checklist for a department that operates on a more electronic basis are included on the CD that accompanies this book.

EXHIBIT 1-1 provides an example of a self-assessment skill checklist that can be used by a director of the MSSD to identify areas of strengths or weaknesses. This example is based on responsibilities and tasks of someone at the manager or director level. Similar self-assessment checklists can be developed for other categories of staff. The self-assessment checklist can be useful in the process of evaluating the performance of staff by having the employee conduct a self-assessment, followed by the evaluation of the employee by the manager. This type of process leads to an open discussion about the differences in perception of strengths and weaknesses between the manager and the employee. It provides a good foundation for the development of continuing education plans and career development action plans.

Evaluation of Staff

Periodic evaluations of staff performance must also be conducted. For new employees, most organizations require an evaluation at the end of the probationary period. Annual performance evaluations must be conducted as well.

It is important to be objective and to evaluate each staff member on how he or she meets the performance criteria or competencies defined in the position description. A critical aspect of performance evaluation is to make sure that the employee is aware of the performance and behavioral expectations required on which he or

Exhibit 1-1 Sample Skills Assessment Checklist

Director—Medical Staff Services Department

Instructions: For each identified skill or task, indicate your level of knowledge/skill with the task.

Skill/Task	Do routinely	Have done	Know how to do	Somewhat familiar	No knowledge
Accreditation Knowledge					
Know standards (e.g., Joint Commission, NCQA)					
Operationalize standards					
Prepare for survey					
Participate in survey					
Develop action plans					
Computer Literacy/Use of Technology					
Basic word processing					
Database management					
Evaluate and select software					
Write reports from software					
Make recommendations for redesign of processes based on available technology					
Credentials Process					
Establish process/procedures for staff to follow					
Write policies and procedures					
Conduct primary source verification					
Prepare files					
Develop and implement quality control system					
Develop and maintain system for monitoring expiring credentials					
Develop and maintain system for reappointment					
Budget and Finance					
Develop operating budget					
Develop capital budget					
Annualize expenses					
Analyze accounting reports					
Monitor budget and adjust operations as needed					

Exhibit 1-1 Sample Skills Assessment Checklist (continued)

Skill/Task	Do routinely	Have done	Know how to do	Somewhat familiar	No knowledge
Human Resources					
Write job descriptions					
Interview candidates					
Hire staff					
Conduct staff training					
Conduct performance evaluations					
Perform counseling/coaching					
Orient staff					
Terminate staff					
Delegate tasks/assignments					
Office Systems					
Organizational skills					
Establish filing systems					
Establish work flow					
Manage projects					
Develop project plans					
Maintain staff schedules					
Medical Staff Services					
Prepare draft bylaws language					
Prepare draft policies/rules					
Research issues for medical staff					
Meeting preparation (agenda, notice)					
Meeting facilitation					
Document minutes of meetings					
Understand peer review process					
Facilitate medical staff in peer review process					
Action Plans/Learning Needs:					

she will be evaluated. This information should be provided to the employee at the time of hire for new staff or periodically throughout the year for existing staff. The MSSP in the management role must be sure to document any counseling session or other interaction taken to improve performance. A strong knowledge and understanding of the organization's human resources policies is necessary for any MSSP in a supervisory position.

Organization

Good organizational skills are required, as the MSSP must maintain important records of the activities of the organized medical staff. Filing systems (whether paper or electronic), credentials files, meeting minutes, and other activities must be readily accessible and maintained in an orderly manner. In larger offices where numerous staff may perform the work, the director must be able to establish processes for assuring that records are maintained appropriately and that each staff member follows the same process. In an MSSD with more than one staff member, the department director or supervisor must not only manage his or her own work, but must also oversee the work of subordinates. This task is made easier if the office is well organized and driven by clearly defined and articulated policies and procedures.

Time Management

The MSSP must be able to manage multiple projects at the same time, which means that good time-management skills are essential. The MSSP will discover that a great deal of work performed is project related. Whether the task at hand involves a rewrite of medical staff bylaws, the implementation of an electronic content management system, or the upgrade of a software program, the use of basic project management techniques will be helpful. Knowledge of the use of project management tools such a Gantt charts, flow diagrams, timelines, or other computerized project management programs is a bonus.

Attention to Detail

Attention to detail will allow the MSSP and the MSSD to fulfill the requirements for medical staff documentation and credentials verification, to name just a few responsibilities. Challenges to the medical staff peer review process, credentialing decisions, or bylaw interpretations can be addressed more easily if the MSSP has maintained detailed, organized documentation that supports the medical staff's actions.

Work Independently

Although clear-cut reporting hierarchies exist within the hospital setting, the MSSP must be able to perform required functions independently. Professionals at the coordinator and director levels must use their own judgment in prioritizing work, delegating tasks, managing projects, and setting their own deadlines. The chief of staff, vice president of medical affairs, or hospital administrator needs to have confidence that the MSSP can perform the job with minimal direction or supervision. The typical MSSP is faced with daily challenges to meet deadlines. It is not unusual to experience interruptions throughout the day or to have sudden shifts in priorities. The MSSP must be able to adapt to changing priorities, reestablish deadlines, and get the work done!

Judgment

The knowledge of when to ask for feedback or direction from a supervisor is a skill that will develop over time as the MSSP and his or her supervisor become more comfortable with each other's style. The MSSP must also use judgment in relaying information to hospital administration that becomes available to him or her through interaction with the medical staff. Is the information vital to the chief executive officer? Will it keep members of the administration from being caught unaware in a meeting? Does the administration need the information to better prepare for new programs or services, or to respond to issues raised by the medical staff?

The preceding discussion is not meant to imply that the MSSP's goal is to gather intelligence for the hospital. Rather, it is intended to emphasize the key role played by the MSSP and the MSSD in facilitating open, effective communication between the medical staff and the hospital administration. The hospital and medical staff should be working toward a common goal—providing excellent patient care. The MSSP plays a large role in facilitating the medical staff's achievement of that goal.

Maintaining Confidentiality

During the performance of their duties, MSSPs have access to sensitive information that must be maintained in confidence. Types of information received may include physician-specific professional liability claims histories, details of previous disciplinary actions, physician health issues, or license sanctions imposed on physicians. Other sensitive information is received from the quality department related to the clinical work of the physician, including peer review actions. Trended data on patient care outcomes such as mortality rates, infection rates, or surgical complication rates are also available. The utilization management department may provide information to the department regarding resource utilization and practice efficiency of individual physicians. All of these data elements are necessary in the preparation of the reappointment profile for each staff member.

The MSSP must assure that the confidentiality of all of this information is maintained. Care must be taken to store such information in secure, locked areas. Access to information held on computerized systems should be limited, with the restrictions being enforced by password protection. Policies should be in place that define who has access to such information. In addition, the MSSP must always refrain from discussing sensitive information with staff members who are not otherwise privy to that information.

Communication Skills

One of the most important skills required of the MSSP is the ability to communicate effectively. Whether in written or oral formats, clear, concise communication is necessary in this role. The MSSP must be able to communicate to a variety of audiences as well. These audiences may include physicians, board members, representatives from accrediting agencies, and peers within the hospital, to name a few. The MSSP must be able to interpret standards, governing body directives, policies, and so on, and communicate them effectively to the medical staff.

Delegation

MSSPs—and especially those working in a leadership capacity in a department with more than one staff member—must be able to delegate effectively. Delegation does not simply mean giving the job or task to another person to perform. Rather, it includes providing clear, concise instructions to follow, establishing timelines, and determining the frequency of progress reports that are needed. For some staff members, the MSSP may simply delegate the function and request a report when the work is done. For others, the MSSP may need to provide directions and request status reports at various steps in the project. The MSSP who is filling the coordinator or director role must be able to evaluate the work style of his or her employees to determine the delegation style that will be most effective for each person.

Interpersonal Skills

In all hospitals, the medical staff make up a highly diverse population, encompassing many types of personalities and often many cultures. As a consequence, the MSSP must be able to work effectively with many different kinds of people. The ability to work professionally with administrators and physicians is a must. To be most effective, the MSSP must be able to maintain emotional balance even in the most stressful situations. Relationships should be kept on a professional level. The MSSP must be able to facilitate discussions between physicians and administrators (without their being aware of the intervention). He or she must also be able to give feedback as well as receive it. For the MSSP who serves as a supervisor of staff, the ability to provide positive or negative feedback to employees is an essential skill.

Computer Literacy

Good computer skills are essential for the MSSP. In today's work environment, the use of word processing software, databases, and spreadsheets as management tools is critical for anyone in a supervisory level. The ability to use statistical analysis tools is also required—particularly as they relate to interpreting quality outcomes during the reappointment process. For all these reasons, the MSSP should keep abreast of industry trends related to use of electronic media. For example, many facilities use electronic mail (e-mail) for internal communication. Which types of safeguards for confidential information should be in place in this circumstance? The MSSP should play a key role in the development of guidelines for electronic transmittal of confidential, medical staff peer review information.

Knowledge of information systems is valuable when working to automate the data collection required for physician profiling. Hospitals typically have more than one computer system. For example, there may be a billing system, a registration system, and an electronic patient charting system. The ability to identify which data elements are necessary for profiling and where they reside in the many hospital computer systems is important. The MSSP with information systems knowledge can work with the appropriate information systems staff to link the databases and generate physician profiles.

Having a working knowledge of the hospital financial system will assist the MSSP in determining the efficiency of a physician's practice. Efficiency data are one criterion that should be taken into consideration at the time of reappointment in addition to quality and peer review data.

Job Titles

The MSSD within a hospital will have a designated leader or supervisor. This person could have the title of Director, Medical Staff Services; Administrative Director, Medical Staff Services; or Coordinator, Medical Staff Services. The title should clearly identify the administrative responsibility of the role. Sample job descriptions are included on the CD that accompanies this book.

Depending on the size of the organization, the MSSD may include one or more staff members who function at different levels of responsibility.

Medical Staff Services Clerk

An employee at the clerk level performs basic tasks that may or may not require previous experience in the medical staff services field. For example, a clerk may be utilized to update a computer database or to scan or file licenses and other documents in credentials files or credentials software system as they are received. The skills necessary for the clerk include organization, the ability to follow directions, understanding filing systems, and knowledge of computer systems.

Medical Staff Secretary

A staff member functioning at the medical staff secretary level should have the same skills as those of the clerk. In addition, the medical staff secretary should have a basic understanding of committee support functions such as agenda planning, taking minutes, preparing minutes, and completing follow-up after the meeting is concluded. The medical staff secretary should have effective interpersonal and communication skills, as this level of staff has many more opportunities for interaction with physicians and other hospital staff.

Medical Staff Assistant

The medical staff assistant needs to have the skill sets of both the medical staff secretary and the clerk. In a small- to medium-sized facility, this position may perform all the required functions in a one-person office. The assistant then should have knowledge of the credentials process, accreditation standards and compliance, and medical staff laws. In a larger facility, the medical staff assistant may have job functions that deal primarily with committee support and medical staff liaison activities such as orientation.

Credentials Specialist

In a large MSSD, the duties and responsibilities might be assigned according to functions. For example, one staff member might manage meetings, while another might be assigned to accomplish the credentials verification process. The credentials specialist is responsible for following established procedures for verifying physicians' credentials and preparing the application for review by the appropriate clinical department chairmen and committees. A person in the credentials specialist role should have a basic knowledge of the credentials process, including the rationale for performing verification, sources for verification, and medical staff law as it pertains to credentialing. Professional certification, such as possession of the Certified Professional Medical Staff Management (CPMSM) or Certified Professional Credentialing Specialist (CPCS) credential, may be required for this position. As mentioned earlier in this chapter, such certifications are available through the NAMSS.

The credentials specialist should have the ability to work independently, while following set procedures. Many challenges faced by the medical staff are those that result from credentialing decisions. The credentials specialist must assure that the procedures are followed meticulously and consistently for each applicant. He or she must have strong documentation skills and be organized. Depending on the size of the organization, the credentials specialist may also provide support to the credentials committee. Consequently, he or she should understand the hospital policies, procedures, and bylaws as they relate to credentialing procedures. The specialist also needs to understand relevant state law. In this role, the credentials specialist is in a position to guide the credentials committee and department chair in decisions related to credentials verification.

Medical Staff Coordinator

In many medium-sized hospitals, the title assigned to the MSSP is Medical Staff Coordinator. The coordinator has responsibility for "coordinating" the activities of the organized staff. These activities may include all aspects of the services provided by the department, including accreditation compliance, credentials verification, medical staff committee support, policy and procedure, and bylaws development. If the MSSD consists of more than one staff member, the coordinator may be responsible for interviewing and hiring employees, initiating disciplinary actions, conducting evaluations, and coaching staff. In addition, the coordinator prepares the budget, writes departmental policies and procedures, and manages the day-to-day activities of the department.

Director, Medical Staff Services

The director of medical staff services is typically the head of a large, multiperson department. He or she is responsible for hiring, coaching, disciplining, and terminating employees. The director must provide orientation and training to enable staff to perform the functions to which they are assigned. He or she must also be financially astute, because developing budgets and maintaining fiscal accountability are major roles for the department director. The director must understand the processes involved in performing the department's work. These processes must then be translated into procedures to be followed by all staff. The director, working with the facility's human resources department, writes job descriptions and performs evaluations of the work done by subordinates. In addition, he or she establishes work standards and quality controls.

Database Manager

A growing trend in MSSDs is to have a dedicated database manager. This individual has a large body of knowledge related to computer software and system interoperability. The database manager would typically function as system administrator for the medical staff database. In addition, he or she would work with other departments to link data systems and generate reports for use by the medical staff in competency assessment and clinical privileges delineation and renewal.

Other Staff Members

Depending on the size of the facility, the MSSD could also include a continuing medical education coordinator and graduate education coordinator. It is not unusual for the medical library function or the institutional review board (IRB) function to rest with the MSSD in small and large facilities. Regardless of the functions residing in the department, there should be strong direction, organization, and established policies and procedures for performing the work.

■ The Medical Staff Services Department

Regardless of the size of the organization and the number of staff in the department, the MSSD functions as the administrative center for the organized medical staff. This office is the "home base" for the elected officers of the medical staff. In many facilities, a decision is made to locate the department in close proximity to the medical staff lounge. This physical location encourages interaction between the

MSSD staff and the physicians. Services provided by the MSSD almost always include management and coordination of activities related to credentialing and medical staff organization committees and departments. In addition, many MSSDs support the medical staff organization's continuing medical education program, the medical staff library, and the IRB, and play a role in the residency training programs if the organization is an academic facility or is affiliated with one. Other activities that occur sporadically, but tend to be time-consuming, include accreditation preparation activities and support for corrective actions, investigations, and fair hearings.

Organizational Structure

The MSSD typically reports to the hospital administrator or to a vice president of medical affairs. In addition to the formal reporting structure for the MSSP and his or her supervisor, there is an informal reporting structure for the MSSP and the elected officers of the medical staff organization. FIGURE 1-1 is a sample organization chart for the MSSD. FIGURE 1-2 depicts how the typical MSSD is positioned in the hospital organizational structure.

Relationship with Other Hospital Departments

The MSSD does not stand alone in the organization. Due to the relationships that are established between the medical staff members and the MSSD staff, many hospital departments and/or functions rely on the MSSD to facilitate communication with the physicians.

Administration

The MSSD interacts with various members of the administrative team. It communicates hospital policies and procedures to the medical staff. The MSSD also assists the administration in meeting accreditation standards and apprises the various leaders of key medical staff issues.

Director of Nursing/Chief Nursing Executive

The director of nursing/chief nursing executive (CNE), as well as various nursing units, rely on the MSSD for notification of new medical staff members. The MSSD maintains the official medical staff roster and records related to clinical privileges. Consequently, it must establish a mechanism for assuring that nursing staff has access to current privileges information. The department must also establish systems to notify nursing units when physicians join or leave the staff, when privileges are suspended or revoked, and when temporary privileges are granted. In addition, the MSSP must work with the CNE on the clinical privilege delineation for allied health professionals such as advanced practice nurses.

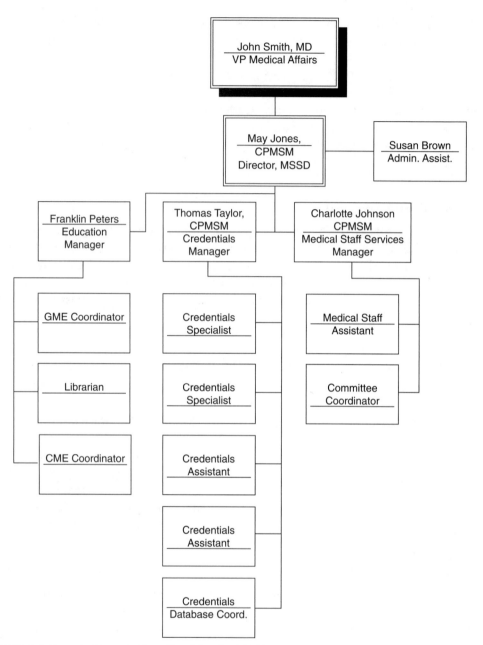

FIGURE 1-1 Sample Organization Chart for the MSSD

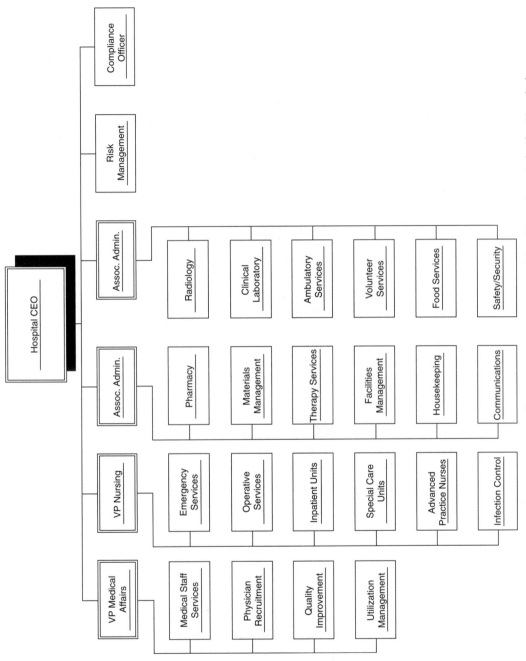

FIGURE 1-2 Relationship of the Medical Staff Services Department to Other Departments in the Hospital

The Medical Staff Services Department

Health Information Management Department

Accurate and timely completion of medical records is an important function that the medical staff must perform. This function is carried out in conjunction with the health information management (HIM) department. The HIM department enlists the assistance of the MSSD in enforcing policies for completion of records. As medical record suspensions may be one of the criteria for reappointment, suspension of clinical privileges for failure to complete records must be done in coordination with the MSSD. The MSSD relies on the HIM department for accurate reports on the number of suspensions for each physician. It also relies on the HIM department for accurate volume data for each physician. The volume data (e.g., number of admissions, discharges, consultations, surgical procedures) serve as the denominator for many of the reappointment criteria.

Quality Assurance or Improvement Department

The MSSD works collaboratively with the quality department, which also plays a key role in supporting medical staff organization functions. The data collected by the quality department are the most important information used in the ongoing professional performance evaluation, focused professional performance evaluation process, and privilege renewal/reappointment process. The clinical department chair, prior to making a decision to reappoint a physician, must review surgical complication rates, mortality rates, and other outcome data. Timely sharing of these data between departments is critical. The quality department also gathers data that may trigger the medical staff peer review process.

The MSSD and the quality department must work closely together and should identify procedures for information sharing. The MSSD relies on the data collected by the quality department; in turn, that department depends on the MSSD to notify it of any new staff physicians, changes in clinical privileges, new or changes to procedures, clinical pathways, or changes in accreditation standards that have an impact on the medical staff quality program. When medical staff organization functions require support from individuals with a clinical background, individuals from the quality management department often fill this role. Regular collaboration between the MSSD and quality management is necessary to support medical staff organization activities.

Utilization Management

As mentioned previously, individuals performing utilization management (called case management department in many hospitals) maintain information on the efficiencies and costs related to specific physicians' practice. These data are also reviewed during the reappointment process. The same type of cooperative relationship that exists between the quality department and the MSSD must also exist between the MSSD and the staff who perform utilization management. In many hospitals, quality improvement, risk management, utilization management, and social services are all functions that may be performed under the umbrella of a single integrated department.

Social Services

The social services or social work function interacts with physicians on a daily basis. There is a need for social work staff to know about newly appointed physicians and changes to medical staff status and privileges. The medical staff may develop policies and procedures that affect the work of the social services staff. The MSSD can facilitate this kind of policy and procedure development in a collaborative way. There should be a mechanism in place within the MSSD so that those departments that may be affected by the changes can review proposed medical staff policies. Social work staff also identify issues related to community resources for various patient types, and the MSSD may be instrumental in enlisting the medical staff organization's assistance in working with community organizations to address these needs.

Emergency Services

In many hospitals, the MSSD is the keeper of the "call schedules" that provide for specialty physician backup coverage for emergency patients. These schedules are necessary for the functioning of the emergency services department. The MSSD must share this information in a timely fashion. The emergency services department also needs to know about new physician members of the medical staff, changes in status or privileges, and suspensions from the medical staff.

Patient Relations

Patient relations staff are responsible for addressing the concerns and complaints lodged by patients. The MSSD should be aware of the policies and procedures related to this function, as he or she may be asked to respond to complaints related to physicians. At the very least, the MSSP must communicate with the appropriate clinical department chair to seek resolution of the complaint. Patient relations staff can provide aggregate data to the MSSD regarding complaints filed for each physician, which are another type of data used in the reappointment evaluation.

Marketing and Business Development

If the hospital has a separate department for marketing and business development, the MSSD will interact with this department regularly. The business development department may produce announcements for new staff, so it will rely on the MSSD to notify it of new medical staff members. In many organizations, a professional "sales staff" of physician relations liaisons is part of the marketing department. These liaisons have the potential for recruiting physicians to join the medical staff. It is necessary for the MSSD to understand the role of the physician relations staff—

just as it is important for the physician relations staff to understand basic medical staff procedures, such as how to apply for medical staff privileges.

Another function performed by the marketing and business development office may be that of contract negotiation or recruitment of new physician employees. Recruitment efforts should always be performed in conjunction with the MSSD. Close cooperation is necessary to assure that the medical staff's criteria for membership as well as all licensing and credentialing standards are met. In the area of contracting, the MSSD director should have the opportunity to review contract language that relates to delegated credentialing, for example.

Public Relations

The public relations (PR) department can provide many services for the MSSD. Editorial services for the medical staff newsletter, continuing education series for physicians and their office staffs, announcements of new staff, and print advertisements for new physicians and services are just a few areas where collaboration is possible. The MSSD can utilize the expertise of the PR staff in the areas of editing and writing.

Physician–Hospital Organization

In larger facilities, the presence of a physician–hospital organization (PHO) requires clear definition of the roles of the MSSD. Will the MSSD serve as an internal credentials verification body for the PHO? Will it share information regarding licensing, credentialing, and peer review? The MSSD staff needs to understand the type of relationship desired by this organization, and establish clear policies and procedures to be followed. If the relationships are not clear, the MSSD should ask for clarification so that the organizational intent can be supported and confidential information protected.

Admissions Department

The hospital admissions department depends on the medical staff services office for an accurate, up-to-date medical staff roster. Most MSSDs control the input of physician data into the hospital registration systems. As a consequence, the admissions department is a primary customer of the MSSD. There should be a cooperative relationship between admissions and medical staff services; the admissions department should contact the MSSD whenever questions arise about a physician's ability to admit and care for patients.

Risk Management

There should be a strong link between the risk management function and the MSSD. The MSSD relies on the legal expertise of hospital counsel or the risk manager when dealing with issues related to bylaws and policy development. In addition, risk management is an important source of claims information necessary for physician reappointment. The MSSD should have in place a system for communicating potential liability or risk issues to risk management.

Medical Staff Attorney

MSSPs are often the conduit through which medical staff leaders have access to legal counsel for medical staff organization activities. Ideally, the MSSP will develop a close working relationship with an attorney who specializes in medical staff organization legal issues. The MSSP may work with the attorney on medical staff bylaws, policies and procedures, credentialing issues, peer review issues, and related correspondence. In addition, when corrective action is contemplated or actually occurs (e.g., summary suspension, limitation of privileges) or investigations occur that result in reports to the National Practitioner Data Bank and triggering of fair hearing processes, it is critical that the MSSP seek legal guidance and assistance on behalf of the medical staff organization.

Hospital Compliance

Since the mid-1990s, hospitals have established compliance offices.[3] The compliance officer's role is to assess and monitor the organization's compliance with laws and regulations. A large part of the compliance officer's role deals with the requirements of Medicare and the federal government. A key element in every compliance program is education of hospital staff (using the CMS hospital compliance guide). The MSSD can and should act as a liaison between the medical staff and the compliance office.

Staffing and Staffing Analysis

The medical staff services industry has sought a benchmark for the number of staff needed for MSSDs. In response to this need, some MSSPs have developed formulas, ratios, and other approaches to determine the number of staff required to perform specific activities. Because of wide variations in the scope of services provided by the MSSD to support the medical staff organization, plus the use of technology to accomplish certain functions, an industry benchmark standard for staffing MSSDs does not exist. For example, in terms of the credentialing function, some medical staff applications are 7 pages long, others are 15 pages, and still others are available online. Not surprisingly, the time required for data entry in these three cases will vary widely. Some MSSDs use electronic methods for querying verification organizations, whereas others rely solely on manual methods. Use of the latter approach can increase the resources required to complete the task by tenfold or more. Therefore, it is essential to clearly define which methods will be used to deliver services before any attempt is made to develop a staffing standard for the department. It is more important for MSSPs to focus their efforts on developing a sound approach for analyzing staffing needs as opposed to searching the literature for a magic number.

To determine the number of employees needed to accomplish the many functions of the MSSD, the department director must be able to perform a detailed staffing analysis. Each function should be broken down into the number of hours required to complete the process. For example, committee support should take into consideration pre-meeting activities such as agenda planning meetings, agenda preparation, and committee packet preparation (copying and distribution). An organization that relies on a paper-based system will require more staff to accomplish these functions than an organization that uses a protected Web site to post meeting materials. Functions of the MSSD may also include attendance at the actual meeting, minute preparation, and preparation of committee follow-up of action items. TABLE 1-1 provides a checklist for the support needed for one committee meeting; the information provided by the checklist should facilitate staffing analysis.

Table 1-1	Competency Checklist
	Meeting Preparation
Step to Complete	**Skill or Competency Required**
Reserve meeting room	• Know whom to contact within the organization to reserve the room
	• Know which form to use reserve room/audiovisual equipment
Arrange for food service	• Know whom to contact within the organization to arrange refreshments
	• Know what form to use to arrange food services
Prepare agenda	• Organization—Maintain list of pending items, old business, new business, correspondence, etc.
	• Know basic meeting rules (e.g., *Robert's Rules of Order*) to determine order of meeting agenda
	• Facilitation—Make sure that appropriate individuals have input on agenda content
	• Word processing skills
Develop meeting notice	• Word processing/typing
Prepare meeting packet organized in the order of the agenda	• Use photocopy equipment
	• Collate materials
	• Operate binding machine
Distribute meeting notice and packet	• Know who the committee members are
	• Generate mailing list from software system
	• Know the organization's mailroom procedures
	• Know which packets to hand deliver

The following formula is then used to determine the number of full-time employees (FTEs) needed to support one committee. (Each committee requires analysis of its support. This illustration cannot be used as a benchmark standard for all medical staff meetings.)

6 hours of staff time is used × 12 months (The committee meets monthly)
= 72 hours (total hours per year needed to support the committee) ÷ 1800 (the number of hours one full-time person actually works/year)
= .04FTE needed to support the committee

Functions

The MSSD performs many functions for the hospital and medical staff. Brief descriptions of some of the key functions follow.

Committee Support

Many medical staff organizations have established a committee structure to assist them in meeting the many accreditation requirements. The MSSD staff must have a good understanding of the committee structure. Typically, only the medical executive committee (MEC) is allowed to take actions; other committees of the medical staff make recommendations for action to the MEC. Some medical staff organizations delegate some decision-making authority.

It is imperative that the MSSD personnel assist the medical staff in maneuvering through the committee structure. To do so, the MSSD should develop a system for transmitting agenda items and recommendations from committees and departments up to the MEC. Similarly, systems should be in place to demonstrate when actions were taken. The department should also maintain a follow-up system to assure that the actions agreed upon are completed in a timely fashion (see Chapter 14).

In addition, the MSSD staff should have a good understanding of the group process. Committees can be effective tools if their members work toward a common goal and if the members understand and agree on the purpose of the committee. The ability to recognize when a committee has become dysfunctional is a valuable skill. Medical staff services personnel can then assist the chair in bringing the group back to common ground.

The MSSD staff represent a key resource for the various accreditation standards related to medical staff. The staff's understanding of accreditation standards requiring documentation of specific medical staff functions is critical. Accreditation agencies, for example, rely on this kind of documentation to demonstrate that the various functions are being performed.

The MSSD maintains the minutes of meetings and follow-up materials for medical staff organization groups. The ability to summarize and document committee proceedings is an acquired skill. It takes practice to learn how to discern what is important to the meeting documentation. MSSPs are able to identify the issue being discussed, the reasons why it is being discussed, important aspects of the discussion, conclusions drawn by the committee, and any actions taken.

The key to an effective committee meeting is good preparation and agenda planning. The MSSP serves to assist the chairs in agenda development and follow-up. Effective agenda planning includes the reasons for presentation of an issue, any supporting documentation, and the desired outcome.

Medical Staff Liaison

The MSSD acts as the liaison to the medical staff. Department staff members have daily contact with many members of the medical staff and can assist them in various ways. For example, issues brought up by physicians are routed to the appropriate committee or administrator via the MSSD. Members of the medical staff should be able to rely on the MSSD for information about the hospital and its services as well as information about policies and procedures that may affect patient care. Additionally, the MSSD may provide special services for the physicians such as use of fax machines, copy machines, and so on.

Orientation

The MSSD is often responsible for assuring that the newly appointed physician receives an orientation to the hospital and the medical staff organization. In conjunction with the medical staff organization, this department establishes orientation objectives and identifies the information that a physician needs to receive prior to caring for patients in the hospital. Working with many other departments, such as human resources, the MSSD develops and implements the orientation program. Recognizing that the physician's time is valuable, many MSSDs have developed orientation programs using the latest technologies. For example, a videotaped orientation program that can be viewed by the physician in his or her office or at home is one way to assure the information is provided in a useful format. Other formats include computer-based learning or links to the orientation content through the MSSD's Web page.

Credentials Verification

One of the most important functions of the MSSD is to complete the verification of physician and other licensed independent practitioner credentials for initial appointment and reappointment. Working within the framework established in the medical staff bylaws, the department establishes complementary policies and procedures to assure a consistent approach to the process. Such procedures include reviewing the application for completeness when received, determining the source of verification for the credentials elements, outlining how the application is prepared for clinical department review and committee review, and so on. Procedures should also address how the MSSP responds to "red flags" in the credentials process (see Chapter 6).

Procedures related to the reappointment process outline the time frame for distributing the reappointment application, determining the source of verification for the credentials elements, identifying the sources for the profiling information (e.g., utilization management, quality and peer review, risk management), and procedures for updating medical staff databases. It is critical that the procedures established for the credentials verification function be followed consistently. It is also critical that the staff members in the department responsible for carrying out the process are trained in how the procedures are carried out and why.

Accreditation Support

Regardless of the accreditation held by the hospital, the MSSD and the MSSPs play key roles in the survey process used to gain such accreditation. The MSSD assists the medical staff organization in ensuring their compliance with relevant standards. The documentation from the various medical staff committees and departments is maintained in the department, which also maintains all of the credentials files. By virtue of the information under its control, MSSD personnel should be included in the survey preparation efforts as well as the actual survey.

An effective role for the department director is as a member of the accreditation preparation task force. This task force usually consists of key administrative personnel (CEO, director of nursing, administrator responsible for ambulatory services, quality director, and the medical director) as well as the MSSP. The task force's duties include communicating changes in standards to the hospital departments as well as for all survey preparation activities. Survey preparation activities can range from mock surveys to in-service education for hospital and medical staff members. During the actual survey, the MSSP should accompany the physician member of the survey team.

Support of Medical Staff Leadership

In many hospitals, the medical staff leaders are elected to their positions and must accomplish the responsibilities of their offices while maintaining heavy patient care loads. The MSSD can assist these leaders in fulfilling their duties in a variety of ways. For example, this department can prepare correspondence for the review and signature of the leader, arrange meetings on behalf of the leadership, establish a quiet space within the department for the leaders to use for meetings, perform committee follow-up, and so on. The MSSP can also assist the leaders by keeping them up-to-date on the activities of the medical staff. Reports on the number of times temporary privileges have been granted or the failure of a committee to adequately perform its functions will facilitate the leaders in identifying opportunities for improvement in the medical staff organization structure. In addition, the MSSD should apprise the leadership of any issue raised in committee or by an individual medical staff member that may be controversial and require a joint medical staff and administrative response. This notification enables the leader to gather additional information and prepare his or her response to the issue.

In that most medical staff leaders are elected and serve limited terms, the MSSP plays a valuable role in continuity of medical staff organization activities (see Chapter 3).

Policy and Procedure Development

The MSSD can also assist the medical staff leaders in identifying topics for policy and procedure development. Policies and procedures (or rules and regulations, depending on the specific medical staff structure) should be limited to issues that may lead to a credentialing action (such as failure to complete medical records documentation) or that outline how a particular standard is to be met. The MSSD is in a position to identify the need for new policies and procedures. In particular, review by the MSSD of trends in complaints or issues raised by other departments can trigger the development of a policy. Following thorough research of standards, laws, or regulations, the MSSD staff may draft policies for consideration of the medical staff leadership. Once policies are developed, the MSSD may establish a mechanism for periodic policy review and revision.

The governing body should approve critical policies and procedures, because these items establish authority and responsibilities of the MSSP as well as physicians and administration. The type of policies that need governing body approval may include those related to credentialing, peer review, and clinical privilege delineation. Other policies that establish key processes or address how the organization complies with statutes or regulations may also require governing body approval. At times, the MSSP may be caught in the middle of competing interests. In these circumstances it is helpful to have the governing body define the accountabilities of the various parties in policy.

Resource Center

The MSSD should establish a resource center for the medical staff leaders and hospital administrators. The information contained in this center should focus on medical staff issues. Examples of documents that should be available include the following:

- *Joint Commission standards manual.* The appropriate Joint Commission accreditation manual provides a detailed listing of the various standards that an organization must meet to obtain and maintain accreditation status. In addition to each standard, the manual outlines specific elements of performance that must be evident in the organization's processes for meeting standards. Accreditation manuals are available for a variety of healthcare settings, including hospitals, home health, ambulatory care, and health networks. The Joint Commission standards are available through the Internet as well, so the MSSP should be able to provide the medical staff leadership with access to the Internet.

- *CMS's Conditions of Participation.* The CMS's Conditions of Participation (COP) outline the requirements that hospitals must meet to participate in the federal healthcare payment programs. The COP cover such areas as governing board structure, medical staff, anesthesia services, and quality of care.
- *Current medical staff bylaws.* The organization's medical staff bylaws provide the framework for the self-governing medical staff organization. Bylaws typically include a description of how the medical staff is organized, qualification for membership, responsibility of membership, committee and department structure, and so on.
- *Current medical staff policies, rules, and regulations.* If the medical staff bylaws provide the framework of the medical staff organization, the policies and procedures or rules and regulations provide the operational processes for conducting medical staff business.
- *Hospital policies and procedures.* Hospital policies and procedures detail the rules and processes that must be followed on a variety of issues that affect the entire organization. For example, hospital policies might address informed consent, human resources matters such as dress codes, or benefit time. Physicians on the medical staff must be aware of the hospital policies with which they must comply.
- *Current state statutes regarding licensure and peer review.* These statutes include state laws or regulations that govern the practice of medicine in the state and state laws or regulations that outline the protection from discoverability for quality and peer review–related activities.

■ Performance Improvement in the MSSD

Many healthcare organizations have adopted a management philosophy that encourages continuous quality improvement. The MSSD should participate in the hospital quality improvement program by establishing a department-specific plan. A simple process can be followed to establish a performance improvement process for the MSSD.

1. Identify the department's customers: physicians, patients, insurers, other hospital departments. What are their expectations of the department? Do they expect committee support, timely processing of their applications for membership, an accurate medical staff roster, or something else?
2. Identify the department's major services. These might include credentials verification, committee support, accreditation coordination, serving as medical staff liaison, or maintaining the medical staff database.
3. Identify any standards that must be met by the department. These items might be external to the department, such as accreditation standards, or they might be internal, such standards for turnaround times for application processing

or response times for requests for verification of staff membership. The department staff should establish internal standards in a collaborative manner.
4. Determine how department staff members know whether the customer's needs and expectations are being met. What is being measured to determine compliance?
5. Establish measurement systems: What will be measured? Also, identify frequency of data collection: How often will the data be collected? Will it be collected continuously or by a sampling method? Who will collect the data? Which tools will be used?
6. Determine the usefulness of the information. Will the data generated be useful in identifying opportunities for improvement within the MSSD? If not, then the collection of those particular data may not be a priority. The overall goal of the department performance improvement plan is to collect general, useful information to help increase efficiencies or improve customer satisfaction. Collecting data simply for the sake of collecting data is a waste of time.

An example of a simple measurement tool is a run chart that documents process time for each application completed. A telephone log can be used to document that calls are returned within whatever time standard has been set by the department. Once these decisions have been made and the data collected, the results must be analyzed. The department must determine who will analyze the data and how the findings will be reported. Keep in mind the end user of the data. Who will see the report—the medical director? The credentials committee? Administrators? Or is the report intended for internal use by the department director only? A sample department performance improvement plan and a sample PI reporting form are included on the CD that accompanies this book.

Customer Satisfaction Survey

A key element to any performance improvement plan is how customers feel about the services provided by the department. MSSDs are no different. The customers of the MSSD are many, as previously noted in this chapter. For the purpose of determining customer satisfaction, the MSSD should focus on the primary customer: the medical staff. When conducting a satisfaction survey, the medical staff can be divided into three components:

- Newly appointed members
- Medical staff leaders (officers, medical directors, department and committee chairs)
- All other medical staff members

Each of these groups can provide useful information on specific areas of the MSSD's responsibility. Newly appointed staff members should be asked to assess the responsiveness, helpfulness, and communication style of the MSSD staff during the application process. Medical staff leaders can assess the responsiveness, committee support, research efforts, document preparation, and so on. Finally, the remaining members of the medical staff can assess overall communication, responsiveness, and professionalism of the MSSD staff.

Conducting a Survey

Once the customers have been identified, the MSSD staff needs to develop a survey tool. Many types of survey methodologies are available, although use of a survey tool that relies on a Likert scale is the most commonly employed approach. A sample survey tool is shown in EXHIBIT 1-2. Ideally, the same survey tool will be used during each survey period. That way, the MSSD can examine the data for patterns or trends. Using a different tool for each survey eliminates the possibility of having historical comparative data.

Once a tool is developed, it is distributed to the survey population. The number of surveys sent out is recorded, as this information is necessary to calculate the response rate. An internal deadline for receipt of responses is set. When the deadline is reached, the response rate is calculated to determine whether it is statistically significant. Most groups consider that at least 30 responses must be received for the results of the survey to be statistically significant. The response rate is calculated by dividing the number of responses received by the number of surveys distributed. For example, if 35 responses are received out of a possible 150, the response rate is 23.3%.

If the response rate is not statistically significant, you may want to send out the survey a second time.

If the response rate is statistically valid, then the data are organized so that they can be easily viewed and analyzed. Excel spreadsheets and Access databases are two popular ways of storing the data for easy analysis.

Once the data are entered into the system, analysis can begin. The most commonly undertaken analysis seeks to determine the percentage for each response to each question. If the survey tool allowed respondents to add specific comments or suggestions, then the types of comments received can be classified into broad categories.

Once the data analysis is complete, the results are displayed and include a comparison to historical data. Managers can draw conclusions and develop action plans in response to the survey findings. A sample report of satisfaction data is shown on the performance improvement report in FIGURE 1-3.

■ Expanded Roles

In today's changing healthcare environment, there may be opportunities for MSSDs and MSSPs to assume expanded roles within the organization. These roles may offer

Exhibit 1-2: Sample Performance Improvement Survey Tool Satisfaction Survey—Medical Staff Services Department

Indicate your level of agreement with the statement below	Excellent/Fully Agree	Satisfactory/Somewhat Agree		Disagree/Poor	N/A
New Applicants	5	4	3	2	1	N/A
Application sent promptly upon your request						
Instructions for the credentials process were accurate and thorough						
Staff answered your questions completely						
Staff kept you informed of status						
Requests for additional information were made courteously						
Overall, my satisfaction with the process						
Overall, my satisfaction with the MSSD staff						
Medical Staff Leadership	5	4	3	2	1	N/A
MSSD staff are responsive to my requests						
Documents prepared are accurate, complete, and professional in appearance						
Staff anticipate my needs						
Staff maintains confidentiality of sensitive information						
Overall, the staff meets my needs						
Overall, I am satisfied with the service provided by the department						
Medical Staff Member	5	4	3	2	1	N/A
MSSD staff are responsive to my requests						
Staff are professional						
Staff are courteous						
Overall, I am satisfied with the department						

Comments:

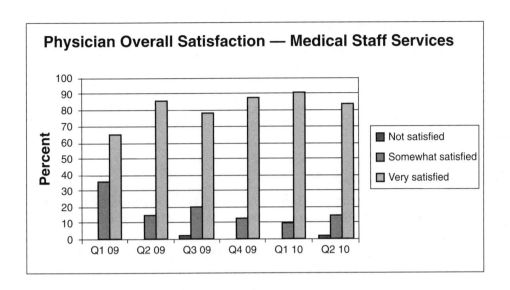

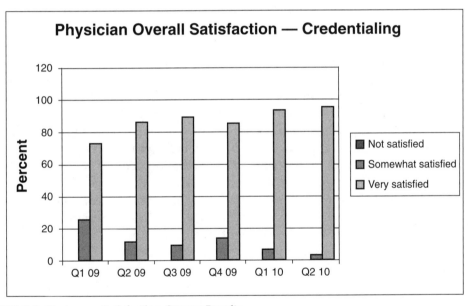

FIGURE 1-3 Customer Satisfaction Survey Results

a chance to assume greater responsibility within the organization or may provide the department an avenue for revenue generation. The department director should approach each opportunity carefully and prepare carefully thought-out business plans for consideration by the organization's leaders.

Integrated Delivery Systems

The up-to-date MSSD will have procedures in place to perform credentials verification. In an integrated delivery system, the MSSP may have the opportunity to centralize certain functions for the organization. These functions might include credentials verification, maintenance of credentials files, or managing the enrollment of physicians in managed care plans. See Chapter 9 for additional information.

Delegated Credentialing

When a managed care company enters into an agreement with a hospital or group practice, part of the standard contract language includes the manner in which physicians will be credentialed to be enrolled in the plan. The concept of delegated credentialing is recognized by managed care companies as a way to avoid duplication of processes. The managed care company can delegate the credentialing of a group practice or select faculty members to the hospital; in essence, the managed care company agrees to accept the credentials verification work already done by the hospital. This saves the physician and the managed care plan considerable time and avoids duplication of efforts.

When entering into a delegated credentialing agreement, the managed care company will do a pre-agreement site visit. At that visit, select credentials files are reviewed, the application forms are reviewed, and medical staff bylaws and medical staff services policies and procedures for the performance of the credentials process are evaluated. It is important to note that the managed care company is evaluating these processes to assure compliance with National Committee for Quality Assurance (NCQA) standards. If it is determined that the procedures meet the NCQA standards, a delegation agreement may be executed.

Once the delegation agreement is in place, the managed care company must show oversight of the process. This is accomplished by the performance of an on-site audit each year. This audit entails review of a select number of credentials files and policies and procedures. If standards continue to be met, the delegation can continue. If the standards are not being met, however, an action plan may be required from the MSSD outlining how the department will change its procedures to meet these standards.

A delegated credentialing arrangement can be very effective. It reduces the paperwork required by physicians and can expedite the enrollment process. The hospital MSSD should establish procedures detailing how to deal with requests for delegation, from contract language review, to scheduling of on-site audits, to providing updates to the managed care company as needed. With the appropriate policies in place, delegation compliance can be accomplished in an efficient manner. For more details, see Chapter 9.

Credentials Verification Organization

In some health systems or integrated delivery networks, several facilities may duplicate credentials verification for the same practitioners. MSSDs have the most experience with the credentials verification process and have established procedures for this task in place. There is logic in centralizing the credentials verification procedures performed at all facilities under the existing MSSD. By establishing an organization-wide CVO, the MSSD can save the organization the costs associated with staffing an office at each location. For more details, see Chapter 10.

Physician Referral Service

Some hospitals have established physician referral services. These telephonic and electronic services offer patients the opportunity to find a physician affiliated with the hospital who meets patient-specific parameters (e.g., is located within a specific ZIP code, is located on a bus line, accepts Medicare payment, speaks Spanish). This strategy is an effective way to build physician loyalty to the hospital. Many MSSDs take a leading role in managing this service.

Quality Improvement

As hospitals look toward reengineering or continuous quality improvement strategies, opportunities may arise to consolidate departments. The merger of the medical staff department and the quality department is a reasonable approach in many organizations. Often, the medical staff services and quality departments have been working closely for years in assuring that physician peer review is accomplished and reported for reappointment. As the emphasis in quality improvement shifts toward process improvement and away from traditional peer review, the MSSD can assume the responsibilities for medical staff peer review. It is not necessary to have a clinical background to manage a quality department. Quality departments typically consist of nurses and other clinicians who can provide the nonclinician director with necessary input. Additionally, the hospital usually identifies a physician liaison who works closely with the quality department and assists with clinical matters. The knowledge and skills held by an MSSP will permit him or her to provide effective leadership of additional hospital departments.

Physician Relations

The use of physician relations representatives to market the hospital and its services to physicians has proven to be an effective strategy for ensuring appointment of quality physicians. By virtue of their knowledge of the healthcare system and the way that the hospital functions, MSSPs are prime candidates to fill the role of physician relations representative. The MSSP demonstrates two key skills that are essential for this position—good interpersonal skills and the ability to communicate effectively with a diverse audience.

Healthcare Compliance

Many hospitals and health systems have established corporate compliance programs and departments. In many cases, this move has come in response to increased scrutiny by the federal government regarding compliance with rules and regulations related to Medicare and Medicaid. As compliance programs grow within the organization, the MSSP may want to consider opportunities in this field. The typical MSSP has the skills required for this position, including understanding of rules, regulations, laws, and statutes, as well as being detailed oriented.

■ Conclusion

The activities of the MSSP are as diverse as the elements found in today's healthcare environment. The MSSP provides essential services to the healthcare facility. His or her unique role as resource person and facilitator enables the hospital and medical staff organization to work toward a common goal—providing quality care for patients. The responsibilities of the MSSP and MSSD are numerous, and the provision of quality patient care can be directly linked to the work performed in the department. To fulfill its responsibilities, the MSSD must have strong leadership, established policies and procedures, and a clear reporting relationship within the administrative structure. Medical staff services can be a challenging and rewarding field.

■ Notes

1. Smits HL. "Quality Management and Consumer Protection Under the President's Health Reform Plan." *Qual Letter Healthcare Leaders.* 1994;5:2–6.
2. U.S. Department of Health and Human Services, Centers for Medicare and Medicaid Services. *Quality Improvement Roadmap: Executive Summary.* Washington, DC: U.S. Department of Health and Human Services; 2005.
3. Troklus D, Warner G. *Compliance 101.* Philadelphia, PA: Health Care Compliance Association; 2001.

CHAPTER 2

Healthcare Organization Accreditation

Cindy A. Gassiot, CPMSM, CPCS
With contributions on international accreditation by
Mary A. Baker, CPMSM, CPCS, DHA

■ Introduction

To receive reimbursement from insurance companies and the federal government's insurance programs, healthcare facilities must be accredited. A plethora of organizations accredit healthcare organizations. In fact, one or more major accrediting groups exist for each type of healthcare organization—hospitals, ambulatory care and surgery centers, long-term care centers, rehabilitation facilities, and managed care organizations, to name a few. Accreditation or certification is also available for activities such as utilization review, home health agencies, and even healthcare Web sites. Each accrediting group evaluates a healthcare organization's compliance with published standards. Additionally, healthcare organizations that are not accredited by one of the voluntary accrediting groups must be approved by the Centers for Medicare and Medicaid Services (CMS) to receive reimbursement for treating patients covered by the Medicare and Medicaid programs. These surveys are conducted by state health departments to determine whether the facilities meet the CMS's Conditions of Participation (COP).

■ Hospital Accreditation

The Joint Commission

The Joint Commission has been the dominant player in accreditation of healthcare organizations for more than 50 years. It was the only hospital accrediting organization guaranteed by statute[1] to have Medicare "deeming" authority; that is, hospitals accredited by the Joint Commission are deemed by CMS to meet the Medicare COP. When the Medicare and Medicaid programs were established in 1965, Congress didn't have much experience in health care and deferred to the expertise of the Joint Commission, a professional accreditation organization that had been in existence since 1951. Congress recognized that voluntary accreditation was one way that hospitals could demonstrate compliance with Medicare' hospital COP and mandated that accreditation by the Joint Commission was equivalent to meeting these conditions. The first Medicare COP was modeled after the Joint

Commission standards as then written. But by giving the Joint Commission statutory deeming authority, CMS had limited oversight of the Joint Commission. Even if problems were identified, CMS could not limit or remove the Joint Commission's accreditation authority.

CMS Takes Charge

In recent years, Congress has become increasingly critical of the Joint Commission's performance. Since the publication in 1999 of the Institution of Medicine's report that attributed nearly 98,000 deaths annually to errors in health care,[2] the nation has become more and more aware that some hospitals are not very safe places. Additionally, in a July 2004 report, the Government Accountability Office (GAO) concluded that 78% of the time the Joint Commission survey process did not identify serious deficiencies that were found by state hospital survey agencies. The GAO recommended that "given the serious limitations in [the Joint Commission's] accreditation program and that efforts to improve this program through informal action by CMS have not led to necessary improvements, Congress should consider giving CMS the same kind of authority over its hospital accreditation program that it has over all Medicare accreditation programs."[3]

In 2008, Congress passed a bill repealing the Joint Commission's special status for deeming authority, effective 2010. Its accreditation program was also placed on a 180-day probationary period and the Joint Commission was ordered to revise its accreditation standards to meet the Medicare COP. In September 2008, CMS also approved a new hospital accrediting organization, Det Norske Veritas Healthcare (DNV). The Joint Commission will have to apply for deeming status—just like all other healthcare accreditation organizations—in the future, and it has some serious new competition in the hospital accreditation arena.

By taking these actions, CMS has signaled that it is now the driving force in healthcare accreditation and will not tolerate deviations from the Medicare COP. In response, the Joint Commission has revised all of its accreditation standards so that they are consistent with the Medicare COP; it was in the process of reapplying for deeming status at the time of this book's writing. Many individuals believe the Joint Commission standards are too prescriptive and that Joint Commission accreditation is too expensive.

History of Joint Commission

Even though the Joint Commission has had its automatic deeming authority removed and now has serious new competition in hospital accreditation, it is the forerunner of healthcare accreditation in the United States and has an interesting history. The Joint Commission evolved from a program initiated by the American College of Surgeons.

In 1910, a physician named Dr. Ernest Codman had an idea for an "end-result system" in hospitals that he explained to Dr. Edward Martin. This system would have hospitals tracking the outcome of patient treatment; if the treatment was not effective, it would find out why so that the hospitals could correct any deficiency identified for future patients. Martin took this idea one step further and decided that an American College of Surgeons should be established, which would incorporate the end result system in a hospital standardization program.[4]

At this time conditions in hospitals were very poor. Hospitals were more or less almshouses. Patients were not properly examined, medical records were not kept, and necessary equipment often was not available; there was no attempt to look into the qualifications of physicians, and no efforts were made to determine the outcomes of treatment.[5] In short, there was no accountability in hospitals.

At the same time, progress was being made in recognizing the significance of asepsis in medical care, and surgery performed in hospitals was becoming safer. Coupled with improvements in management theory and in the science of medicine, hospital administrators and those involved in medicine were hopeful about the future. At a meeting of the Congress of Surgeons of North America in November 1912, Dr. Franklin Martin proposed that an American College of Surgeons be formed. Immediately following his address, Dr Edward Martin proposed the following resolution:

Be it resolved by the Clinical Congress of Surgeons of North America here assembled, that some system of standardization of hospital equipment and hospital work should be developed, to the end that those institutions having the highest ideals may have proper recognition before the profession, and that those of inferior equipment and standards should be stimulated to raise the quality of their work. In this way patients will receive the best type of treatment, and the public will have some means of recognizing those institutions devoted to the highest ideals of medicine.[6]

Thus a hospital standardization program became a major focus of the American College of Surgeons (ACS) when it was founded in 1913. During those first few years, a majority of applications from hospitals had to be rejected because they did not meet the requirement for 50 case records on which to base a review of clinical competence. Efforts continued on a hospital standardization program. In 1918, the ACS published a "Standard on Efficiency" in its *Bulletin of the American College of Surgeons* journal, which hospitals would have to meet to become accredited. Field trials were held in 1919, and it was announced that out of 692 hospitals with 100 beds or more that had been surveyed, only 89 hospitals met the standards.[7] These results were shocking: Although the results were published, the list of hospitals surveyed was burned in the basement of the Waldorf Astoria Hotel in New York. Subsequently, 109 hospitals corrected their deficiencies and their initial surveys were later approved. In December 1919, the ACS published new standards, known as the *Minimum Standard*, which became the forerunner of the standards that exist today.[8]

Table 2-1   The Minimum Standard

1. That physicians and surgeons privileged to practice in the hospital be organized as a definite group or staff. Such organization has nothing to do with the question as to whether the hospital is "open" or "closed," nor need it affect the various existing types of staff organization. The word *staff* is here defined as the group of doctors who practice in the hospital inclusive of all groups such as the "regular staff," the "visiting staff," and the "associate staff."

2. That membership upon the staff be restricted to physicians and surgeons who are (a) full graduates of medicine in good standing and legally licensed to practice in their respective states or provinces, (b) competent in their respective fields, and (c) worthy in character and in matters of professional ethics, that in this latter connection in the practice of the division of fees, under any guise whatsoever, be prohibited.

3. That the staff initiate and, with the approval of the governing board of the hospital, adopt rules, regulations, and policies governing the professional work of regulations, and policies governing the professional work of the hospital; that these rules, regulations, and policies specifically provide:

    (a) That staff meetings be held at least once each month. (In large hospitals the departments may choose to meet separately.)

    (b) That the staff review and analyze at regular intervals their clinical experience in the various departments of the hospital, such as medicine, surgery, obstetrics, and the other specialties; the clinical records of patients, free and pay, to be the basis for such review and analyses.

4. That accurate and complete records be written for all patients and filed in an accessible manner in the hospital—a complete case record being one which includes identification data; complaint; personal and family history; history of present illness; physical examination; special examinations, such as consultations, clinical laboratory, X-ray, and other examinations; provisional or working diagnosis; medical or surgical treatment; gross and microscopical pathological findings; progress notes; final diagnosis; condition on discharge; follow-up and, in case of death, autopsy findings.

5. That diagnostic and therapeutic facilities under competent supervision be available for the study, diagnosis, and treatment of patients, these to include at least (a) a clinical laboratory providing chemical, bacteriological, serological, and pathological services; (b) an X-ray department providing radiographic and fluoroscopic services.

Source: Reprinted with permission from the *Bulletin of the American College of Surgeons*, Vol. 8, p. 4 ©1924.

By 1950, the hospital standardization program had grown to the point that ACS could no longer support it on its own. In 1951, the American College of Physicians, the American Hospital Association, the American Medical Association, and the Canadian Medical Association joined the ACS in forming the Joint Commission on Accreditation of Hospitals, which began to accredit hospitals in 1953. From its program to accredit hospitals, programs to accredit other types of healthcare organizations have evolved over the years. Many iterations of the standards have been realized over the years, and staff in Joint Commission–accredited healthcare organizations sometimes grow weary of the many changes and additions to the requirements.

The Joint Commission Today

The 29-member Joint Commission Board of Commissioners consists of representatives of the American College of Physicians, the American College of Surgeons, the American Dental Association, the American Hospital Association, and the American Medical Association. The Joint Commission accredits the following types of organizations:

- General, psychiatric, children's, and rehabilitation hospitals
- Critical access hospitals
- Medical equipment services, hospice services, and other home care organizations
- Nursing homes and other long-term care facilities
- Behavioral healthcare organizations and addiction services
- Rehabilitation centers, group practices, office-based surgeries, and other ambulatory care providers
- Independent or freestanding laboratories[9]

At the time of this writing, the Joint Commission had accredited more than 16,000 healthcare organizations and programs in the United States.

In 1994, Joint Commission International was launched, with offices being established in Italy and France in 2004. More than 220 healthcare organizations in 33 countries are accredited by Joint Commission International.[10]

Standards

The standards have expanded over the years from the minimum five to hundreds. Joint Commission standards address the organization's level of performance in key functional areas, such as patient rights, patient treatment, and infection control. The standards focus not simply on an organization's ability to provide safe, high-quality care, but on its actual performance as well.[11]

Performance Measures and Patient Safety

Beginning in 1997, accredited hospitals were required by the Joint Commission to participate in its ORYX initiative and later in providing data related to a set of core measures. The ORYX requirement calls for healthcare providers to collect and send performance data to the Joint Commission on acute myocardial infarction, heart failure, pneumonia, pregnancy and related conditions, hospital-based inpatient psychiatric services, children's asthma care, surgical care improvement projects, and hospital outpatient measures.[12] In 2002, accredited hospitals began collecting data on standardized—or "core"—performance measures. In 2004, the Joint Commission and the CMS began working together to align measures common to both organizations. These standardized common measures, called Hospital Quality Measures, currently include acute myocardial infarction, heart failure, pneumonia, and surgical care improvement projects. In addition, the Joint Commission has core measure sets for pregnancy and related conditions and children's asthma care.[13] Findings from these measures are integrated into the priority focus process that the Joint Commission uses to develop its on-site survey evaluation activities. Additionally these data are publicly reported on the Joint Commission Web site via Quality Check (www.qualitycheck.org). Public availability of performance measure data allows users to compare hospital performance at the state and national levels.

Patient Safety and Sentinel Events
The Joint Commission places a high priority on patient safety, and each year new national patient safety goals (NPSG) are published to help organizations address specific areas of concern related to this issue. Compliance with these goals is factored into the Joint Commission's accreditation decision for healthcare organizations. Safety goals are updated annually and can be reviewed on the Joint Commission's Web site.[14]

Along with the focus on improving the quality of health care provided to the public, The Joint Commission reviews organizations' responses to sentinel events as part of its accreditation process.

> *A sentinel event is an unexpected occurrence involving death or serious physical or psychological injury, or the risk thereof. Serious injury specifically includes loss of limb or function. The phrase "or the risk thereof" includes any process variation for which a recurrence would carry a significant chance of a serious adverse outcome. Such events are called "sentinel" because they signal the need for immediate investigation and response.*[15]

When a sentinel event occurs, the healthcare organization must conduct a root-cause analysis and propose an action plan in an effort to determine what caused the event and to put preventive measures in place to ensure that it does not happen again. Sentinel Event Alerts are available on the Joint Commission's Web site as well as information on lessons learned from previous sentinel events. How well an organization responds to recommendations made through Sentinel Event Alerts is a part of the scoring process in accreditation decisions.

The Survey Process
Surveys for the Joint Commission accreditation have occurred on an unannounced basis in hospitals since 2006 and are conducted approximately every three years. In 2004, the Joint Commission implemented a redesign of the survey process to shift from a process focused on survey preparation and score achievement to one

of continuous systematic and operational improvement. The surveys now focus more on the provision of safe, high-quality patient care, treatment, and services.

In-depth information is collected about healthcare organizations and used to help focus the survey. This is accomplished through an electronic request for application and the Priority Focus Process. In this process, data about an organization are gathered from multiple sources (ORYX data, previous accreditation data, MedPar data, and application for accreditation data, among others). These data are analyzed using a set of defined, automated rules, which turn the data into information the surveyors can use to tailor the survey to the needs of that organization. This process enables the Joint Commission to identify the top four clinical or service groups of patients. Surveyors then use this information to guide their choice of actual patients who are traced through the facility. Surveyors track the care provided to those patients by going to any areas in which the individuals received care, treatment, or services throughout the organization. Along the way, they speak to the staff members who provided the care and assess how well the care was provided. If a compliance issue is identified, surveyors can pull additional patient records to identify whether the issue is isolated or whether it is a harbinger of a bigger system issue. Each tracer can take from one to three hours to complete. The average three-day survey will include 11 individual tracer patients.

In addition to tracing patients who receive care throughout the organization, surveyors assess specific systems related to care. For example, systems of medication management, infection control, and data use have been analyzed in some recent surveys. Topics of system tracers may change from year to year as the healthcare environment changes.

The changes include a more continuous accreditation process that will facilitate an organization's incorporation of the standards into daily operations. For example, a Periodic Performance Review (PPR) must be performed by the organization at the mid-point of its three-year accreditation cycle. This makes the accreditation process more continuous, reduces organizations' tendency to undertake last-minute efforts before the on-site survey, and promotes continuous organization compliance with the standards. PPR findings result in a plan of action for areas of noncompliance, which is reviewed and finalized by telephone with a Joint Commission staff member. The PPR findings and the plan of action will not affect the organization's current accreditation decision. The PPR process is supported by newly developed software that substantially minimizes the work burden.

The hospital survey lasts from two to five days, depending on the number of beds and the extent of hospital patient care activities. Smaller hospitals may be assessed by two surveyors (a physician and a nurse), whereas larger hospitals are examined by three surveyors (a physician, a nurse, and an administrator). A life safety surveyor was added in 2009. Most surveys include an opening conference and orientation with key leaders; a survey planning session; surveys of individual tracer activity, system tracer activity, and proficiency testing validation (laboratory only); special issue resolution; a daily briefing; review of the organization's competency assessment process, medical staff credentialing and privileging process, human resources review, environment of care session, and building tour; and the CEO exit briefing and organization exit conference. The surveyors use laptop computers to enter results of their surveys so as to expedite completion of the final report.

The organization's accreditation decision is based on how well it complies with the elements of performance for the standards, and each standard is judged either compliant or noncompliant. For any standard with which the hospital is found to be not compliant, the organization will receive a "requirement for improvement," which must be addressed in an "evidence of standards compliance" report within 45 days of the survey. If an organization is compliant with all standards at the time of the on-site survey, it will be accredited at that time. An appeals process is available for hospitals that wish to challenge the decision to deny accreditation.[16]

Health Facilities Accreditation Program

A viable alternative to the Joint Commission, the Health Facilities Accreditation Program (HFAP), was created in 1945 to accredit osteopathic hospitals. Today, it accredits more than 200 acute care and critical access hospitals and more than 150 other healthcare organizations in the United States. Accreditation is not limited to osteopathic facilities; HFAP also accredits allopathic acute care facilities. HFAP's Web site emphasizes that it is one of only three national voluntary accreditation programs authorized by CMS to survey hospitals for compliance with the Medicare COP, that it has maintained its deeming authority continuously since the inception of CMS in 1965, and that it meets or exceeds the standards required by CMS.[17] Some allopathic hospitals are now seeking HFAP accreditation rather than Joint Commission accreditation because it is less costly and the standards are more specific, making it clearer what an organization must do to achieve compliance.

HFAP accredits the following types of facilities:

- Hospitals and their clinical laboratories
- Ambulatory care/surgical facilities
- Mental health facilities
- Substance abuse facilities
- Physical rehabilitation facilities
- Clinical laboratories
- Critical access hospitals
- Stroke centers[18]

Standards

HFAP standards are cross-referenced to the Medicare COP for each type of facility. This approach means anyone reading the HFAP standards manual can clearly see how each standard ties directly to a Medicare COP. Forty percent of the HFAP standards reflect Medicare standards, 27% relate to patient safety, 29% to quality improvement, 26% to environmental safety, and 47% to patient treatment. Compliance with HFAP requirements assures compliance with Medicare standards.[19]

Quality Assessment and Performance Improvement

HFAP participates in a Clinical Quality Measurement Program with CMS that provides hospitals with periodic quality summary reports. Using aggregated data from CMS for quality-of-care measures for acute myocardial infarction, heart failure, pneumonia, and surgical infection prevention, the program makes it possible to compare a facility's quality data with data from the rest of the nation, the state, and other HFAP-accredited hospitals. HFAP uses this information to provide educational opportunities and workshops, develop accreditation standards, and improve the accreditation process.[20]

The Survey

Surveys are conducted every three years within the HFAP accreditation system. Surveyors are experienced healthcare professionals, and all surveys are unannounced. The survey team usually consists of a hospital administrator, a nurse, and a physician. The survey process entails an application, an on-site survey, a deficiency report, a plan of corrections, and the accreditation action. Three levels of accreditation exist:

- *Full accreditation,* which requires resurvey within three years, indicates that a healthcare facility meets the HFAP accreditation requirements in all performance areas.
- *Interim accreditation* indicates that a facility generally meets the standards, but that certain areas have been identified as needing additional work to be compliant. Interim accreditation will not exceed 12 months.
- *Denial of accreditation* indicates that a healthcare facility has been denied accreditation because it does not meet HFAP requirements.

An appeals process is available to organizations that wish to dispute the HFAP's decision.[21]

National Integrated Accreditation of Healthcare Organizations

In September 2008, CMS granted deeming authority to Det Norske Veritas (DNV) as a national hospital accrediting organization. Established in 1864, DNV is an independent foundation whose purpose is to safeguard life, property, and the environment. DNV's Web site states, "Increasing patient safety and reducing errors in healthcare is an important part of that purpose."[22] DNV has issued 1200 International

Organization for Standardization (ISO) certificates to healthcare facilities worldwide, including hospitals, outpatient clinics, diagnostic centers, laboratories, nursing homes, and home care centers.

DNV's accreditation program, known as National Integrated Accreditation of Healthcare Organizations (NIAHO), is the newest alternative in hospital accreditation and is the first new program approved for deeming authority by CMS in 40 years. It is also the first hospital accreditation program that incorporates the ISO 9001 quality management system requirements with the Medicare COP. To date, NIAHO has accredited 27 hospitals in 22 states.[23] The healthcare industry has been excited by its introduction, and views the advent of another hospital accrediting organization as good news and a welcome alternative to the Joint Commission.

Standards

The NIAHO standards look very much like the Medicare COP. The quality management standards require organizations to become compliant with ISO 9001 standards within two years of initial NIAHO accreditation. In the interim, the facility must establish and maintain a program with measurable quality objectives and analyze the results.

ISO 9000 is a family of standards for quality management systems and is administered by a variety of accreditation and certification bodies. At the time of this writing the requirements in ISO9001 include the following provisions:

- Adhering to a set of procedures that cover all key processes in the business
- Monitoring processes to ensure they are effective
- Keeping adequate records
- Checking output for defects, with appropriate and corrective action where necessary
- Regularly reviewing individual processes and the quality system itself for effectiveness
- Facilitating continual improvement[24]

The Survey

NIAHO conducts annual surveys to avoid the "fire drill" effect that sporadic surveys create in organizations.[25] Survey teams consist of administrators, nurses, physicians, and quality managers, all of whom are experienced in the life safety code, and information technology specialists. All survey team members are trained in the ISO 9001 quality management system. The on-site survey includes observation of care provided, patient and/or family interviews, staff interviews, and medical record review. Many documents are also reviewed, and a credentials file review is performed. Like the Joint Commission, NIAHO uses a patient tracer methodology, which had been in place with ISO 9001 long before it was adopted by any accreditation organization.[26]

If the organization elects to obtain NIAHO accreditation and ISO 9001 compliance or certification at the same time, the surveys usually take place according to the following schedule:

Year 1: NIAHO accreditation survey and ISO 9001 pre-assessment survey

Year 2: NIAHO accreditation survey and ISO 9001 compliance or certification survey

Year 3: NIAHO accreditation survey and ISO 9001 periodic survey

Year 4: NIAHO accreditation survey and ISO 9001 periodic survey

Year 5: NIAHO accreditation survey and ISO 9001 compliance or recertification survey

Year 6 through year 8 and beyond: Continue to repeat the processes for years 3 through 5

If the organization chooses to delay ISO 9001 compliance or certification for up to two years, ISO 9001 compliance or certification must be obtained no later than during the NIAHO accreditation survey conducted in the third year. Failure to obtain this ISO compliance or certification in this time frame will result in accreditation jeopardy status for the accredited organization.[27]

■ International Healthcare Accreditation

Due to a near-universal desire for quality health care and the fact that in many parts of the world, more people are choosing to cross international borders to access health care, there is a growing interest in international healthcare accreditation.[28] Medical tourism (global health care) is becoming increasingly important as people seek health care outside their own country for a variety of reasons, such as affordability, long waiting lists at home, cost, and confidentiality. Global health care represents a growing, multi-billion-dollar (or euro or pound sterling) business of increasing importance to the economies of many countries such as Singapore, Thailand, India, Hong Kong, Malaysia, and the Philippines.[29] The following quotation, taken from the Web site of Partners Harvard Medical International, crystallizes the increasing relevance of international healthcare accreditation:

> *Internationally, the growth of the health care industry has resulted in increased competition, leading hospitals to attempt to differentiate themselves through accreditation and certification by internationally recognized health care evaluators. Recognition from these organizations is a powerful symbol of a health care organization's commitment to high-quality health care, continuous improvement across all aspects of patient care and services, and patient safety.*

Accreditation and other measures of quality vary widely across the globe. There are risks and ethical issues that make the method of accessing medical care controversial.[30] Accreditation schemes that are well recognized as providing services in the international healthcare accreditation field include the following options:

- Trent Accreditation Scheme (or Trent), which is based in the United Kingdom/Europe, Hong Kong, the Philippines, and Malta (http://www.trentaccreditation-scheme.org/). Trent was the first organization to accredit a hospital in Asia, when it did so in Hong Kong in 2000.
- Joint Commission International (JCI), which is based in the United States (http://www.jointcommission.org/). The first hospital to be accredited in Asia by JCI was Bumrungrad International Hospital in 2002.
- Australian Council for Healthcare Standards International (ACHSI), which is based in Australia (http://www.achs.org.au/ACHSI/).
- Accreditation Canada (formerly the Canadian Council on Health Services Accreditation [CCHSA]), which is based in Canada (http://www.accreditation.ca).
- India: National Accreditation Board for Hospitals and Healthcare Providers (http://www.qcin.org/nabh/index.php).
- New Zealand: Quality Health New Zealand (QHNZ). QHNZ quality standards are based on those used in Australia and Canada. QHNZ is accredited by the international umbrella organization, the International Society for Quality in Healthcare.
- France: Haute Autorité de Santé (HAS).

The International Society for Quality in Health Care (ISQua) is an umbrella organization for organizations providing international healthcare accreditation (http://www.isqua.org/). Based in the Republic of Ireland, ISQua is a nonprofit, independent organization with members in more than 70 countries. It provides services to guide health professionals, providers, researchers, agencies, policymakers, and consumers to achieve excellence in healthcare delivery to all people, and to continuously improve the quality and safety of care. ISQua does not actually survey or accredit hospitals or clinics itself.

The United Kingdom Accreditation Forum (UKAF) is a U.K.-based umbrella organization for organizations providing healthcare accreditation (http://ukaf.org.uk/). Based in London, UKAF—like ISQua—does not actually survey and accredit hospitals itself.

The Joint Commission International (JCI) has accredited hospitals in Asia, the Middle East, Europe, the Americas, and Africa.[31] While JCI does not accredit medical personnel (it accredits only healthcare organizations, such as hospitals, polyclinics, and other service delivery facilities), it has built into its accreditation standards a number of requirements that reduce the risk of having unqualified professionals. Not unlike the Joint Commission, JCI standards require healthcare organizations to do the following:

- Verify each credential with the primary source—the organization that awarded the diploma, certificate, or other credential.
- Assign privileges to ensure that doctors practice only within their competency sphere. These privileges must limit doctors to practicing only in areas where they received training.
- Ensure that nurses and other professionals are assigned according to their credentials and demonstrated competencies.
- Have an ongoing professional performance review instead of a periodic review, which will quickly identify those whose actions render patients unsafe.

Although JCI standards are similar to those of the Joint Commission, there are subtle differences, from a credentialing perspective. The first obvious difference is that the Joint Commission requires reappointment every two years, whereas JCI reappointment is performed every three years. The Joint Commission (Standard MS.06.01.03) requires "the hospital to verify...the applicant's current license at the time of initial granting, renewal, and revision of privileges, and at the time of license expiration."[32] In contrast, JCI (Standard SQ.9) requires verification at the time of appointment, reappointment, and expiration.[33] The Joint Commission requires hospitals to query the National Practitioner Data Bank (NPDB) when clinical privileges are initially granted, at the time of renewal of privileges, and when a new privilege is requested,[34] while JCI is silent on use of NPDB. Of course, this should not prevent or deter a foreign hospital from querying the NPDB for practitioners who migrate to their hospital from the United States.

While the Middle East has become an oasis of expansion for health care, fraudulent credentials for healthcare professionals continues to be a major issue endangering patients in this region. For more information on physician, nurse, and other professional credentialing, visit the Staff Qualifications and Education (SQE) standards found in the third edition of JCI's *Accreditation Standards for Hospitals* (pages 204–212 in the printed version, including detail, or on pages 28–29 on free access to standards only).[35]

■ Long-Term Care Accreditation

The Joint Commission accredits long-term care facilities, including licensed nursing homes, but excluding intermediate care facilities specializing in care for individuals with mental retardation and other developmental disabilities; long-term care units in hospitals, but excluding beds belonging to a long-term acute care hospital and hospital swing beds; skilled nursing facilities; and long-term care facilities operated by a governmental entity, such as the Department of Veterans Affairs or a state authority. The standards are published in the *Comprehensive Accreditation Manual for Long Term Care* and address important functions relating to the care of residents and the management of healthcare organizations.

Surveys are conducted approximately every three years by experienced long-term care professionals. Long-term care facilities must participate in the ORYX initiative or another external performance measurement system. Accreditation decisions and the appeals process are the same as those for hospitals.

Managed Care Organization Accreditation

National Committee on Quality Assurance

The National Committee on Quality Assurance (NCQA) was founded in 1990. NCQA accredits health plans, managed care organizations (MCOs), managed behavioral healthcare organizations, new health plans, preferred provider organizations (PPOs), disease management programs, and quality plus, a quality measurement program for health plans. It offers certification programs for credentials verification organizations, physician organizations, health information products, utilization management and credentialing, disease management, and physician and hospital quality. NCQA also has the following physician recognition programs: back pain recognition, diabetes recognition, heart/stroke recognition, physician practice connections, and patient-centered medical home care.

The NCQA board of directors includes representatives from employers, physicians, public policy experts, consumer groups, and health systems. NCQA's mission is to improve the quality of health care. Its vision is to transform healthcare quality through measurement, transparency, and accountability. NCQA's activities center on accreditation or certification and performance measurement.

Health Plan Accreditation

NCQA health plan accreditation is designed to help employers and consumers distinguish between health plans based on their quality. The accreditation standards for MCOs and PPOs have been aligned into a unified set of standards for all health plans.

Health plan accreditation evaluates not only the core systems and process that make up the health plan, but also the actual results that the plan achieves on key dimensions of care and service. The review process is rigorous, consisting of on-site and off-site evaluations conducted by survey teams of physicians and managed care experts. The Review Oversight Committee (ROC), a national oversight committee of physicians, analyzes the teams' findings and assigns an accreditation status based on a plan's compliance with NCQA standards and its performance, relative to other plans, on selected Healthcare Effectiveness Data and Information Set performance measures, such as immunization and mammography rates and member satisfaction.[36]

The Survey

NCQA uses an online process as part of its accreditation survey. Its interactive Web-based system guides participants through a survey, provides feedback along the way, and saves time previously spent preparing paper documentation for the survey. Each organization requesting accreditation completes an online survey tool indicating compliance with each standard and attaches electronic copies of materials to its application to support its claims of standards compliance. Following off-site review of an organization's completed survey tool, a survey team makes an on-site visit to the facility. Surveyors typically spend two days on site validating key information and interviewing senior management staff of the organization being surveyed.

Following the completion of the survey, managed care plans may receive full accreditation for three years, one-year accreditation, provisional accreditation, or denial of accreditation, depending on their quality improvement programs and their level of compliance with the standards. NCQA levels of accreditation are specified as Excellent, Commendable, Accredited, Provisional, or Denied. An appeals process is available to MCOs that have been denied accreditation.

Performance Measurement: HEDIS and Quality Compass

NCQA's performance measurement tool for managed care is the Healthcare Effectiveness Data and Information Set (HEDIS), a set of standardized measures used to compare health plans. NCQA collects HEDIS data and accreditation information in a national database known as Quality Compass. Using Quality Compass, NCQA can generate national and regional averages on specific measures and identify benchmarks that are useful for comparative purposes. HEDIS assesses how effectively health plans care for acute and chronic illnesses, and it includes measures that address many of the nation's most serious health problems, such as breast cancer screening and advising smokers to quit.[37]

Beginning in 1999, MCOs seeking NCQA accreditation were required to implement HEDIS and submit audited HEDIS performance results to NCQA. Like hospital accrediting agencies, NCQA considers performance results as a part of the accreditation process. To ensure that quality and performance are maintained between on-site surveys, health plans are required to submit independently audited HEDIS results to NCQA annually. Should these results suggest a lapse in quality, NCQA may elect to resurvey the health plan.

In addition to HEDIS activities, health plans must conduct Consumer Assessment of Health Plans (CAHPS) surveys. CAHPS is kit of survey and report tools that provides information on consumer satisfaction with health plans; it was developed by the Agency for Healthcare Research and Quality (a government agency). NCQA began requiring the submission of CAHPS data in 1999. Like HEDIS, CAHPS provides reports that compare survey results to benchmarks.

URAC

Another managed care accrediting organization, URAC, was originally called the Utilization Review Accreditation Commission, but has now shortened its name to only the acronym. URAC accredits health plans and health networks, credentials verification organizations (CVOs), utilization review programs, and numerous other healthcare-related organizations. Founded in 1990, its initial focus was on standardizing utilization review procedures. In 1994, URAC acquired the American Accreditation Program, which accredits PPOs. URAC then expanded its managed care accreditation program to include health maintenance organizations (HMOs), physician–hospital organizations (PHOs), independent physicians associations (IPAs), independent delivery networks, management service organizations, and single specialty networks. URAC also accredits utilization review, worker's compensation, disease management, health call centers, case management programs, and claims processing programs; it even has a program for accreditation of health-related Web sites. Representatives of managed care associations, healthcare providers, and members of the public make up the URAC board of directors.

URAC has a modular accreditation system, which allows for a diverse range of healthcare organizations to apply for its accreditation. Organizations (with the exception of health-related Web sites) must meet core standards and may meet standards for various other modules, depending on the type of organization and its needs. Core standards address organizational structure, policies and procedures, staff qualifications, staff management, clinical oversight, quality improvement management, and consumer protection, among others. Organizations may then add modules for other functions such as case management, disease management, credentialing support or provider credentialing, and so on, depending on the organization's current needs and business goals.

The survey process consists of desktop review (review of documents) and an on-site survey; the final decision on accreditation is made following committee review. URAC's accreditation awards include two-year accreditation, conditional accreditation, and provisional accreditation. Organizations that are unable to meet URAC standards may be assigned corrective action status, or may choose to withdraw from the accreditation process.

■ Ambulatory Care Accreditation

Accrediting agencies for ambulatory care facilities include the American Association for Accreditation of Ambulatory Surgery Facilities, the Accreditation Association for Ambulatory Health Care, the Joint Commission, and HFAP.

American Association for Accreditation of Ambulatory Surgery Facilities

The American Association for Accreditation of Ambulatory Surgery Facilities (AAAASF), founded in 1980, has accredited more than 1000 single-specialty and multispecialty ambulatory surgery facilities, including centers that perform minor surgical procedures using local, regional, or topical anesthesia, and centers that perform major surgical procedures using sedation or general anesthesia by intubation. Its board of directors consists of physicians, nurses, and an attorney. The AAAASF accreditation standards address the following areas: equipment, operating room safety, and personnel and surgeon credentials.

Surveys are conducted every three years and consist of an application process, an inspection, and a decision by an accreditation committee. Surveyors are board-certified or board-qualified surgeons from AAAASF-accredited surgical facilities. The surveyors assess how well the facility complies with the standards as well as the scope of procedures being performed at the facility to ensure the surgeons have comparable hospital privileges.

Facilities may be awarded accreditation, provisional accreditation, or denial of accreditation. The accreditation is valid for three years, though facilities must complete a self-evaluation during the second and third years of each accreditation cycle. AAAASF has deemed status from Medicare.[38]

Accreditation Association for Ambulatory Health Care

The Accreditation Association for Ambulatory Health Care (AAAHC) was formed in 1979 and has accredited more than 4000 ambulatory healthcare facilities and organizations, including ambulatory and office-based surgery centers, MCOs, and Native American and student health centers, among others. Members of the governing board of the AAAHC are appointed from a number of professional medical academies and societies as well as college and community health centers. The AAAHC has deemed status from Medicare.

Core standards cover patient rights, governance, administration, quality of care provided, quality management and improvement, clinical records and health information, and facilities and environment. The following adjunct standards may apply depending on the type of organization:

- Anesthesia services
- Surgical and related services
- Overnight care and services
- Dental services
- Emergency services
- Immediate/urgent care services
- Pharmaceutical services

- Pathology and medical laboratory services
- Diagnostic imaging services
- Radiation oncology treatment services
- Employee and occupational health services
- Other professional and technical services
- Teaching and publication activities
- Research activities; managed care organizations
- Health education and wellness

The survey includes a self-assessment by the organization and an on-site survey that can last up to two days, depending on the size and type of organization. Facilities are granted three-year accreditation, one-year accreditation, or deferred accreditation.[39]

Joint Commission Ambulatory Care Accreditation

The Joint Commission has accredited more than 1600 freestanding ambulatory care facilities. These facilities include outpatient surgery centers, rehabilitation centers, infusion centers, clinics, teleradiology operations, and group practices, among others. The standards for ambulatory care facilities cover the environment of care, emergency management, human resources (credentialing and privileging standards are located here), infection control, information management, leadership, life safety, medication management, national patient safety goals, performance improvement, provision of care treatment and services, record of care treatment and services, rights and responsibilities; transplant safety, and waived testing. Surveys are conducted every three years; the surveyors are ambulatory care professionals with advanced medical or clinical degrees. The types of accreditation decisions are the same as those described for hospital surveys.

HFAP Ambulatory Surgery Center Accreditation

HFAP has deeming authority to accredit ambulatory surgery centers. Its program requirements incorporate the CMS COP along with other quality-related and patient safety standards. Unannounced surveys are conducted every three years. The survey process and accreditation levels are the same as those for hospitals.

■ Rehabilitation Facility Accreditation[29]

The Joint Commission accredits rehabilitation hospitals under its hospital accreditation program, and the Commission on Accreditation of Rehabilitation Facilities (CARF) accredits the rehabilitation program of the hospital. CARF also accredits outpatient rehabilitation programs. Since 1997, CARF and the Joint Commission have conducted their surveys concurrently in a combined process.

■ Commission on Accreditation of Rehabilitation Facilities

CARF was established in 1966 and accredits medical rehabilitation programs in comprehensive integrated inpatient rehabilitation hospitals, outpatient medical rehabilitation services, home- and community-based rehabilitation programs, residential rehabilitation programs, vocational services, pediatric and amputation specialty programs, brain or spinal cord injury programs, pain rehabilitation programs, occupational rehabilitation programs, health enhancement programs, and medical rehabilitation case management programs.[40] This organization's board of directors is composed of representatives of 26 medical academies and associations, as well as at-large trustees.

Medical rehabilitation programs must meet CARF standards related to their core values and mission; input from the persons served and other stakeholders; individual-centered planning, design, and delivery of services; rights of the persons served; quality and appropriateness of services; continuity of care; leadership, ethics, and advocacy; planning; financial management (including risk management); human resources; accessibility; health and safety; outcomes management and performance improvement; and infrastructure management.[41]

Surveys are conducted every three years. CARF surveyors have expertise in the areas they survey. Rehabilitation programs may receive three-year accreditation, one-year accreditation, provisional accreditation, nonaccreditation, or preliminary accreditation from CARF. There is an appeals mechanism for those organizations that are denied CARF accreditation.

■ Centers for Medicare and Medicaid Services

Title XVIII of the Social Security Act, Health Insurance for the Aged, is commonly known as Medicare. This legislation was originally passed in 1965 and went into effect in 1966. The Department of Health and Human Services' Centers for Medicare and Medicaid Services (CMS) operates the Medicare program.

Hospitals receiving Medicare reimbursement must satisfactorily comply with the COP, which are federal regulations delineating standards for healthcare delivery. As stated earlier, hospitals accredited by the HFAP or NIAHO are "deemed" to meet the conditions and the Joint Commission is in the process of reapplying for deeming status. State-level Departments of Health conduct CMS surveys validating the voluntary accreditation agency survey findings; they may also perform unannounced surveys of hospitals in response to a patient or family complaint. These surveys can be very rigorous and thorough—frequently more so than the voluntary accreditation program surveys, especially if the survey is performed in response to a complaint about patient care or treatment. A number of small rural hospitals do not seek voluntary accreditation but are surveyed by state agencies on behalf of CMS and are accredited by CMS so that they qualify for reimbursement for treatment of Medicare and Medicaid patients.

CMS has recently flexed its muscles concerning compliance with the COP. It is imperative that all healthcare organizations comply with these standards. The conditions for hospitals cover the following issues:

- Compliance with federal, state, and local laws
- Governing body
- Patients' rights
- Quality assessment and performance improvement program
- Medical staff
- Nursing services
- Medical record services
- Pharmaceutical services
- Radiological services
- Laboratory services
- Food and dietetic services
- Utilization review
- Physical environment
- Infection control
- Discharge planning
- Organ, tissue, and eye procurement
- Surgical services
- Anesthesia services
- Nuclear medicine services
- Outpatient services
- Emergency services
- Rehabilitation services
- Respiratory care services
- Special provisions applying to psychiatric hospitals
  - Medical record requirements
  - Staff requirements
- Special requirements for hospital providers of long-term care services[42]

Interpretive guidelines for complying with the COP can be found at the following Web site: http://dhi.health.state.nm.us/elibrary/hflcregs/AP-a.pdf.

CMS Quality Initiatives

In an effort to improve the quality of hospital care, CMS has partnered with several accreditation organizations in the Hospital Quality Measures program, and hospitals now regularly report their findings for these activities to CMS. CMS also sponsors Hospital Compare, which is a consumer-oriented Web site that provides information on how well hospitals deliver the recommended care to their patients. On this site, the consumer can see the recommended care that an adult should get if being treated for a heart attack, heart failure, or pneumonia or having surgery. The performance rates on the Web site generally reflect care provided to all U.S. adults with the exception of the 30-day risk adjusted death measures, which include only Medicare beneficiaries hospitalized for heart attack and heart failure.[43]

CMS also has instituted a policy that it will no longer reimburse hospitals for reasonably preventable medical errors. The conditions for which Medicare will no longer reimburse hospitals for treatment include falls; infections of the mediastinum, which can develop after heart surgery; urinary tract infections that result from improper use of catheters; pressure ulcers; and vascular infections that result from improper use of catheters. In addition, the nonreimbursable conditions include three "never events": objects left in the body during surgery, air embolisms, and blood incompatibility.[44]

■ International Organization for Standardization

ISO standards are developed by international groups of experts from business, government, and other organizations. In 1979, a technical committee was approved by ISO to address quality management and quality assurance. Twenty member countries became active in the work of this committee, and an additional 14 countries followed the work of the committee as observers. When the committee started work on generic quality management standards for worldwide application, contributions were made by a substantial foundation of national experience, particularly from the United Kingdom and Canada. Other countries with strong quality management practices, such as Japan, were also very interested in the work of the committee. The first standards for quality management and quality improvement were published in 1987, and were known as the ISO 9000 series. Today 69 country members and 18 observer countries participate in the work of this committee.

Some hospitals are now using the ISO 9001 quality management standards and are seeking certification by that organization in lieu of the Joint Commission accreditation. As mentioned earlier, the newest accrediting organization, NIAHO, has incorporated the ISO 9001 quality management standards into its accreditation process. These standards are adaptable to multiple types of business settings, including hospitals. They represent an international consensus on good management practices and address what the organization must do to manage processes that influence quality. Healthcare organizations that seek this type of certification believe that it is more relevant to improving performance in the organization.

Eight quality management principles are defined in ISO 9000:

- Principle 1: Customer focus
- Principle 2: Leadership
- Principle 3: Involvement of people
- Principle 4: Process approach
- Principle 5: System approach to management
- Principle 6: Continual improvement
- Principle 7: Factual approach to decision making
- Principle 8: Mutually beneficial supplier relationships

Healthcare organizations can implement and benefit from ISO quality management standards without seeking certification of conformance with the standards. Those that do seek certification undergo an audit and are then registered with ISO.[45]

■ Reviewing Credentials Files in an Accreditation Survey

The review of credentials files is a major part of all healthcare organization accreditation surveys. In most surveys, practitioner files are identified for review as part of the tracer methodology. In other words, the surveyors review files of the practitioners caring for the patients identified as tracer patients. Some surveyors supplement this material with a list of other credentials files they want to review. It is common for surveyors to review several allied health professional files (usually physician assistants and advanced practice nurses), but some surveyors also request files of medical staff leaders and practitioners who have been disciplined or who have requested additional privileges. Because the credentialing or medical staff services department does not get much notice about which files will be reviewed, it is very important to maintain all credentials files in good order at all times. With unannounced surveys, there can be no slacking for two or more years and then a mad scramble a few months or weeks before the anticipated survey.

In addition to looking for documentation of current licensure, the surveyor checks credentials files for adequacy of and institution-specific privilege delineation as well as appropriate source verification of education, training, and experience. Reappointment documentation is checked to determine whether the reappointment has occurred within the required reappointment period. The surveyor will also determine whether there is evidence of ongoing professional practice evaluation that supports the clinical privileges exercised by the staff member. Surveyors frequently ask for documentation supporting a practitioner's competence to perform a specific clinical privilege.

Minutes of medical executive committee meetings may be reviewed if a question or issue is identified in the process of the tracer patient methodology and the surveyors want to investigate a problem or issue. It is important that these minutes are maintained in an organized, professional manner.

Notes

1. 42 U.S.C. §§1395bb(a).
2. Koln, LT, Corrigan JM, et al. *To Err Is Human: Building a Safer Health System*. Washington, DC: Institute of Medicine; 1999.
3. U.S. General Accounting Office, Medicare. *CMS Needs Additional Authority to Adequately Oversee Patient Safety in Hospitals*. GAO-04-850. Washington, DC: Author; July 2004. Available at: http://www.gao.gov/new.items/d04850.pdf.
4. Robert JS, Coale JG, Redman RR. "A History of the Joint Commission on Accreditation of Hospitals." *JAMA*. 1978;258:936–940.
5. Robert et al., note 4.
6. Davis L. *Fellowship of Surgeons: A History of the American College of Surgeons*. Chicago, Ill: American College of Surgeons; 1973.
7. Davis, note 6.
8. Robert et al., note 4.
9. The Joint Commission. "Facts about the Joint Commission." Available at: http://www.jointcommission.org/AboutUs/Fact_Sheets/joint_commission_facts.htm. Accessed June 16, 2009.
10. Joint Commission International. "About Joint Commission International." Available at: http://www.jointcommissioninternational.org/about-jci/. Accessed June 16, 2009.
11. The Joint Commission, note 9.
12. The Joint Commission. "Facts about ORYX for Hospitals." Available at: http://www.jointcommission.org/AccreditationPrograms/Hospitals/ORYX/oryx_facts.htm. Accessed June 16, 2009.
13. The Joint Commission. "Facts about ORYX® for Hospitals, Core Measures and Hospital Quality Measures." Available at: http://www.jointcommission.org/NewsRoom/PressKits/AnnualReport/ar_facts_oryx.htm. Accessed June 16, 2009.
14. The Joint Commission. "Facts about the National Patient Safety Goals." Available at: http://www.jointcommission.org/PatientSafety/NationalPatientSafetyGoals/npsg_facts.htm. Accessed June 16, 2009.
15. The Joint Commission. "Sentinel Event." Available at: http://www.jointcommission.org/SentinelEvents/. Accessed June 16, 2009.
16. The Joint Commission. "Facts about the On-Site Survey Process." Available at: http://www.jointcommission.org/AboutUs/Fact_Sheets/onsite_qa.htm. Accessed June 19, 2009.
17. Healthcare Facilities Accreditation Program. "About HFAP." Available at: http://www.hfap.org/about/faq.aspx. Accessed June 18, 2009.
18. Healthcare Facilities Accreditation Program, note 17.
19. Healthcare Facilities Accreditation Program, note 17.
20. National Association for Healthcare Quality. "E-News Spotlight." Available at: http://www.nahq.org/enews/pdfs/0608_spotlight.pdf. Accessed June 18, 2009.
21. Healthcare Facilities Accreditation Program. "The Accreditation Process." Available at: http://www.hfap.org/AccreditationPrograms/accreditationProcess.aspx. Accessed June 18, 2009.
22. Det Norske Veritas. "Advantages of DNV Accreditation." Available at: http://www.dnv.com/industry/healthcare/hospital_accreditation/niaho_advantages/index.asp. Accessed June 18, 2009.
23. Det Norske Veritas, note 22.

24. International Organization for Standards. "Quality Management Principles." Available at: http://www.iso.org/iso/iso_catalogue/management_standards/iso_9000_iso_14000/qmp.htm. Accessed June 18, 2009.
25. International Organization for Standards, note 24.
26. Det Norske Veritas. "Introduction to DNV Healthcare and NIAHO." Available at: http://www.dnv.com/industry/healthcare/hospital_accreditation/resources/index.asp. Accessed June 18, 2009.
27. Det Norske Veritas. "NIAHO Accreditation Process." Available at: http://www.dnv.com/binaries/NIAHO%20Accreditation%20Process-Rev%2011_tcm4-338749.pdf. Accessed June 18, 2009.
28. Lovern E. "Accreditation Gains Attention." *Mod Healthcare*. 2000;30(47):46. Available at: http://findarticles.com/p/articles/mi_hb6375/is_/ai_n25535702. Accessed June 27, 2009.
29. Ramanna M. "Medical Tourism and the Demand for Hospital Accreditation Overseas." (2006). Available at: http://www.law.uh.edu/healthlaw/perspectives/2006%5C(MR)MedicalTourismFinal.pdf. Accessed June 27, 2009.
30. Gahlinger PM. *The Medical Tourism Travel Guide: Your Complete Reference to Top-Quality, Low-Cost Dental, Cosmetic, Medical Care and Surgery Overseas*. North Branch, MN: Sunrise River Press; 2008.
31. Placid Way. "Understanding JCI Credentials." (n.d.). Available at: http://www.placidway.com/article/55. Accessed July 5, 2009.
32. The Joint Commission. *2008 Hospital Accreditation Standards*. Oakbrook Terrace, IL: Author; 2008:146.
33. Joint Commission International. *Accreditation Standards for Hospitals* (3rd ed.). Oakbrook Terrace, IL: Joint Commission International: 2008:305.
34. The Joint Commission, note 32, p. 147.
35. Joint Commission International, note 33, p. 204.
36. National Committee for Quality Assurance. "Health Plan Accreditation." Available at: http://www.ncqa.org/tabid/689/Default.aspx. Accessed June 19, 2009.
37. National Committee for Quality Assurance. "HEDIS and Quality Compass." Available at: http://www.ncqa.org/tabid/187/Default.aspx. Accessed June 19, 2009.
38. American Association for Accreditation of Ambulatory Surgery Facilities. "About Accreditation." Available at: http://www.aaaasf.org/surgicenters.php. Accessed June 23, 2009.
39. Accreditation Association for Ambulatory Health Care. "About AAAHC." Available at: http://www.aaahc.org/eweb/dynamicpage.aspx?site=aaahc_site&webcode=about_aaahc. Accessed June 23, 2009.
40. Commission on Accreditation of Rehabilitation Facilities. "2009 Medical Rehabilitation Program Descriptions." Available at: http://www.carf.org/pdf/MedProgDesc.pdf. Accessed June 23, 2009.
41. Commission on Accreditation of Rehabilitation Facilities. "Medical Rehabilitation Accreditation and Standards." Available at: http://www.carf.org/Providers.aspx?content=content/Accreditation/Opportunities/MED/AccreditationStandards.htm. Accessed June 23, 2009.
42. 2004 CFR Title 42, Chapter IV, Part 482. Available at: http://www.access.gpo.gov/nara/cfr/waisidx_04/42cfr482_04.html. Accessed June 23, 2009.
43. Centers for Medicare and Medicaid Services. "Hospital Compare." Available at: http://www.cms.hhs.gov/HospitalQualityInits/11_HospitalCompare.asp#TopOfPage. Accessed June 23, 2009.
44. Centers for Medicare and Medicaid Services. "Details for: Eliminating Serious, Preventable, and Costly Medical Errors—Never Events." Available at: http://www.cms.hhs.gov/apps/media/press/release.asp?Counter=1863. Accessed June 23, 2009.
45. International Organization for Standardization, note 24.

CHAPTER 3

The Medical Staff Organization

Cindy A. Gassiot, CPMSM, CPCS
Vicki L. Searcy, CPMSM

"A hospital medical staff organization is created by the hospital's corporate bylaws to care for patients and to be its agent in the functions of peer review and credentialing."

C. Wesley Eisele, MD[1]

■ Introduction

Most laypersons are not aware that there is an "organization" within the hospital for the physicians and other professionals who practice there. (Indeed, many hospital workers are not well informed about this fact, either.) Many people believe that physicians are employees of a hospital. That is not true in the majority of cases, although employment of physicians by hospitals is becoming more common. In any event, whether they are employees or not, physicians must apply to become members of the hospital's medical staff organization and request privileges to practice in the hospital. When first learning about the medical staff organization, most people are amazed that its structure is so complex and are surprised to learn of the many checks and balances that are built into the system. Although these measures do not always work as well as they should, they do exist and can be made to work well by a dedicated medical staff and knowledgeable hospital support staff.

It is sometimes difficult to organize medical staff members and coordinate their activities. Physicians are not inherently organizationally oriented people. They are trained to be individual thinkers, and some are unfamiliar with working in an organizational setting. There are always some, however, who rise to the occasion and make superb medical staff leaders. These individuals make the medical staff services professional's work especially satisfying and rewarding.

More than just individuals who treat patients in a hospital, the medical staff is a structured organization with elected officials and a set of bylaws used to govern

---

Portions of this chapter are revised and updated from *Principles of Medical Staff Services Science* by Cindy Orsund Gassiot and Patricia Starr, National Association Medical Staff Services, 1987.
© Cindy Orsund Gassiot and Patricia Starr.

itself. To function effectively, the medical staff services professional (MSSP) must have a thorough understanding of this structure and the purposes and functions of the medical staff organization. The MSSP should also understand how the medical staff organization fits into the overall management structure of the hospital (see Chapter 1).

■ The Medical Staff Organization

The Joint Commission on Accreditation of Healthcare Organizations (Joint Commission), an accrediting organization for hospitals, characterized the medical staff as follows in an earlier version of the Medical Staff Standards:

> *The organized medical staff has a critical role in the process of providing oversight of quality of care, treatment, and services.... The tasks of the medical staff are numerous and require a dedicated and organized leadership to adequately perform their duties.*
>
> *The standards further define the organized medical staff.... Individual members of the medical staff care for patients within an organization context. Within this context, members of the medical staff, as individuals and as a group, interface with, and actively participate in, important organization functions....*
>
> *The hospital has an organized, self-governing medical staff that provides oversight of care, treatment, and services provided by practitioners with privileges; provides for a uniform quality of patient care, treatment, and services; and reports to and is accountable to the governing body.*[2]

Each medical staff has the following characteristics: It includes fully licensed physicians (doctors of medicine [MD] and osteopathy [DO]), and may include other licensed individuals permitted by law and by the hospital to provide patient care services independently in the hospital. Those individuals may include physicians, oral and maxillofacial surgeons, dentists, podiatrists, and, in some states, clinical psychologists. In most hospitals, allied health professionals such as physician assistants and advanced practice nurse practitioners are granted clinical privileges. The latter practitioners are usually not members of the medical staff, but they do have clinical privileges to practice in the hospital, sometimes with minimal physician supervision. For example, in Arkansas, only physicians and dentists can be members of the medical staff. In contrast, in California, the medical staff may comprise physicians, dentists, podiatrists, and clinical psychologists. In Texas, its composition may include physicians, dentists, and podiatrists. The membership allowed differs from state to state.

To determine the types of practitioners eligible to be members of the medical staff, the organization should research its state law (regulations related to the make-up of the medical staff are usually contained in the hospital state licensing standards or requirements). The Medicare Conditions of Participation Interpretative Guidelines (updated October 17, 2008) contains the following information related to membership on the medical staff.

Interpretive Guidelines §482.12(a)(1)

The governing body must determine, in accordance with State law, which categories of practitioners are eligible for appointment to the medical staff.

The medical staff must, at a minimum, be composed of physicians who are doctors of medicine or doctors of osteopathy. In addition, the medical staff may include other practitioners included in the definition in Section 1861(r) of the Social Security Act of a physician:

- Doctor of medicine or osteopathy;
- Doctor of dental surgery or of dental medicine;
- Doctor of podiatric medicine;
- Doctor of optometry; and
- A Chiropractor.

In all cases, the practitioners included in the definition of a physician must be legally authorized to practice within the State where the hospital is located and providing services within their authorized scope of practice. In addition, in certain instances the Social Security Act and regulations attach further limitations as to the type of hospital services for which a practitioner may be considered to be a "physician." See 42 CFR 482.12(c)(1) for more detail on these limitations.

The governing body has the flexibility to determine whether other types of practitioners included in the definition of a physician are eligible for appointment to the medical staff.

Furthermore, the governing body has the authority, in accordance with State law, to appoint some types of non-physician practitioners, such as nurse practitioners, physician assistants, certified registered nurse anesthetists, and midwives, to the medical staff.

Practitioners, both physicians and non-physicians, may be granted privileges to practice at the hospital by the governing body for practice activities authorized within their State scope of practice without being appointed a member of the medical staff.

■ Accountability

The governing body of the hospital is the source of all legal authority and may not delegate the ultimate responsibility for the overall quality of care delivered in the hospital. The governing body does, however, delegate responsibility to the medical staff to perform credentialing and peer review activities. In carrying out these functions, the medical staff organization acts as an agent of the governing body and must be accountable for its performance. By adopting its own bylaws, the medical staff organization becomes self-governing, but as a creation of the hospital corporate bylaws, the medical staff organization derives its authority to act from this source. The medical staff organization reports directly to the governing body of the hospital through the president or chief of the medical staff.

The membership of the governing body of a hospital usually consists of hospital senior management representatives, representatives of the local business community, and physicians.

■ The Traditional Model Medical Staff Organization

Purpose

It is generally agreed that the medical staff organization has two major purposes: (1) to establish mechanisms for controlling the quality of care rendered by medical staff members and other practitioners granted clinical privileges and (2) to provide a structure whereby physicians have input into decision making within the institution.

Functions

In carrying out its purpose, certain functions are performed by the medical staff organization:

- Establishing professional standards
- Providing for continuous surveillance to see that standards are met
- Taking a leadership role in performance improvement and patient safety
- Making regular reports to the governing body on the quality of medical care
- Making recommendations to the governing body on appointments, reappointments, and clinical privileges
- Ensuring compliance with medical staff bylaws, rules, regulations, and hospital policy
- Taking disciplinary action (enforcement of professional standards) when necessary
- Participating in hospital and strategic planning
- Providing continuing medical education for medical staff members

Membership Categories

The medical staff organization is also divided into membership categories. Staff categories are not working units of the medical staff organization, but rather clarify the activity level of the individual member as well as his or her potential involvement in participation in medical staff organization functions and activities. Although they vary depending on the hospital, membership categories typically include active, provisional, courtesy, consulting, honorary, and affiliate or nonadmitting members. Some medical staff organizations are finding that these typical categories are no longer relevant and, in an effort to simplify them, have restructured their categories to include only voting and non-voting members.

Active Members

Active members are the practitioners who actively admit to or work in the hospital. The bylaws accord the active members voting and officer candidacy rights. Medical staff committees are generally composed of active members, and there are sometimes meeting attendance requirements for active staff members.

Provisional Members

Provisional membership is actually a membership status rather than a staff category. However, many hospitals use "provisional" or "associate" as a staff category. In the past, the Joint Commission required all newly appointed members to serve a provisional period of time. This is no longer the case, however, and there is no mention in current Joint Commission standards related to a provisional period. Regardless of what it is called, this is typically the category into which all newly appointed medical staff members are placed. The length of the provisional period may vary from hospital to hospital, but is usually one year. Because membership and privileges are granted based on a review of paper credentials, the staff member's competence is further assessed during the provisional period through close observation and review of work (in Joint Commission–accredited hospitals, this validation of competency would be through focused professional practice evaluation).

Courtesy Members

The courtesy category is usually composed of staff members who use the hospital less frequently than active staff members. These members are not accorded voting or officer candidacy rights, and they generally are not required to attend medical staff meetings.

Consulting Members

The consulting category is composed of practitioners who perform consultations for other categories of staff members. These members sometimes do not admit patients to the hospital but assist other practitioners in caring for them. Consulting members usually do not have voting rights, nor are they required to attend medical staff meetings.

Honorary Members

This staff category implies emeritus status and may be reserved for practitioners who no longer actively practice medicine or members who hold teaching positions at medical schools. Honorary staff members do not have admitting or clinical privileges.

Affiliate or Nonadmitting Members

This staff category has been created by some medical staff organizations to accommodate practitioners who refer patients to the hospital for treatment by other medical staff members but do not admit patients on their own. Many of these are office-based practitioners who no longer treat hospitalized patients for various reasons. In many cases, affiliate staff members do not have admitting or clinical privileges.

Structure

The medical staff organization usually is structured with three components or working units:

- Medical staff officers
- Clinical departments
- Medical staff committees

FIGURE 3-1 is a sample organizational chart for the traditional medical staff organization.

Medical Staff Officers

Although there is variation from hospital to hospital, the usual officers of the medical staff are the president or chief of staff, the vice president or vice chief, and the secretary-treasurer. Some medical staff organizations include the immediate past president/immediate past chief of staff as an officer.

The president of the staff is elected or selected to act as head of the medical staff and is accountable to the governing body for all activities of the medical staff organization. The president is usually chair of the executive committee of the medical staff. The medical staff bylaws must specify the method of selection, tenure, and qualifications of all officers.

Each clinical department is represented by a chair (or chief) in a departmentalized medical staff organization. The method of selection of each department chair is specified in the bylaws and may include election by the department or appointment. The chair's responsibilities include being accountable for all professional and administrative activities within the department and continuing surveillance of the professional performance of all members of the department. He or she is also responsible for implementation of a program to monitor and evaluate the quality and appropriateness of patient care provided by members of the department.

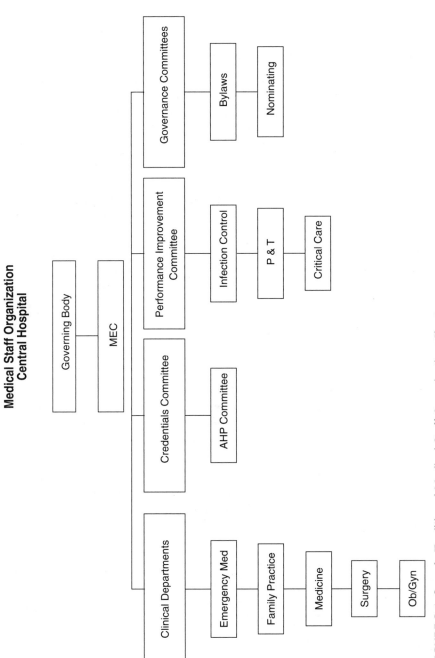

FIGURE 3-1 Sample Traditional Medical Staff Organization Chart

The Traditional Model Medical Staff Organization

Medical Staff Departments

Most hospitals with large numbers of medical staff members in a variety of specialties have departmentalized medical staffs. That is, the staff is organized into groups of practitioners with similar specialties, such as surgery, medicine, family practice, obstetrics/gynecology, and pediatrics. Large hospitals with hundreds of medical staff members may have ten or more clinical departments, which may be further subdivided into sections or services within those departments. For example, urology and ophthalmology may be sections within the department of surgery. Alternatively they may be free-standing departments if there are large numbers of these specialists. Although the trend has been to reduce the number of departments or sections by combining some of them, many medical staff organizations persist in having a large number of departments. Also, in many teaching hospitals, the medical staff departments mirror the organizational units of the teaching program.

Each medical staff member must be assigned to one department. Members can, however, have clinical privileges in more than one department.

Many medical staffs have restructured their organizations in the past ten years, reducing the frequency of departmental meetings from monthly to bimonthly or even quarterly. There must be some forum for communication among department members and means for them to consider the findings of the monitoring and assessment of patient care provided by members of the department. Traditionally, holding departmental meetings was the method used to meet this communication requirement and to conduct department business. Other means may also be used to review outcomes of care provided, such as each person reviewing the findings individually and then conducting a conference call discussion. These findings must be distributed in a way to ensure confidentiality, as it is essential that peer review deliberations and findings be kept confidential.

When the medical staff is departmentalized, the active medical staff members usually meet at least annually (often receiving annual reports, approving bylaws amendments, and electing officers). Some medical staff organizations meet on a quarterly basis.

Nondepartmentalized Medical Staffs

When the hospital is small and the number of medical staff members is small, the medical staff is usually nondepartmentalized. A nondepartmentalized medical staff may have a medical executive committee, or the active members may act as a whole to perform the required functions.

Medical Staff Committees

In addition to departments, medical staff committees are working units of the medical staff organization. While the Joint Commission requires only one medical staff committee—the medical executive committee—there are usually numerous others. Both the Joint Commission standards and CMS state that the executive committee must be made up of fully licensed doctors of medicine or osteopathy who are actively practicing in the hospital. (It should be noted that CMS does not require a medical executive committee, but the Conditions of Participation [COP] state that if there is a medical executive committee, the majority of members must be MDs or DOs.) Over the years, committees have often been formed to perform the functions required by the Joint Commission, even though the Joint Commission does not formally require a committee. One or two individuals can perform many of these functions.

Most medical staff organizations have committees to perform the functions of credentials review, operative procedure review, pharmacy and therapeutics review, medical records review, performance improvement, peer review, and so on. The COP requires that a committee be designated responsibility for utilization review. Departments also sometimes form committees to perform administrative or oversight functions. Examples include operating room committees or critical care committees. Committees are generally designated as standing, special, or ad hoc (task oriented).

Restructuring has occurred in many medical staff organizations, reflecting the trend toward reducing the number of medical staff committees and increasing the assignment of functions to individuals. However, old habits and traditions die hard in some facilities, and many medical staff organizations still abound with committees.

The Medical Executive Committee

As mentioned previously, the medical executive committee (MEC) is the only medical staff committee required by the Joint Commission. It is the chief policy-making and action committee of the medical staff. This committee acts as the overseer of all functions performed by the medical staff. The executive committee of the medical staff is also a focal point for changes in the medical staff, be they organizational, functional, or attitudinal. This committee should be the element of the medical staff organization that exercises the greatest influence on the organization as a whole.

The MEC is usually composed of the medical staff officers and department chairs, with representatives from administration and nursing management (this composition varies from hospital to hospital, although the Joint Commission standards require that the chief executive officer or his or her designee be an ex officio member with or without voting privileges). The MEC typically meets on a monthly basis to receive and act on reports of departments and committees that report directly to the MEC. This body holds the medical staff accountable to the governing board for the quality of care rendered within the hospital. It is also the vehicle for medical staff input into hospital planning to meet community needs.

■ Developing Medical Staff Leaders

The key to a well-functioning medical staff organization is its leadership and support. For leaders to function at the highest level, they should be educated to their roles. This preparation should include an orientation to the purposes and functions of the medical staff organization as well as a job description specific to the particular position. (A sample job description for a medical staff leader can be found on the CD that accompanies this book.) Many organizations hold orientation for leaders in-house, bring consultants in to present the information, or sponsor attendance of key leaders at outside educational sessions specifically designed for leadership training. Several excellent leadership training seminars are presented by various organizations. If funds are not available to send leaders away for training, a good orientation can be organized and presented locally by hospital staff.

Support by an educated and competent MSSP is also essential to building a high-performing medical staff organization. Medical staff leaders look to the MSSP as a resource and for guidance and support in many of the functions that are the responsibility of the medical staff organization (see Chapter 1).

■ Medical Staff Bylaws

Like any other organization, the medical staff must have a set of guiding principles by which to operate.

> *Medical staff bylaws are the blueprints for medical staff organization. They constitute the glue that holds the parts of the medical staff organization together.... The major emphasis of the bylaws must be to coordinate all the efforts of all members of the medical staff in the fulfillment of institutional goals. At the same time, they serve to formalize ways in which each staff member can be assured that his or her constitutional rights are protected.*[3]

For the MSSP, the bylaws (and related manuals) should serve as a road map to the medical staff services department in carrying out its daily operations. In addition to outlining the organizational structure of the medical staff, bylaws or policies should contain specific procedures for appointment, reappointment, and granting of clinical privileges. The provisions in the bylaws for corrective action, due process, and appellate review are of great importance. The manner in which officers are elected or selected and functions of committees are to be found in the bylaws. In short, the answers to questions about authority, responsibilities, functions, and rights of medical staff members should be contained in the bylaws. See Chapter 4 for additional information on medical staff bylaws.

■ Relevance of the Medical Staff Organization

Critics of traditional medical staff organizations contend that the way medical staff organizations function is antiquated and out of step in today's healthcare environment. The point out that modern-day health care requires thoughtful—but rapid—decision making as well as restraint in using the time of busy practitioners for activities that are often perceived to have little or no value. These critics believe that medical staff organizations are largely ineffective in establishing systems to ensure practitioner competency, and they suggest that medical staff organizations have become so mired in tradition, politics, and bureaucracy that their chance of making the transition to more meaningful, effective, and efficient ways of handling medical staff organization business and functions is miniscule.

In many organizations, this is all too true. Many medical staff organizations have cumbersome committee structures, with ill-defined responsibilities, accountabilities, and a lack of any positive outcomes. Others have officers and department chairs that cannot or will not do the jobs for which they were elected or appointed. Still other organizations have problem practitioners and fail to take actions to protect patients.

Stories abound about endless medical executive committees, meetings that have to be rescheduled because a quorum wasn't present, meetings that start 30 to 45 minutes late, and so on. Some chiefs of staff appear for medical executive committee meetings without the benefit of having even glanced at the agenda for the meeting. And what about those occasions when candidates come to be interviewed by the credentials committee—but the majority of credentials committee members don't attend the meeting? Is there any wonder that the relevance of the medical staff organization is being judged—and found wanting?

Short of blowing up the current organization structure, what can be done?

■ Barriers to Success with the Traditional Medical Staff Organization

Traditional medical staff organization structures worked better in the past than they do in today's healthcare environment. What is the difference between then and now? Here are a few ideas about what is happening that has diminished the effectiveness of current medical staff organizations:

- Physicians have less time. Physicians are busier than ever, and finding physicians who are willing to take on leadership positions (or will even serve on a committee) is becoming harder.
- In many areas, physicians are not "loyal" to a hospital, as they might have been in the past.

- Reimbursement systems may require that physicians maintain privileges at more hospitals, further reducing their available time to serve in any type of leadership position.
- Many physicians are angry at hospitals. Hospitals are perceived by physicians as forcing them to take emergency calls and "donate" their time to activities that are not financially rewarding.
- Serving as a medical staff leader doesn't bring the same honor and respect that it did in the past. Today's medical staff member is likely to believe that serving as a medical staff leader will be onerous (e.g., dealing with behavior issues, competency problems, attending hours of meetings), rather than something he or she will look back on with pride and satisfaction.
- Many physicians perceive that the medical staff organization exists to help the hospital meet the Joint Commission requirements—and physicians are tired of hearing about the latest and greatest changes in standards requirements and survey methods.
- Hospital administrators are busier than ever, and they may deliver a message through their behavior (such as by being late to meetings or not appearing at all) that the work performed by the medical staff organization is unimportant.
- There are more paid positions, such as physician administrators, and medical staff members may believe that if the hospital wants the work done, it should give the work to the physicians who are being paid to do it.
- Sometimes medical staff leaders are paid (i.e., a stipend for the chief of staff, department chairs), but it is the rare medical staff organization that couples a stipend for a position with a relevant job description. If there is, in fact, a job description, there is rarely any type of meaningful performance evaluation associated with it.

■ Alternatives to the Traditional Medical Staff Organization

Are there alternatives to the traditional medical staff organization? Is there some outside force that requires our ongoing support for these often ineffective structures?

First, the CMS's COP requires that the medical staff organization perform specific functions (credentialing, privileging) and adopt and enforce bylaws, but there is no absolute requirement for a medical executive committee (or any other medical staff organization committees). The Joint Commission standards require a self-governing medical staff organization, bylaws, credentialing and privileging, quality oversight, and a medical executive committee. The Joint Commission is much less prescriptive about how the medical staff organization carries out its responsibility

Exhibit 3-1: Evaluation Tool for Understanding Committees and Their Roles

Committee Meeting: _____
Analysis Prepared by: _____
Date: _____

Issue	Comments

Committee Purpose
- What is the purpose of the committee?
- Is the purpose clearly defined in writing?
- Where is the purpose of the committee described?
- Do the committee members know the purpose?
- How do we determine if the purpose is being fulfilled?

Committee Members
- Who are the members of the committee?
- In which documents are the members specified (and their roles, if any)?
- Is it clear which members are voting members versus nonvoting or ex-officio members?

Minutes
- Where are the complete sets of minutes and records maintained?

Frequency of Meetings
(Review Attendance Records)
- How often is the committee supposed to meet?
- How often did the committee meet during the past 12 months (go back two years, if possible)?
- Was a meeting ever canceled because of a lack of quorum?
- Was a meeting ever held despite not having a quorum?
- Do physicians regularly attend this meeting?
- What percentage of meetings are attended by each physician? Other key individuals?

Committee Relationships
- How does this committee relate to other medical staff organization (or nonmedical staff organization) committees?

than it was in years past. The focus of the Joint Commission is on functions—not committees.

Some consultants who regularly work with medical staff organizations believe that, in the future, physicians will be paid to perform specific functions. For example, a physician (or two) could be paid to function in a credentialing capacity to act in lieu of a "volunteer" credentials committee. There are already precedents for "outsourcing" and paying for peer review activities.

There are downsides to use of paid physicians to complete these functions, however. These disadvantages tend to be emphasized by physicians who believe that making changes to current medical staff organization structures will have a negative effect on the quality of care provided by a healthcare organization. Unfortunately, the physicians who object to moving to a more contemporary way to carry out necessary functions and activities rarely have solutions for fixing what currently doesn't work.

The MSSP should do all he or she can to support the work of the medical staff organization in an efficient and effective manner. Credentialing, privileging, peer review, and other responsibilities assigned to this structure are critical functions to ensure patient safety, and the MSSP must remember that fact during the dark hours when physicians and medical staff leaders fail to step up to the plate to assume their roles and responsibilities. Here are a few things that MSSPs can do to make current organization structures more effective:

1. Don't encourage physicians to have meetings when a lack of substantive agenda items makes having a meeting a waste of everyone's time.
2. Don't propagate retaining ineffective structures because "it has always been done that way" or because there is a (usually mistaken) belief that an accreditation/regulatory agency requires a specific committee.
3. Do as much work outside committee meetings as possible.
4. Encourage physicians who have new ideas about methods to get a particular function done.
5. Do an analysis of current committees to ascertain their effectiveness and the costs of doing business.
6. Always encourage physicians to be prepared for meetings in advance. Don't let poor planning on your part (i.e., writing an agenda at the last minute) be the reason for poor committee performance.

It is clear that medical staff organizations will not disappear anytime soon. Any number of physician-led professional organizations (such as the American Medical Association) would lobby hard to prevent, for example, a decreased emphasis by the Joint Commission on the roles and functions of the organized medical staff. Nevertheless, some medical staff organizations are slowly restructuring themselves into more effective models. These models usually have fewer committees and fewer departments, and they assign responsibilities to individuals and small groups rather than to standing committees. They are typically found in organizations where the "rank and file" medical staff members trust their elected officers to lead the organization and make decisions on behalf of the members. In other words, these organizations don't believe that each active member must vote on every issue. They provide for alternative and creative ways for members to have input into medical staff organization business without having endless committee meetings.

MSSPs who enjoy being part of a dynamic organization structure should seek out those opportunities and be part of a growing cadre of professionals who are eager to accept the challenge of change and create new ways to design and implement functions that are essential to providing safe patient care.

■ Notes

1. Eisele CW, Fifer WR, Wilson TC. *The Medical Staff and the Modern Hospital.* Englewood, CO: Estes Park Institute; 1985;3.
2. Joint Commission on Accreditation of Healthcare Organizations. *Comprehensive Accreditation Manual for Healthcare Organizations.* Oakbrook Terrace, IL: Author; 2004.
3. Williams KJ, Donnelly PR. *Medical Care Quality and the Public Trust.* Chicago, IL: Pluribus Press; 1982:86.

Medical Staff Bylaws and Related Documents

CHAPTER 4

Christina W. Giles, CPMSM, MS

These will be your Bible—do not go anywhere with out them!

Truer words were never said with regard to medical staff bylaws—this is best practice advice for all medical staff services and credentialing professionals.

Although in most organizations, bylaws are referred to as a necessary evil—a document described as legalistic, lengthy, unclear, and difficult to understand—the reality is that you will not be successful in your job if you do not have useful, well-written bylaws and related documents, policies, and procedures. If you have been working in medical staff services for any period of time, you know that eventually many key issues discussed at medical staff committee and department meetings or questions from medical staff leaders can be answered by researching the bylaws, rules and regulations, or related documents.

The bylaws, rules and regulations, and policies and procedures provide a written outline of the medical staff's structure and function, along with the medical staff's responsibility in accomplishing the goals, mission, and vision of the organization.[1] These documents contain the different components and specificity of the medical staff structure. The policies and procedures contain detailed how-to's providing the medical staff services professional (MSSP) with an opportunity to follow procedures that have been well established and that are compliant with the relevant accrediting agency standards, as well as with state, federal (Centers for Medicare and Medicaid [CMS]), and hospital requirements.

■ Definitions

Defining the names given to each kind of document will help identify what each contains.

- *Bylaws* are a governance framework document that establishes the roles and responsibilities of a body and its members.[2]
- *Medical staff bylaws* are regulations and/or rules adopted by the organized medical staff and the governing body of an organization for internal governance

and for defining rights and obligations of various officers, persons, or groups, within the organized medical staff's structure.³

- A *policy* is defined by *Webster's Dictionary* as a statement of fact that refers to a standard to be maintained; management or procedure based primarily on material interest; or a definite course or method of action selected from among alternatives and in light of given conditions to guide and determine present and future decisions; or a high-level overall plan embracing the general goals and acceptable procedures of a governing body.⁴
- A *procedure* is defined by *Webster's Dictionary* as a set of instructions on how the policy will be achieved; a particular way of accomplishing something; a series of steps followed in a regular definite order; a traditional or established way of doing things.⁵
- A *rule* is a prescribed guide for conduct or action, a written regulation governing procedure or controlling conduct.⁶
- A *regulation* is an authoritative rule dealing with details or procedure.⁷

Some medical staffs also have separate departmental rules and regulations. These documents typically contain the specifics of treating patients in that particular specialty, specialty specific privileging criteria, and/or state and federal requirements.

Based on various court interpretations, there continues to be uncertainty as to whether the bylaws constitute a contract—a document binding on the parties that agree to them—between the medical staff and the hospital or healthcare entity that approves and signs them. The AMA's policy states, "The medical staff bylaws are a contract between the organized medical staff and the hospital."⁸ The Joint Commission standards require that the medical staff bylaws create a system of rights and responsibilities between the organized medical staff and the governing body and between the organized medical staff and its members."⁹ Joint Commission standards also currently require that the governing body approve of and comply with the medical staff bylaws. Neither body may unilaterally amend the medical staff bylaws or rules and regulations.¹⁰ One may infer from this standard that because neither the medical staff nor the governing body can amend the bylaws or rules and regulations without the other group's input, these documents form a contract that cannot be changed by just one party. There have been various court cases representing both sides of this issue. (See Chapter 16 for more information on relevant court cases.)

■ Medical Staff Bylaws and Related Manuals

The Joint Commission outlines in its hospital accreditation standards what the medical staff bylaws should include. The CMS also outlines what should be included in medical staff bylaws in the hospital COP. Both documents should be maintained in the office as resource material. A table that provides a comparison of CMS and

Joint Commission requirements concerning the content of medical staff bylaws as well as the National Committee for Quality Assurance's (NCQA's) requirements for content of policies and procedures can be found on the CD that accompanies this book.

Many medical staffs have separated the bylaws document into multiple documents: a credentials manual, an organization manual, a fair hearing plan, rules and regulations, and policies and procedures. If more than one document is developed, all of the documents should be defined in the initial definition of the medical staff bylaws as "related documents or manuals" of the bylaws. For example, the definition of medical staff bylaws may appear as follows:

> *Medical staff bylaws or bylaws means the bylaws of the medical staff. Related manuals means any one or more of the following documents as appropriate to the context and shall be considered as included in the bylaws:*

- Medical staff credentials manual
- Medical staff fair hearing plan
- Organization manual
- General rules and regulations—policies and procedures of the medical staff

The reasoning behind separating the documents is based on the time and effort it takes to amend them. Traditionally, medical staff bylaws required that the active medical staff (or all those members designated as having the right to vote) must vote on any and all revisions. Some bylaws even require one or two "readings," and the medical staff must receive the proposed revisions 30 to 45 days prior to voting on the changes. By separating the bylaws content into different manuals, the revision process may become both more timely and easier to achieve. For example, credentialing procedures, which may be influenced by state, federal, and accrediting body requirements, and the organizational structure, such as the numbers of departments/divisions and medical staff committees, could be delineated in manuals in which the amendment process is achieved in a more timely manner, such as presentation to the medical executive committee for voting and then to the governing body.

Until 2005, it appeared that the Joint Commission was willing to accept this alternative approach of creating multiple documents with some of them containing a shorter, more direct amendment process. Since 2005, however, the Joint Commission has conducted multiple task force meetings leading to several revisions of the bylaws standards—specifically, what is to be included in the bylaws and what can be placed in policies and procedures. As of September 2009, the final revised Joint Commission language had not been established. In the absence of agreement on the Joint Commission bylaws standards, the MSSP should always have available the CMS standards concerning bylaws [§482.22 (c)].

An example of the "multiple manual" approach might include the following items:

- The bylaws containing the "nuts and bolts" of the medical staff organization
- The credentials manual containing the specifics about the appointment, reappointment, and privileging processes
- The organization manual containing the listing of departments/divisions and committees
- The rules and regulations containing the specifics about how to admit, transfer, care for and discharge patients, and any operating room requirements and medical records requirements

The policies and procedures would cover such issues as licensed independent practitioner health and well-being, code of behavior, medical staff peer review, practitioner interview, sedation/analgesia, and so on. Some medical staffs want the fair hearing and appellate procedures included in the bylaws; others would prefer that a separate document be established. Either way, the two sections/documents that would still be voted upon by the whole medical staff are the bylaws and the fair hearing and appellate review procedures.

FIGURE 4-1 depicts a traditional bylaws table of contents. There is no specific method for separating these topics into manuals, but many legal counsels who support the idea of separation of the documents would be able to advise which items to include in which documents.

CMS and accrediting body requirements for what needs to be in the medical staff bylaws should be reviewed annually to determine if there have been any revisions to the requirements. FIGURE 4-2 is a sample table of contents for medical staff rules and regulations.

After reading this chapter, take some time to review your institution's medical staff bylaws and identify the CMS requirements as well as any accrediting body standards relevant to medical staff bylaws with which you must comply. This step will familiarize you with your documents, and assist you in reviewing them for compliance with external standards. In addition, obtain a copy of the hospital's bylaws and compare the language in the medical staff section of the hospital bylaws to the relevant wording in the medical staff bylaws—there should not be any discrepancies. The medical staff bylaws are typically revised more often than the hospital bylaws, and discrepancies can often occur within the two documents.

The most important thing to remember about bylaws and related manuals is that they must always reflect the current structure and practice of the medical staff. They should be considered "living" documents, in that they will be used by many people on a continual basis; therefore, they must always be up-to-date and reflect compliance with state, federal, and accrediting body requirements as well as current practice in the hospital.

ARTICLE	TITLE	PAGE
	Definitions	3
I	Purpose	6
II	Name	7
III	Responsibilities of the Medical Staff Organization	8
IV	Membership	10
V	Medical Staff Categories	13
VI	Appointment and Reappointment	18
VII	Delineation of Clinical Privileges	26
VIII	Officers	29
IX	Clinical Departments	35
X	Committees	41
XI	Corrective Action	46
XII	Procedural Rights	54
XIII	Confidentiality, Immunity, and Releases	66
XIV	General Provisions	69
XV	Adoption and Amendment of Bylaws	72

FIGURE 4-1 Sample Medical Staff Bylaws Table of Contents

■ Medical Staff Bylaws and Related Manuals Revision Project

The revision process should be handled by taking a project management approach. Most medical staffs have certain key committees as part of their formal structure, and a bylaws committee is typically one of them. Oftentimes members include past presidents or leaders of the medical staff who are familiar with the medical staff's roles and responsibilities and the need to maintain a current set of bylaws. First

14.1 RULES AND REGULATIONS

The medical staff shall initiate and adopt such rules and regulations as it may deem necessary for the proper conduct of its work and shall periodically review and revise its rules and regulations to comply with current medical staff practice. Recommended changes to the rules and regulations shall be submitted to the medical executive committee for review and approval. Following approval by the medical executive committee, rules and regulations shall be submitted to the board. Such rules and regulations shall become effective following approval of the board, which approval shall not be withheld unreasonably, or automatically within 60 days if the board takes no action. Applicants and members of the medical staff shall be governed by such rules and regulations as are properly initiated and adopted. If there is a conflict between the bylaws and the rules and regulations, the bylaws shall prevail. The mechanism described herein shall be the sole method for the initiation, adoption, amendment, or repeal of the medical staff rules and regulations. Neither the medical executive committee nor the board may unilaterally amend the rules and regulations.

14.2 MEDICAL STAFF ORGANIZATION AND FUNCTIONS MANUAL

The medical executive committee shall review and recommend to the board for approval, a manual on committees and medical staff functions. Following approval by the medical executive committee, the committees and functions manual shall be submitted to the board. The committees and functions manual shall become effective following approval of the board, which approval shall not be withheld unreasonably, or automatically within 60 days if no action is taken by the board. If there is a conflict between the committees and functions manual and the bylaws, the bylaws shall prevail. The mechanism described herein shall be the sole method for the amendment or repeal of the medical staff organization and functions manual. Neither the medical executive committee nor the board may unilaterally amend the organization and functions manual.

FIGURE 4-2 Excerpted Language from Bylaws Explaining Related Manuals

the key stakeholders in this process should be identified: bylaws committee members, key medical staff leaders, the whole medical staff, hospital administration, the MSSP and other internal administrative managers or directors, the governing body, and legal counsel. Typically, the medical staff organization is allowed a great deal of creative freedom in developing the medical staff documents. Some medical staffs prefer "vague" language that allows more freedom when making decisions when issues arise. Other medical staffs prefer very specific language that clearly spells out what to do in a particular situation. Most medical staff service professionals favor the latter approach because it is helpful to have a definitive bylaw, rule, regulation, or policy statement to refer to when a particular issue is raised.

As noted earlier, the bylaws provide a description of the current structure and practice of a particular medical staff. Each institution and its medical staff organization also has its own culture. Oftentimes it is possible to "see" within the document language the type of relationship that exists among the medical staff, hospital administration, and board of trustees.

Medical staff bylaws generally reflect the "culture" of the medical staff. While many standard provisions are typically included in bylaws, certain other provisions—not necessarily legal but essential to the functioning of the medical staff—will generally be included as well. The degree of governing body control, the role of legal counsel, the level of medical staff authority or representation on board committees, and the approach to medical staff corrective action all provide indications of the institutional culture. No specific approach or culture is preferable, but different cultures will generally result in different bylaw provisions.[11]

Typically the MSSP is charged with the responsibility of assisting the medical staff in its job of reviewing and revising the medical staff documents. Often, the MSSP is the person who actually drafts proposed language and then presents the new language to the bylaws committee and legal counsel, who may revise it as necessary.

A major bylaws revision project is quite an undertaking and requires many weeks or months of work. Some hospitals prefer to hire a consultant and outside legal counsel to draft the documents and assist the medical staff in working through the new language. Because there are so many legal issues involved in medical staff activities today, it is always helpful to have legal counsel assistance or at least review prior to finalizing any revisions.

A major revision project is also an opportunity to consider changing or revising not only language, but perhaps the structure or organizational details of the organized medical staff as well, especially if the organization has become too bureaucratic or complicated. Such changes might include a reduction in the number of departments, medical staff committees, or staff categories; a lengthening of the medical staff officer's and department chairs' terms of office; reduction in meeting attendance requirements; or simplification of the bylaws amendment process. The redesign of the medical staff has to take place first; the preparation of revised documents that describe the redesign would be the last step in the process.

The effects of the proposed changes should be identified, examined, discussed, and negotiated with key members of the medical staff, hospital administration, and governing board. "Working" the proposed revisions in this manner should preclude any unexpected opposition.

Medical staff professionals should maintain an ongoing bylaws and medical staff document revision file in which all relevant articles or findings that need to be discussed by the bylaws committee or medical staff officers are maintained. Any recommendations for changes from a medical staff member, department, or committee should also be maintained, researched, and then presented to the committee for consideration. Members of the governing body may also submit requests for bylaws revisions that must be considered by the medical staff.

The MSSP and medical staff leaders have to be constantly aware of changes in state and federal law and in the accrediting agency's and CMS hospital requirements that might affect the medical staff organization, its structure, and the way in which it currently functions. The MSSP should develop appropriate liaisons and conduct monthly research on helpful Web sites or use healthcare-related newsletters to capture these prospective changes and issues (e.g., contacts at the local or state medical societies, state hospital association, state association of medical staff services, and the National Association of Medical Staff Services). In addition, monthly checks with the *Federal Register* for changes in federal law should become part of the work process (www.acess.gpo.gov). The American Health Lawyers Association (www.healthlawyers.org) has a helpful Web site, as do Horty, Springer and Mattern, P.C. (www.hortyspringer.com—go to health law library); the American Hospital Association (www.aha.org); and the American Medical Association (www.ama-assn.org).

■ Reviewing the Amendment Process

The bylaws amendment process should be defined in the bylaws. Amending the document typically requires a review and recommendation from the bylaws and medical executive committees, advance notice of proposed revisions to the active medical staff (or those with voting prerogatives), specific voting procedures as outlined in the bylaws document (which may include a voice, secret ballot, mail ballot, show of hands, or proxy vote), a majority vote of those allowed to vote, and approval by the governing board.

Review your institution's bylaws amendment process and identify any opportunities for improvement in this process. For example, can this process be simplified?

- Consider changing the time frame for providing notice of proposed revisions to the whole medical staff to 15 days, instead of 30 or 45 days.
- Consider changing the required vote from a majority of the members able to vote to a majority of the members able to vote and present at the meeting held for the purpose of acting on revisions.
- Consider allowing for a mail ballot, to be distributed 14 working days prior to the voting deadline. An affirmative vote may be cast by marking the ballot "yes" or by discarding the ballot. A negative vote may be cast by marking the ballot "no" and returning. To be adopted, an amendment must receive a majority of the votes cast.
- Consider allowing the MEC to have the power to adopt amendments that involve technical or legal modifications or clarifications, reorganization or renumbering, or amendments made necessary because of punctuation, grammar, or spelling errors. Such amendments can become effective immediately and will be permanent if not disapproved by the medical staff or the board within 60 days of adoption by the MEC.

Major Considerations for a Medical Staff Bylaws Revision Project

- Right people
- Right tools
- Medical staff support
- Administrative support
- Legal counsel assistance

The Right People

The members of the bylaws committee should be carefully chosen and appointed. It is often helpful to have past presidents or medical staff leaders serve on this committee, as they will have experienced many situations that require the use of the bylaws and related documents to help them handle the difficult situations. They have a good idea of what these documents contain, why, and which revisions would make the documents more useful.

In the past, the bylaws committee was typically controlled by one or two physicians who had an interest in the legal document and in protecting the medical staff. They actually drafted the bylaws language. Today, the level of interest has to be much broader. The physicians serving on this committee need to be able to recognize the external changes to health care and to understand how those changes have or will affect the healthcare institution. They need to be aware of state, federal, and accrediting agency requirements and changes, and should embrace the "change mode." Much of the old medical staff structure still exists; however, the old medical staff structure is not always the best way to handle current and future problems—change is inevitable, but the members of this committee have to be able to search it out, not try to avoid it.

Another consideration is the politics of the bylaws. Recognizing that it is a very important document, some physicians may try to use their membership on this committee to assist in achieving their own or specialty-specific agendas. The physicians on this committee have to be fair-minded, remain objective, and always be ready to listen to proposed changes, as the current practice and function of the medical staff is constantly changing. It is also very helpful to have at least one medical staff member who is well respected by the other members and who has strong leadership qualities. This person will take on the responsibility of "working" proposed revisions through with key medical staff leaders, to help them understand the reasons for the changes and to get their support for the changes. EXHIBIT 4-1 provides a sample bylaws committee description.

Exhibit 4-1 Bylaws Committee Description

4. Bylaws Committee

4.1 Purpose

The purpose of the Bylaws Committee is to assure the medical staff and the governing board (board of supervisors) that medical staff organization foundation documents (bylaws, rules and regulations, and so on) are in compliance with licensing, regulatory, and accreditation requirements; that the aforementioned documents are consistent with each other; that they reflect current practice; and that the documents are reviewed and updated as necessary.

The Bylaws Committee is not required by any regulatory or licensing agency. However, in carrying out the responsibilities that have been delegated to it by the Medical Executive Committee, the Bylaws Committee must be aware of the following:

Regulatory Body	Specific Citations	Comments
Title 22 (California state law)	Governing Body: 70701 (a)(8) and (9) Organized Medical Staff: 70703 (b), (d) and (e)	Describe requirements related to the content of medical staff bylaws and responsibility for bylaws adoption and approval (governing body and medical staff).
Medicare Conditions of Participation for Hospitals	§482.12 Condition of Participation: Governing Body (a) (3) and (4) §482.22 Condition of Participation: Medical Staff (c) (1) through (6)	Describe requirements related to the content of medical staff bylaws and responsibility for bylaws adoption and approval (governing body and medical staff).
Joint Commission	Medical Staff: MS.01.01.01. and MS.01.01.03	These sections of the Joint Commission standards define the requirements for medical staff bylaws and the content of the medical staff bylaws.
Health Care Quality Improvement Act		See *National Practitioner Data Bank Guidebook*

Exhibit 4-1 Bylaws Committee Description (continued)

4.2 Composition

Voting Members	How Appointed
Chief of Medical Staff	Appointed by virtue of elected office
Chief of Medical Staff-elect	Appointed by virtue of elected office
Past Chief of Medical Staff	Appointed by virtue of elected office
Medical Director	Appointed by virtue of position

Invited Guest	How Appointed
Compliance Officer	Appointed by virtue of position
Legal Consultant	Appointed by hospital administration
Medical Staff Services Professional	Appointed by virtue of position

Bylaws Committee Support

Overall responsibility for the content of agendas is the responsibility of the chair and the medical staff coordinator.

Support for meetings (e.g., securing a room, meeting notices, completion of minutes) is the responsibility of the medical staff coordinator.

The Bylaws Committee chair is the chief of medical staff-elect. The chief of medical staff-elect and/or Bylaws Committee may request that additional individuals attend on an "as needed" basis, without a vote. These persons may include individuals with specific expertise needed by the committee.

Three voting members of the Bylaws Committee constitute a quorum.

4.3 Reporting Relationships

The Bylaws Committee reports to the Medical Executive Committee.

4.4 Duties

(a) Responsible to be aware of licensing, regulatory, and accreditation requirements related to the content of medical staff bylaws and associated documents.
(b) Conduct a periodic review of the medical staff bylaws, credentialing procedures manual, rules and regulations, medical staff committees and functions manual, rules and regulations of medical staff departments, and other related documents.
(c) Assure that documents listed in (b) are in agreement with one another.
(d) Assure that the documents listed in (b) reflect current practice.
(e) Make recommendations to the Medical Executive Committee for changes in documents listed in (b) to be in compliance with licensing, regulatory, and accreditation requirements, to reflect current practice or to eliminate discrepancies between documents.

Exhibit 4-1 Bylaws Committee Description (continued)

4.5 Meetings

The Bylaws Committee shall meet as needed to fulfill its functions. Meetings are called by the committee chair.

4.6 Related Documents
- Medical Staff Bylaws
- Credentialing Procedures Manual
- Medical Staff Rules and Regulations
- Medical Staff Committees and Functions Manual
- Rules and Regulations of Medical Staff Departments
- Documents that impact provisions of medical staff bylaws and related rules, regulations, and so on

The Right Tools

The MSSP can be very helpful to the bylaws committee by providing the committee with the right tools for the revision project: current documents, copies of proposed revision language, supporting documentation for the revisions, changes in accreditation agency standards or state or federal legislation, and new approaches to these documents based on what others are doing in the region or across the country. The bylaws committee should not be asked to "pen the revised language." Rather, revised language should be presented to the bylaws committee for consideration and discussion. If the committee members do not feel that the draft language is appropriate or acceptable, then the MSSP should collect their concerns and ideas and come back to the next meeting with revised language. Many resources are available through the AMA, state medical societies, and healthcare legal firms and consultants that can provide sample bylaws language addressing new and upcoming issues.

Use of a simple and clear format for presenting proposed revisions is often helpful to keep the discussion on track. A sample format for introducing revisions to the bylaws committee is included on the CD that accompanies this book. This same format can also be used to present revisions to the MEC and then to the whole medical staff.

The bylaws document as well as any related manuals should be maintained in the MSSD. A historical chronology of amendments to the bylaws and related manuals must be maintained, because MSSPs are often asked to reproduce a set of bylaws that may have been in place 10 to 15 years ago. Thus it is ideal if an electronic copy is maintained; if not, paper copies are essential.

Medical Staff Support

The bylaws and related manuals are the medical staff's documents. They describe the organization, structure, and responsibilities of the medical staff. For that reason, you never want a bylaws revision project to appear to be underway without full support from the appropriate medical staff leaders and members of the bylaws committee. Although many forces or reasons may drive the revisions to these documents, the medical staff always has to be fully involved. They will not support any activity that is led by or fully controlled by any other group in the hospital. As noted earlier, ensuring that a well-respected past medical staff leader is on the bylaws committee will assist greatly when the proposed revisions have to be discussed. This individual can work behind the scenes to communicate with other medical staff leaders about the proposed changes.

Administrative Support

Although the bylaws are medical staff documents, the governing body must approve them. The hospital chief executive officer (CEO) represents the governing body, and he or she should also be involved in the project. Many CEOs want to attend every bylaws committee meeting; others just want periodic reports on the process. Either way, it would be beneficial for the MSSP to discuss with the CEO (or his or her designee) what level of participation he or she plans to have and which specific goals or requirements he or she would like to see achieved. The MSSP should never undertake a revision project by working with medical staff leaders alone; hospital administration needs to be aware of the meetings and agenda for change for the documents.

Legal Counsel Assistance

Each hospital uses its legal counsel differently. The relationship with the hospital legal counsel and the medical staff is key in how the attorney is perceived. Sometimes the medical staff may decide they want their own attorney to work with them in revising the bylaws. If this is the case, the MSSP needs to ensure that the hospital CEO or designee is kept fully informed of such a decision. The hospital legal counsel is someone who is paid by the hospital and, therefore, would view the document from the hospital's perspective; however, such individuals are also typically advocates for the medical staff and want to ensure that revisions are acceptable to both the medical staff and the institution's governing board.

The worst-case scenario occurs when there is an adversarial relationship between the medical staff and hospital administration. In such a case, the legal counsel has the difficult job of maintaining a balance in his or her perspective and the way in which the revisions are approached.

Some medical staffs believe that they need to have their own legal counsel, separate and apart from the hospital's legal counsel. The goal should always be that the two counsels attempt to work together for the development of a document that will protect the patient, the practitioner, and the institution.

■ Distribution of New Documents

After the governing board has endorsed and accepted the revisions to the medical staff documents, the MSSP is responsible for ensuring that all members of the medical staff are informed of those changes and receive copies of or access to the revised documents. Many hospitals still print paper copies of the documents and distribute them to the active staff members after revisions are finalized. A cover memo used for the distribution can highlight the major changes and the effects of those changes on the individual members of the medical staff. (A sample format for distributing a summary of revisions is included on the CD that accompanies this book.) A copy of the cover memorandum or revisions format should be retained with a copy of the revised document. This will provide documentation that the new documents were provided to the medical staff.

Alternative methods of distribution include posting the medical staff documents on the hospital's Web site and notifying the members via e-mail or blast fax that the revised documents are now available on the Web site. Always offer to provide members with paper copies if they should require or wish to receive them. If the hospital does not have a Web site, then the documents can be distributed on CDs. Any of these alternative approaches should be pursued and adopted to reduce the cost of making hundreds of paper copies of these documents.

Whatever process is used for distribution, the MSSP must ensure that all members of the medical staff are provided with current information and documents, noting the recent amendments and their effects on the individual medical staff member.

■ Conclusion

The medical staff bylaws and related manuals are the most important documents that an MSSP works with. These documents define the medical staff structure, organization, and responsibilities and reflect current practice in the hospital. Maintaining documents that reflect current practice and are also compliant with federal, state, and accrediting agency requirements is a time-consuming task but one that should rank very high on the MSSP's priority list.

It is important to have the right people using the right tools during a bylaws revision project, as key issues must be addressed and shared with other members of the medical staff prior to presenting the documents for a vote. The bylaws document should define the amendment process, and that process must be carefully followed. The MSSP is responsible for maintaining a chronological history of all the documents and revisions. Although the medical staff does not have to perform an annual review of the medical staff documents, the MSSP should continually assess these documents to ascertain their level of compliance with accrediting agency standards and current practice. If no changes are required, then no revisions are made, but the collection of possible revisions should take place throughout the year.

■ Notes

1. The Joint Commission. *The Medical Staff Handbook: A Guide to Joint Commission Standards.* Oakbrook Terrace, IL: Author; 1999.
2. The Joint Commission. *2009 Hospital Accreditation Standards.* Oakbrook Terrace, IL: Author; 2009.
3. American Medical Association. *AMA Policy Compendium H-235–989.* Chicago, IL: Author; 1997.
4. *Merriam-Webster Online Dictionary.* Springfield, MA: Merriam-Webster; 2005. Available at: http://www.m-w.com. Accessed September 27, 2009.
5. *Merriam-Webster Online Dictionary,* note 4.
6. *Merriam-Webster Online Dictionary,* note 4.
7. *Merriam-Webster Online Dictionary,* note 4.
8. American Medical Association. *Physician's Guide to the Medical Staff Organization's Bylaws.* Chicago, IL: Author; 1999.
9. The Joint Commission. *2009 Hospital Accreditation Standards.* Oakbrook Terrace, IL: Joint Commission MS.01.01.01; 2009.
10. The Joint Commission, note 9, MS.01.01.03.
11. American Medical Association, Department of Organized Medical Staff Services. *Medical Staff Bylaws Update.* Chicago, IL: American Medical Association; 2001.

CHAPTER 5

Physician Executives

Vicki L. Searcy, CPMSM

■ Historical Perspective

Many physicians practicing today have fond memories of less complicated times, before the initiation of current reimbursement systems, before the implementation of the National Practitioner Data Bank, before the malpractice crisis—of times when "marketing" was not a healthcare verb and patients trusted and respected their physicians. The relationship of physicians to their hospitals seemed similarly uncomplicated: A lone secretarial type usually manned the minuscule medical staff office, processing the one- or two-page applications for medical staff membership and keeping a calendar of the meetings.

In those untroubled years, physicians and administration coexisted in a stance of polite nonintimacy, even as they reaped their portions of the green harvest of Medicare charge-based reimbursement. Practitioners performed their healing arts in their hospital "workshops," filling the beds (and often straining the bed capacity), while the administrators kept the shop running. The infrequent contacts between the two groups usually arose from requests by the physicians for more equipment or services, which were usually forthcoming as third-party payers picked up the tab.

Into the 1970s, the organizational structure of the typical medical staff was relatively straightforward, governed by a pyramidal hierarchy consisting of committee chairs, heads of clinical departments, and a chief of staff at the apex. In the community hospitals, top medical staff leaders typically were elected and held office for one or two years.

In most hospitals, this time-tested "laissez-faire" model persisted into the early 1980s. During this decade, however, a number of forces converged to irreversibly alter the delivery of healthcare services in hospital and nonhospital settings, including the physicians' office practices.

■ Hospital Trustee Accountability

Beginning with the landmark *Darling* case in 1965, the U.S. courts and the various regulatory and accrediting bodies have increasingly held hospital governing boards accountable for the quality of care delivered in their institutions. Trustees are no longer simply public-spirited citizens, contributing time and fund-raising abilities to their hospitals of choice. They now typically assume fiduciary roles that encompass the responsibility for the practitioners' performance in patient care. Rarely, however, are trustees medically sophisticated, and they rely heavily on the medical staff not only to deliver an acceptable level of care but also to document and report to the governing body information about the quality and appropriateness of such care. Although the governing board has historically, of necessity, delegated the monitoring of quality to the medical staff, the pattern of "arm's-length" delegation has increasingly become unacceptable: We are now in the age of accountability.

■ Hospital Reimbursement

The institution of the prospective payment system, replete with its diagnosis-related groups (DRGs), in 1983 signaled the end of the financial cornucopia for hospitals. The Medicare and other third-party spigots were tightened, resulting in an abrupt change in hospital admission patterns. As the medical staff learned that "groupers" were not a variety of fish, length of patient stay dropped dramatically. Many procedures previously performed comfortably within the walls of the hospital suddenly became outpatient procedures. The case mix changed as well: The patients admitted were sicker and required greater intensity of care.

To monitor Medicare admissions, a professional review organization (PRO) appeared in every state by congressional mandate. Initially, the PROs monitored only the financial aspects of the admissions, but subsequently the monitors included quality of care (and the name PRO changed to QIO—quality improvement organization). At the same time, there has been progressive "ratcheting down" of the reimbursements, with the result that hospitals must be managed efficiently or risk losing money on their Medicare and Medicaid admissions. The *Medicare Modernization Act of 2003* established the Medicare Recovery Audit Contractor (RAC) program as a demonstration program to identify improper Medicare payments—both overpayments and underpayments. The *Tax Relief and Health Care Act of 2006* made the RAC program permanent and authorized the Centers for Medicare and Medicaid Services (CMS) to expand the program to all 50 states by 2010. In July 2008, CMS reported that the RACs had succeeded in correcting more than $1.03 billion in Medicare improper payments, 96% of which involved Medicare overpayments. The Medicaid Integrity Contractors (MIC) began reviewing Medicaid claims in 2009 to see whether inappropriate payments or fraud may have occurred. The MICs audit Medicaid claims and identify overpayments and areas of high risk for payment error or fraud.

In addition, the proliferation of managed care and the contractual arrangements of health plans with hospitals have resulted in the necessity to manage all hospitalized patients efficiently—not just Medicare patients. In doing so, hospitals must carefully and correctly document all care and services provided.

■ Problems of Traditional Hospital Medical Staff Leadership

Time Commitments

Physicians have typically assumed medical staff leadership positions during their most active practice years. Though the job has always been demanding, the increasing responsibilities and time commitments in recent years have made it very difficult for a practitioner to perform the functions of a chief of staff or departmental or committee chair without the skilled assistance of a full-time or part-time physician executive.

Dual Roles

The dual roles of elected medical staff leaders are often not fully appreciated by the governing board, nor by the elected leaders themselves or the medical staff organization members. In one capacity, the chief of staff is the president or chief executive of the medical staff. As such, the chief of staff exercises the authority and assumes responsibility for the functions of the medical staff. The chief of staff also represents the interests of the staff to the hospital administration and to the governing board.

At the same time, whenever the chief of staff, departmental or committee chairs, or any other officers of the medical staff are performing their official functions, they are acting on behalf of the governing board. As such, they are, in effect, "officers" of that board, with derivative authority, accountability, and fiduciary responsibility.

Lack of Continuity

Elected medical staff leaders characteristically serve in this capacity for only a very few years. One or two years is the usual term for a chief of staff. Typically, by the time this individual has acquired the information and know-how necessary for effective functioning, the term of office is over. The physician then usually returns to his or her neglected practice (often after a stint serving on the medical executive committee as the past chief of staff), rarely surfacing thereafter in the medical staff hierarchy. The physician's administrative expertise and experience are lost, and the successor begins the acquisition process anew.

Information Base

The sheer quantity of information needed to manage the affairs of a medical staff in today's hospitals appears to be growing exponentially. In view of the limited terms of office and the demands of their medical practices, elected leaders often cannot acquire the information base necessary to effectively carry out the many functions of medical staff leadership.

Lack of Managerial Abilities

Rarely have elected medical staff leaders had significant training or experience in managerial functions, even though these skills are essential for the orderly management of the medical staff. Some leaders seem to have been born with executive skills, others acquire them over time, and some never acquire them. Clearly, the basic method of on-the-job-training is not an ideal mechanism given today's enormously complex hospital healthcare delivery systems.

Potential Conflicts of Interest

As practitioners, medical staff leaders have built-in potential conflicts of interest. Official decisions that they may be called on to make will often affect their practices, their referrals, or their economic interests. These dilemmas are commonplace and will call into question the decision-making processes used by the medical staff. In addition, the interests of practitioners are often opposed to those of the institution.

Authority and Accountability

The derivative authority and the attendant accountability of the medical staff leadership concern the quality and appropriateness of patient care. The various monitoring mechanisms involved in this awesome responsibility include quality improvement or performance improvement, utilization review, risk management, and patient safety. Also affecting the leadership are the mandates handed down by multiple accrediting and regulatory bodies, including the Joint Commission, the National Committee for Quality Assurance (NCQA), health plans, and state licensing and federal regulatory agencies. Practicing physicians rarely have the time, the store of information, the skills, or the will needed to fulfill the medical staff's delegated responsibilities regarding quality of patient care.

■ The Physician Executive

The demands of leading the medical staff organization and ensuring that required functions are fulfilled often exceed the ability of practicing physician volunteers to meet those demands. This led to the emergence, in many hospitals, of the position of medical director. For the purposes of the remainder of this chapter, the title "physician executive" will be used to describe this role, as it encompasses the multiple titles currently in use (medical director, vice president of medical affairs, chief medical officer, senior vice president, and others). Initially, the role of the physician executive was to assist the medical staff leadership by bridging the hospital's clinical and administrative operations. However, a new era in health care is rapidly being ushered in—one marked by new trends, issues, and events; one creating new organizations, structures, and methods; and an era that is changing physician executive roles and careers.

The recent changes in the healthcare environment have greatly enlarged the physician executive role in many organizations. Functions that were at one time the focus of a medical director's activities, such as credentialing, are overseen and performed by specialists in those areas, such as medical staff services professionals (MSSPs). As a result, physician executives have a greater role in the overall management of the organization, are part of the executive management team, and are essential players in the strategic planning process.

Depending on the setting in which a physician executive works—such as a hospital or group practice—the title and duties will vary. In managed care, the title may be "executive vice president for medical management," reflecting the physician executive's expanded managerial role. Many physician executive roles are system-wide positions and have been elevated to an executive vice presidency within a healthcare system. The physician executive in any type of organization usually reports directly to the president or CEO and is a member of its executive council.

The physician executive may be a lightning rod for physician anger. He or she tends to be "alone on an island," attempting to strike a balance between the management of the organization, the medical or professional staff, and the physicians. It can be a difficult job, and one in which the physician executive is perceived to be neither totally part of administration nor totally part of the medical staff organization.

According to experts, prerequisites to becoming a physician executive might include the following:

- *A physician background.* The American College of Physician Executives (ACPE) recommends that prospective physician executives become board-certified clinicians and practice for three to five years, if only because physician executives must manage physicians who generally do not like taking instructions from someone lacking a patient care background. Physician executives who have practiced medicine understand medical care from a practitioner's perspective.[1]
- *Certification as a physician executive.* The ACPE sponsors a certification examination (via a not-for-profit affiliate of the ACPE—the Certifying Commission in Medical Management [CCMM]) for physician executives. Since 1997, 1326 Certified Physician Executives (CPEs) have been approved by the CCMM. To

become a CPE, a physician must be board certified in a clinical specialty and have either a graduate management degree or 150 hours of tested management education, including courses in health law, financial decision making, and marketing.[2]

- *Ability to handle criticism.* Physician executives must have "thick skins" so they do not personalize the attacks upon their positions or their decisions. They must also recognize that what they—and the organization—value may not be valuable to the individuals whose support they seek.
- *Good negotiating skills and the ability to compromise.* Despite the need to compromise, physician executives must always put the quality and safety of patient care above concerns of the organization or individual physicians.
- *Political skills.* The ability to communicate and the ability to plan are both important; however, knowing how to manage competing interests may be the single clearest determinant of a physician executive's success or failure. Physician executives must understand their constituencies, which range from physicians to patients, or they will have problems in managing those constituencies.
- *Comfort with change.* Physicians who become physician executives must be able to deal with ambiguity and constant change, two areas that are generally not a strong suit for someone trained in a science.
- *Management training.* Organizations increasingly want their physician executives to have a degree in management. As mentioned previously, management training is a prerequisite for certification as a physician executive.
- *Open to promotion.* Physician executives more frequently have the option of becoming the CEO of an organization. Historically, this has not been a common career path for physician executives, because many of them lacked management training. As more physician executives receive advanced management degrees, it is anticipated that their moving into the role of CEO will become more common.
- *Communication and listening skills.* Physician executives must have excellent communication skills (the ability to make effective presentations is critical), as well as the capability to actively listen (and respond) to various constituencies within a healthcare organization.

A physician executive in a hospital environment is usually administratively responsible for the operation of the medical staff services department, primarily supporting medical staff credentialing and privileging, committee management, and arranging for physician leadership support. The physician executive position has expanded into performance improvement, sometimes limited to the medical staff, although many physician executives are responsible for the departments that support performance improvement throughout the organization.

Departments that commonly report to the physician executive include medical staff services and, sometimes, the quality management and health information management departments, infection control, case management and risk management. Because of the changes in reimbursement systems, many physician executives are heavily involved in clinical documentation improvement programs, and issues that relate to "pay for performance."

Managed care has expanded the physician executive's role to include areas such as contracting, aligning physician groups with the organization, and developing new service lines and sources of revenue.

Modern Physician (*Modern Healthcare*'s sister publication) annually ranks the physicians believed to be the 50 most powerful physician executives in health care. Physicians routinely hold positions in every sector of health care—as chief executive officers (of hospitals, managed care organizations, and other organizations) and directors of large national organizations, such as the U.S. Centers for Disease Control and Prevention, the Public Citizen's Health Research Group, the Medical Group Management Association, and the Joint Commission.

Although physician executives' roles may vary depending on the type of healthcare organization in which they work, the ACPE has identified some potential elements of the position:

- Improve clinical performance
- Oversee conversion to evidence-based medicine
- Head up safety initiatives
- Direct quality assurance
- Direct utilization review activities
- Recruit physicians
- Oversee credentialing and privileging of physicians
- Evaluate physician performance and recommend corrective action, if necessary
- Manage physician performance
- Coordinate activities of the hospital's infection control program
- Serve as a liaison between physicians and administrative personnel
- Serve as a liaison with outside organizations about issues such as marketing, consumer affairs, public relations, and community support
- Develop provider relations
- Resolve member or provider grievances
- Prepare medical expense budgets
- Develop staffing plans
- Assure compliance with corporate policies, bylaws, and mission statement
- Assure that medical staff efforts meet or exceed the standards put forth by the various accrediting and approving bodies
- Assist in design of educational programs for hospital employees
- Perform special projects as assigned by the board of directors

- Mediate professional disputes and interdepartmental problems
- Serve as a member or ex-officio member of the board of directors

Because of the variety and complexity of the potential functions that can be performed by physician executives, many organizations have multiple physician executives. For example, a physician executive might specialize in issues related to utilization and reimbursement. In a large organization, that might be a full-time position. Another physician executive might be an expert in informatics and focus on implementation of electronic patient records and other related data systems.

In summary, physician executives will continue to be an important component of the executive team, and their role will continue to be expanded and redefined. Continuing requisites for the job will be broad shoulders, a thick skin, and a sense of humor.

■ Notes

1. American College of Physician Executives. *Health Care Competency and Credentialing Report: Competency Profiles: Vice President of Medical Affairs*. Tampa, FL: Author; March 1998; and American College of Physician Executives. *Changing Disciplines: Making Sure Your Physician Executive Is Prepared for the Job*. Tampa, FL: Author: November 1997.
2. Romano M. "Certificate of Authenticity?" *Mod Healthcare*. May 23, 2005:24.

CHAPTER 6

The Hospital Credentials Process

Vicki L. Searcy, CPMSM

■ Why Credential? What Are Credentials?

The credentialing process is a vital function performed by the medical staff services department (MSSD). The primary purpose of the credentialing process is to ensure that any healthcare practitioner who wishes to provide patient care services within a hospital or other healthcare facility is qualified and competent to exercise the clinical privileges that have been granted to the individual.

Our healthcare organizations and the public depend on excellent credentialing—which means credentialing performed in a way that assures all of us that when we seek medical care in a hospital we are seen and treated by trained, qualified, and competent practitioners. Medical staff services professionals (MSSPs) typically spend hours confirming the education, background, and credentials of qualified and competent practitioners, looking for the relatively small percentage of practitioners who have misrepresented their backgrounds or who cannot demonstrate that they are qualified and currently competent.

What Is a Credential?

Many terms and definitions are associated with the credentialing function. *Merriam-Webster Online Dictionary* defines a *credential* as follows: "something that gives a title to credit or confidence; testimonials showing that a person is entitled to credit or has a right to exercise official power."[1] A healthcare practitioner's credentials result from education, training, medical licensure, and board certification. Healthcare practitioners also have other qualifications that allow them to practice their profession. A subsequent section will deal with the specifics of each type of credential.

There are numerous reasons why hospitals perform credentialing, including the fact that it is a required and heavily regulated process.

Credentialing Is Required

One reason that hospitals perform credentialing is because it is required by regulatory and accreditation bodies, including hospital licensing requirements (each state may have specific requirements), Medicare Conditions of Participation (COP; applicable to those hospitals that receive federal funds for providing care to Medicare and Medicaid patients), and accreditation organizations, such as the Joint Commission, the Health Facilities Accreditation Program, and DNV Healthcare for those hospitals that seek voluntary accreditation. In addition, many hospitals have relationships with payers that require a credentialing process as a condition of contracting. Insurance companies often require that hospitals have a credentialing process as a condition of being insured.

Credentialing Provides Risk Management

If an individual always performed only what he or she was qualified to do and did it well, there would theoretically be no need for a credentialing process. In the real world, however, we know that some practitioners overstate or falsify their credentials, some practitioners may be competent but have behavior or health problems that affects their competency, and some practitioners simply attempt to provide care or perform procedures for which they are not adequately trained or do not possess current experience. The credentialing process is critical to prevent these scenarios, with the burden being placed on the medical staff and governing body to ensure a careful matching of credentials to privileges.

If practitioners are credentialed in a haphazard manner, not only can patients be harmed, but the healthcare organization may also find itself paying out large sums of money in response to lawsuits due to negligent credentialing. When a patient or family is unhappy with the care received in a hospital, the credentialing and privileging of the practitioner who provided the care will almost inevitably be examined.

Doubters of the necessity for credentialing have but to review any number of significant court cases, noting their impact on hospitals. Chapter 16 describes significant credentialing cases.

Credentialing Protects Patients

Credentialing is essentially a patient-protective activity. As the courts have stated, hospitals and their governing bodies have a duty to the public to ensure that only qualified, competent practitioners are allowed to provide care in their organizations. Physicians and other independent practitioners must be licensed, of course, but hospitals cannot equate competency with the fact that a practitioner has a license. Licensing agencies do not establish competency to perform specific clinical privileges. That is what hospitals do, through their medical staff organizations and governing bodies, as part of the privilege delineation process (the privilege delineation process is covered in detail in Chapter 7).

Credentialing is the foundation of the quality program for the medical staff organization. Quality care begins with making sure that care is directed and provided by practitioners who have the appropriate training and experience, and who have been determined to be currently competent to exercise specific clinical privileges.

■ Key Terms

A **licensed independent practitioner** (LIP) is any individual who is permitted by law and by the organization to provide care and services, without direction or supervision, within the scope of the individual's license and consistent with the individually granted clinical privileges.

Individuals who are credentialed via the medical staff organization, but who are not licensed independent practitioners, are commonly referred to as **allied health professionals** (AHPs). AHPs may include physician assistants and advanced practice registered nurses (APRNs), although whether an APRN can be considered to be a licensed independent practitioner is determined by state law. For purposes of discussion of credentialing, throughout the remainder of this chapter, LIPs and AHPs will be collectively referred to as "practitioners."

Competency (as in current clinical competency) means "a determination of an individual's skills, knowledge, and capability to meet defined expectations."[2]

Credentialing is an umbrella term commonly used to describe a variety of processes or activities, including the initial medical staff appointment, the initial delineation of clinical privileges, and the periodic reappraisal and reappointment of medical staff members. Credentialing actually involves two separate decisions. The first regards membership on the medical staff and the second focuses on the granting of clinical privileges.

Membership on the Medical Staff

Some practitioners are granted membership with no clinical privileges. For example, a physician in an administrative role with a hospital (e.g., chief medical officer) may be a member of the medical staff but have no clinical privileges. Many medical staff organizations have an "honorary" medical staff membership category for those practitioners who no longer practice (and, therefore, have no clinical privileges) but wish to retain their membership. In addition, some hospitals allow practitioners who have office-based practices to obtain membership on the hospital medical staff organization. A staff category that is often used to describe this type of membership is affiliate. Sometimes affiliate staff members have no privileges; in other hospitals, they may be eligible to refer patients to the hospital, but are not eligible for privileges to manage patients.

Criteria for membership on the medical staff, which are separate from the criteria for clinical privileges, should be adopted. Some examples of membership criteria are listed here:

- Completion of a specific level of professional education. For physicians this might be completion of a residency training program in the specialty he or she wishes to practice.
- Board certification. This has become a fairly common membership requirement in some areas and is a customary requirement in teaching hospitals. If this requirement is used, stipulate whether current board certification is required, rather than whether the practitioner was board certified at one time during his or her career.
- Absence of any felony convictions. Sometimes there are some qualifiers attached to this criterion, such as felony convictions that could conceivably have an impact on the practice of medicine.
- No current Medicare or federal or state sanctions.

Granting of Clinical Privileges

Some practitioners may have clinical privileges but not be granted membership on the medical staff organization. See Chapter 7 for additional information on this subject.

■ Key Players and Their Roles

The critical steps in the credentialing process are as follows:

1. *Establish and document the credentialing process.* This step involves making decisions related to the types of practitioners who are eligible to be credentialed and receive privileges (e.g., physicians, dentists, podiatrists) and the basic requirements that must be met by all practitioners (e.g., current licensure, professional liability insurance in the required amount, board certification). Another component of this step involves determining the groups or individuals who will be responsible for evaluation and decision making. Establishing the credentialing process is usually a collaborative effort by medical staff leaders and the governing body. Documentation of these decisions can be found in the governing body and medical staff bylaws as well as credentialing policies and procedures.
2. *Data collection.* Data are collected from applicants through the use of applications, privilege delineation forms, and other documents that must be submitted by an applicant.
3. *Data verification.* Data are verified in accordance with approved policies and procedures.
4. *Evaluation.* Throughout the credentialing process, information is constantly evaluated. Is the information complete? Does the information obtained and verified indicate that there may be a problem? Which information requires

more investigation? When an application is sent through the medical staff organization for recommendation to the governing body, the accumulated information is evaluated so that an appropriate recommendation can be made.

5. *Decision making.* The governing body makes credentialing decisions based on predetermined standards that have been established and recommendations made by the medical executive committee (MEC).
6. *Data management.* Once a practitioner has been credentialed, data about the practitioner must be maintained in a retrievable fashion and updated as information becomes outdated or expires. For example, verification of current licensure is obtained as the license expires, not just at the time of initial appointment or reappointment.

Key players in the credentialing process include the medical staff services department, department chairs, the credentials committee and MEC, and the governing body. The roles of each party are described in the following sections.

Medical Staff Services Department

The MSSD plays several critical roles in the credentialing process. One role is to make sure that the medical staff bylaws clearly define the credentialing process and that the bylaws are in compliance with applicable regulatory, licensing, and accreditation standards.

Policies and procedures should then be written describing specifically how the processes will be implemented. For example, medical staff bylaws commonly require that those practitioners who are credentialed must have professional liability insurance. Credentials policies and procedures will be more specific, identifying the amount of insurance that must be carried, the type of insurance, the type of evidence required to prove that the practitioner actually has the required coverage, and the frequency with which this information will be updated (e.g., at the time of expiration of the current policy, or annually, or at the time of reappointment). The credentials policy and procedure include the application forms to be used (initial application form, reappointment application form, application form for temporary privileges, and so on), privilege delineation forms for all specialties, and forms and methods used to verify information. The MSSD must make sure that appropriate policies and procedures are developed to assure that the credentialing process is adequately described and carried out consistently for all practitioners.

The MSSD then plays a pivotal role in the credentialing process by implementing and coordinating the appropriate policies and procedures. For example, in an initial application process, the MSSD usually performs the following services:

1. Initial screening of a potential applicant to assure that the applicant meets the credentialing standards. For instance, an applicant will not be given access

to an application if he or she has not completed residency training if the organization's requirements include completion of residency training.
2. Make the application materials available to the applicant. This may include mailing out application forms and related documents, such as medical staff bylaws, privilege delineation forms, and so on, or it may involve providing instructions on how to access applicable applications and documents via a Web site.
3. Review the returned application materials to assure that the application meets standards to begin the verification process.
4. Implement the verification process, following established policies and procedures.
5. Prepare the credentials file for medical staff leaders (e.g., department chair or service chief) and committee members (e.g., credentials committee) who will review and evaluate the file. This step often includes preparing a summary of the file and identification of potential adverse or problematic information ("red flags") to assist in the evaluation and decision-making process. The importance of this role, which the MSSD fulfills by analyzing credentials files, cannot be overstated. Most department chairs, credentials committee members, and other medical staff leaders heavily rely on the MSSD to identify credentialing issues for them.
6. Route the file through the review, evaluation, and decision-making process (usually beginning with a department chair and proceeding to the credentials committee, then the MEC, and ending with the governing body). This process often involves communicating with the applicable department chair to review a file (particularly if the file has problems) and presentation of files to the credentials committee. The MSSP assures that documentation of all recommendations is captured in the credentials file and in minutes of committees that are involved in making recommendations.
7. Prepare a transmittal to the governing body related to the MEC's recommendation.
8. Communicate with the applicant during and at the conclusion of the application process, informing the applicant of the governing body's decision. The MSSD is usually responsible for planning and executing an orientation process for new members.
9. Notify hospital departments (if the applicant was approved by the governing body) of essential information related to the applicant, his or her new status at the hospital, clinical privileges that have been granted, and other necessary information.

The MSSD also plays a key role in data management and is almost always the department responsible for maintaining an accurate database of all credentialed and privileged practitioners. The MSSD that is able to deploy selected parts of the database (e.g., a picture of the practitioner, his or her granted privileges, key contact information) throughout the organization adds prestige to the MSSD, and it certainly makes the information more readily accessible and current to those individuals who have a need for it.

Medical Staff Leaders

Medical staff leaders are responsible for collaborating on the design of the credentialing processes. This includes establishing standards for access to the credentialing process as well as for medical staff membership. It also includes establishing mechanisms to assure that standards are uniformly and consistently applied to all practitioners who are eligible to be credentialed.

Credentials Committee and Medical Executive Committee

Neither the Joint Commission nor the Centers for Medicare and Medicaid Services (CMS) requires that a healthcare organization have a credentials committee. Nevertheless, many medical staff organizations—particularly those that are larger—find that a credentials committee contributes significantly to the credentialing and privileging processes. The role of a credentials committee usually includes the following responsibilities:

- Assure the MEC that medical staff bylaws provisions that relate to credentialing processes are being fulfilled, as well as credentialing policies and procedures and other credentialing-related medical staff documents. This committee also monitors compliance with all credentialing policies and procedures.
- Evaluate recommendations made by department chairs. The credentials committee is looking for completeness, thoroughness, and adherence to credentialing and privileging policies and standards. Assure the MEC that department-specific standards for clinical privileges are in compliance with medical staff bylaws and credentialing policies and procedures, and that these standards are uniformly and fairly applied to each applicant.

In doing its work, the credentials committee may focus on the files that have been determined to be problematic (such as those having time gaps, problems with references, and malpractice claims) and assures that all issues have been appropriately addressed and that there is complete and thorough documentation for the recommendations that have been made to the MEC. The credentials committee may also have an important role in coordination of privileging criteria, particularly when privileges are exercised by more than one specialty (see Chapter 7 for additional information).

The MEC evaluates the recommendations that are forwarded by the department chairs and credentials committee and makes a recommendation to the governing body. If any part of the MEC's recommendation to the governing body is adverse (e.g., the recommendation may be to deny membership and/or all or a portion of requested clinical privileges), medical staff bylaws provisions related to fair hearing procedures become applicable. A fair hearing is provided prior to an adverse recommendation being sent to the governing body.

Governing Body

The governing body receives recommendations from the MEC and makes credentialing and privileging-related decisions. See FIGURE 6-1 for steps in routing an application.

■ Applicable Standards

The Joint Commission is the accreditation body most likely to provide accreditation services in the hospital environment, although a number of hospitals seek accreditation from additional sources (see Chapter 2). At the time when this chapter was written, the Joint Commission standards related to credentialing in hospitals were contained in the *Joint Commission Comprehensive Accreditation Manual for Hospitals* in the chapter entitled "Medical Staff." All individuals who have a significant role in credentialing and privileging should carefully review these standards. The standards define the type of information to be documented in bylaws, policies, and procedures; roles and responsibilities in the credentialing and privileging process; elements of current clinical competency; and other requirements related to the credentials process.

Other Joint Commission accreditation programs (e.g., for ambulatory care and long-term care) have similar credentialing and privileging requirements, but standards related to credentialing and privileging are located in chapters related to human resources because there is no requirement for an organized medical staff in these other accreditation programs. The only accreditation program that requires an organized medical staff is the accreditation program for hospitals.

■ Credentialing Documents

Credentialing requirements are described in such documents as the medical staff bylaws and credentialing policies and procedures, as well as in the delineation of privileges forms. In addition, credentialing requirements may be described in general rules and regulations and department-specific rules and regulations.

Caution should be taken to avoid duplication of the same information in multiple documents. Duplication of information often leads to inconsistencies and contradictions as one document gets revised and others do not. If duplication of

Steps in Routing an Application

1. Request for application
2. Pre-application process
3. Medical staff services applies ⟶ Medical staff services applies membership criteria to applicant
4. Application sent to applicant
5. Medical staff services verifies application: licenses, education, training, professional references, hospital affiliations, certification status, professional liability coverage, claims history, NPDB, sanctions.
6. Application reviewed by department chairperson, who makes written report and recommendation for privilege delineation ⟶ False, misleading, or incomplete data ⟶ Further information requested from applicant ↓ Application denied by governing body ⟵ None provided
7. Application reviewed by credentials committee, which makes recommendations for:
   a. Approval with no restrictions
   b. Approval with qualifications or conditions
   c. Denial
8. Recommendation forwarded to executive committee
   a. Recommends appointment
   b. Recommends denial — applicant notified, including right to a hearing — If requested, due process hearing held — Decision affirmed / Decision overturned — Applicant notified, including right of appellate review / Refer back to executive committee for further consideration — If requested, appellate review held — Decision affirmed / Decision overturned — Refer back to executive committee for further consideration
9. Referred to governing body for final action
10. Applicant notified

FIGURE 6-1 Steps in Routing an Application

information is needed, the secondary document should refer to the primary document, rather than repeating the provision or requirement. For example, if the bylaws contain provisions for temporary privileges and there is further documentation in a policy and procedure about temporary privileges, the policy and procedure should refer to the bylaws in the policy. Many medical staff organizations have created significant problems for themselves by not paying close attention to maintaining documents that are consistent and are not contradictory.

Medical Staff Bylaws

Medical staff bylaws (or related documents—see Chapter 4) usually describe the following credentialing-related issues:

- Types of practitioners eligible for medical staff membership and clinical privileges
- Basic criteria for membership and clinical privileges (e.g., current licensure, professional liability insurance, board certification, and any other requirements for membership)
- Medical staff membership categories (e.g., active, associate, courtesy, consulting), including requirements for each category (e.g., serve on committees) and prerogatives for each category (e.g., voting at meetings, ability to hold elected office)
- Information that applicants for membership and clinical privileges must provide
- Initial appointment and reappointment processes
- Elements of a complete application
- Evaluation and decision-making process
- Circumstances under which temporary privileges may be applied for and granted
- Focused professional practice evaluation process for new applicants
- Fair hearing plan

Rules and Regulations

Medical staff general rules and regulations may contain more specific information related to the credentialing and privileging processes. For example, the medical staff bylaws might require professional liability insurance, and the rules and regulations might specify the required amount (e.g., $1 million/$3 million). Or the bylaws may state that an applicant must live close enough to the hospital to provide continuous care to his or her patients, and the rules and regulations might define the specific parameters (e.g., must be able to get to the hospital within 20 minutes).

Alternatively, this information could be included in a credentialing policy and procedure or in department-specific rules and regulations—or as part of the privilege delineation form for each specialty.

Department-Specific Rules and Regulations

Department-specific rules and regulations often contain criteria specific to the privileges recommended by each department. For example, the rules and regulations for the department of obstetrics and gynecology might require that applicants to the department provide documentation of having completed residency training in obstetrics and gynecology or board certification by the American Board of Obstetrics and Gynecology. It is recommended, however, that any standards to be met for clinical privileges be placed on the privilege form itself rather than in a separate document. It is more likely that standards will be understood and that there will be consistent application of the criteria to all applicants if the requirements are located in a place that is clearly visible to applicants and to those involved in evaluation and decision making.

Privilege Delineation Forms

Privilege delineation forms are critical documents and are described in Chapter 7.

Credentials Policies and Procedures

Credentials policies and procedures contain detailed information on precisely how credentialing is to be implemented. Policies and procedures are critical to assuring that credentialing activities are conducted in a fair and consistent manner. These policies and procedures should be developed by the medical staff organization and approved by the governing body. The MSSD is usually responsible for supporting policy and procedures development and is often the instigator of the development of appropriate policies and procedures. Forms used to conduct the credentialing and privileging processes should be incorporated into the appropriate policy and procedure (e.g., forms used to verify education, training, experience, and peer references).

The CD that accompanies this book includes a sample policy and procedure for verification requirements and methods for the initial appointment. Policies and procedures should relate to the governing documents (e.g., medical staff bylaws) as well as be operational in nature by relating to use of the credentialing software utilized in the department, if software is used.

■ The Pre-application Process

Many hospitals have implemented a pre-application process. The purpose of the pre-application process is to screen out candidates who are obviously not qualified for staff membership or clinical privileges. If the candidate does not meet criteria established by the governing body (e.g., licensed in the state in which the practitioner will be exercising clinical privileges, board certification, absence of felony convictions), the applicant is notified and is not provided with an application packet. This saves time for both the MSSD and the candidate—neither will spend time completing and processing forms that cannot result in granting of membership or clinical privileges.

To expedite the application process, many hospitals now conduct this screening by telephone with the candidate, discussing the criteria by telephone and sending the application only upon assurance by the candidate that he or she meets all qualifications. If the application is received and it is apparent that the applicant does not meet applicable criteria, the application is not processed. One alternative plan is to provide application forms upon request, accompanied by documentation that clearly outlines membership and/or privileging criteria. The applicant is instructed to review criteria carefully and to submit the application only if he or she meets all criteria.

Whatever methods are used, it is important to assure that potential applicants meet baseline criteria before the application is accepted for processing.

Criteria for Membership

The requirements for medical staff membership and privileges are stated in the medical staff bylaws. They usually include the following specifications:

- Type of practitioner (e.g., physician, dentist, podiatrist)
- Appropriate professional licensure
- Appropriate educational and training credentials
- Practice in one of the clinical services provided for the community by the hospital or into which the hospital is expanding
- Professional liability insurance coverage in the amount required by the governing body

Occasionally medical staff bylaws require the applicant to agree to reside and maintain an office within a stated distance from the facility. This requirement is made to ensure the practitioner's availability to care for patients in a timely manner, including emergencies.

Requiring board certification is becoming more prevalent as a requirement for medical staff membership (or this requirement may be applied to clinical privileges as opposed to medical staff membership—for instance, an applicant must be board certified by the American Board of Surgery to apply for privileges in general surgery). It is recommended that organizations that require board certification carefully consider the following issues:

- The requirement for board certification must be clearly related to quality of care. Otherwise, it may be construed by some as an attempt to freeze out competition for patients.

- The requirement must be consistent with state law, determination of which may require a legal opinion.

Other considerations related to board certification as a medical staff requirement include the following:

- The requirement must start on the date the governing body approves the medical staff bylaws change or on a date in the future approved by the governing body. At the same time the governing body approves board certification requirements, the decision must be made as to whether all current non-board-certified staff members are to be automatically grandfathered in. Grandfathering is a way that an organization "raises the bar" on criteria for privileges (criteria are usually related to education, training, board certification, and so on), but does not penalize those practitioners who already have the privilege(s) in question by retroactively applying the criteria to those who have been granted the privileges. New criteria that are approved are usually applied to all applicants after board approval of the criteria. For example, a board may decide that, effective on a certain date, all subsequent applicants in a certain specialty must be board certified. The current practitioners in that specialty would not be required to become board certified if they were "grandfathered in." The exception to the "grandfathering" rule is when a clinical activity requirement, continuing medical education requirement, or some other new requirement is added to reappointment requirements (for example, to have obstetrical privileges, all physicians with those privileges must do x number of deliveries every two years). At the time that physicians come up for reappointment, they must meet the new requirement(s).
- If grandfathering occurs, is it to be permanent, or is there to be a reasonable period during which grandfathered individuals must become board certified?
- Is certification required only at the time of initial appointment, or must the certification be maintained during the entire period of medical staff membership? Most specialty board certifications expire within seven to ten years.
- If current certification is required and a practitioner's board certification expires and is not renewed, will the practitioner be automatically suspended or will there be a grace period? If there is a grace period, how long will it last?
- If there is a practice requirement between the completion of a practitioner's formal training and the point at which he or she can sit for the board exams, would this gap prevent the organization taking in a highly qualified practitioner pending his or her taking the board exams? And if the practitioner does not become certified, will he or she have to leave the staff?
- To help ensure the same level (standard) of certification, would physicians have to be certified only by boards approved by the American Board of Medical Specialties? Would another board certification system for physicians be considered (e.g., American Osteopathic Boards)?

- What would be the certification requirements (if any) used for the various types of nonphysician medical staff applicants or members?

■ Application for Membership and Privileges

Application Form

The first serious dialogue between the applicant and the medical staff and governing body is the filing of a completed application form (along with any additional required documentation). A cover letter or instructions outlining membership criteria and requirements for documents that should accompany the application should be included with the initial application form. A sample cover letter can be found on the CD that accompanies the book.

The application form requests all routine background and current information and, in addition, poses some critical questions. Routine information includes the following:

1. Full name of the applicant, date and location of birth, current home and office addresses and telephone numbers, date of application, and professional (practice) affiliation.
2. Undergraduate education information, including the name of the school, its location, dates attended, and degree received.
3. Postgraduate education information, including the name of the school, its location, dates attended, and degree received.
4. Residency (includes internship if not a recent trainee) and fellowship information (if applicable) such as hospital, location, dates of training, and specialty.
5. Previous and current hospitals and other healthcare affiliations, including their names, locations, and dates of employment.
6. Faculty or training appointments.
7. Specialty board certification status, including the name of the board and date of board certification (if not certified, whether the applicant is a current candidate for examination should be indicated). Terms such as "board qualified" or "board eligible" should not be used on the application form; this restriction should be stated on the form so that these terms are not written in.
8. List of all state licenses, with the expiration date of each.
9. Federal Drug Enforcement Administration (DEA) registration certificate number and date of expiration (similarly, any state narcotics certificate number and expiration date should be indicated when the state has such a requirement).
10. Professional references who have personal knowledge of the applicant's recent professional performance and experience. (Peers who have not personally observed the clinical work of the applicant, as well as relatives and business

associates, are usually not acceptable. Most hospitals require two to four professional references.)
11. Information on all previous practice and employment, such as designations as a solo practice or partnership, locations, and dates.
12. Information related to continuing medical education for the past two years.
13. Professional liability coverage information, including carrier, amounts, and dates of coverage.
14. Past and present professional litigation and liability history, including any open cases.
15. Clinical privileges requested (this information will be contained in a privilege request form and consistent with the specialty in which the applicant proposes to practice).
16. Optional items such as the following:
    - A list of publications and major speeches given, along with the pertinent subjects, locations, and dates.
    - A small recent photo. (The bylaws should state that the photo will help identify the applicant at the time of any required interview or a copy will be sent to any training or education program requested to comment on the applicant. The photo is an excellent requirement, but must be used properly.)
    - A list of a specified number of patients treated or procedures performed, and any related records.
    - Any required fee for processing the application, and information about whether it is applied toward annual medical staff dues for successful staff applicants.

Critical Information from the Applicant

The following critical information must be obtained from the applicant for the purpose of detecting previous professional problems, competency, and behavior or health problems:

- Any previous or currently pending challenges to any licensure or registration
- Past and present voluntary and/or involuntary relinquishments of any license or registration
- Past and present voluntary and/or involuntary terminations of any medical staff membership
- Past and present voluntary and/or involuntary limitations, reductions, or loss of clinical privileges
- Information about past and present professional liability actions and any currently pending claims (look for unusual patterns or excessive numbers)
- Information about the applicant's health status

The following are representative of the types of questions that might be asked on an application form in order to obtain the preceding information:

- Have you ever been requested to appear before any licensing or regulatory agency (e.g., the State Board of Medical Examiners, the Drug Enforcement Administration, the Quality Improvement Organization [QIO], or the Inspector General) for a hearing or complaint of any nature?
- Has any professional license of yours ever been denied (on application), suspended, revoked, limited, or otherwise acted against?
- Have you ever been denied (on application) or surrendered a narcotics tax stamp?
- Has any (professional/medical) license of yours ever been denied (on application), suspended, revoked, or limited?
- Has your DEA registration ever been denied (on application), suspended, revoked, or limited?
- Have your clinical privileges (including admitting, consulting, and assisting privileges) or staff membership at any healthcare facility ever been denied, suspended, limited, revoked, not renewed, or otherwise acted against?
- Have you ever been denied membership, or renewal thereof, or had your membership revoked or otherwise acted against, or been subject to disciplinary action, in any medical or professional organization or by any licensing agency of any state, district, territorial possession, or country?
- Have you ever been convicted of a felony or misdemeanor (other than minor traffic offenses)?
- Has any liability insurance carrier canceled, refused coverage, or increased your rates because of unusual risk?
- Are any actions pending for the preceding items?
- Have any judgments or settlements been obtained against or from you in professional liability cases?
- Are any professional liability cases pending against you?
- Have you ever been under treatment for drug addiction or alcoholism? (If so, list any rehabilitation programs, with dates of treatment.)
- Have you ever received psychiatric treatment or care? (If so, list any treatment programs, with dates of treatment.)
- Are you currently under care for a continuing health problem?
- Have you ever discontinued practice for any reason (other than for routine vacation or formal education/training) for one month or more?

If the answer to these questions is yes, the applicant should be asked to furnish further details.

A health status question such as the following should be included:

- Do you feel that your health status is adequate enough to permit you to provide the patient care services for which you are requesting clinical privileges with or without reasonable accommodation? Yes _____ No _____

If the answer is no, the applicant should be asked to furnish further details. The applicant could also be asked to enclose a copy of his or her most recent comprehensive physical examination report or include authorization for release by the examining physician.

The application usually includes an "Immunity from Liability" section as well as a series of pledges by the applicant to do the following:

- Adhere to the generally recognized standards of professional ethics of his or her profession.
- Not participate in fee splitting or "ghost" surgical or medical care.
- Participate, as required, in peer evaluation activities.
- Provide continuous care for his or her patients and delegate the responsibility for diagnosis or care of patients only to a practitioner who is qualified to undertake that responsibility.
- Obtain appropriate informed consent as required for the intervention contemplated.
- Abide by the medical staff bylaws, rules and regulations, and hospital policies affecting the medical staff.
- Complete adequately, and in a timely fashion, the medical and any other required records for all patients he or she admits or in any way provides care for in the hospital.
- Seek consultation whenever necessary.
- Maintain the required amount of professional liability insurance coverage.
- Reasonably assist the hospital in fulfilling its uncompensated or partially compensated patient care obligations within the areas of his or her professional competence and credentials.
- Reasonably cooperate with the hospital in its efforts to comply with accreditation, reimbursement, and legal or other regulatory requirements.

The application should conclude by indicating that one or more interviews may be required and asking if the applicant would be willing to be interviewed at the hospital if requested. The applicant should sign the form. Somewhere on the application form, perhaps below the signature area, a highlighted note should appear, stating that failure to complete any part of the form or the inclusion of false information will delay the application processing and may render the applicant ineligible for staff membership. The bylaws should support this outcome.

A copy of the current medical staff bylaws, rules, and regulations and a relevant privilege request form should accompany the application form for staff membership.

In lieu of sending paper copies of bylaws and other relevant documents, the applicant may be given access to these documents via a Web site.

■ Processing the Application

Once the application form is received and the applicant is seriously pursuing staff membership and clinical privileges, a new-applicant processing checklist should be started that permits the medical staff services professional to know at a glance which information is already captured and which is missing. If the hospital uses credentialing software, the software program can generate this checklist. For the sake of efficiency this software should be used, rather than the manual checklist often affixed to the front of the credentials file. If the electronic checklist is used, all employees in the MSSD will have immediate access to the information. If a paper checklist is used, the credentials file will have to be found should a question come up related to the status of the credentialing process (e.g., if a practitioner calls to find out if his or her file is complete).

The processing checklist automatically includes and focuses on application items that require primary source verification. These data include state licenses, postgraduate degrees (medical, dental, podiatric), residency and fellowship training, specialty board status (to verify any statement made by the applicant as to certification or candidacy for examination), and professional liability insurance coverage. The references provided by the applicant should be sent a letter asking specific questions about the applicant's qualifications and current clinical competency. The CD that accompanies this book includes sample follow-up letters notifying the applicant of any needed additional or missing information and of the status of the application as well as a sample letter notifying the applicant that the application has been voluntarily withdrawn due to failure to respond to requested information.

At the time this chapter was written, the majority of hospitals were still using paper applications and privilege delineation forms. However, it is clear that the healthcare industry is rapidly moving in the direction of eliminating paper records, and the MSSD is not exempt from this trend. A number of healthcare organizations now provide all application materials electronically to applicants for initial appointment, reappointment, requests for new privileges, and so on. Providing application materials electronically lowers costs and results in faster submission of required information.

The Credentials File

Once the application has been received and processing starts, a credentials file is established. It may be either an electronic file (no paper) or a segmented paper file. The trend is to eliminate paper from the credentialing process, and many organizations have been successful in establishing electronic systems. If a segmented paper file is used, how it is set up is a matter of an individual choice. However, some basic advice may help to make the use of a paper file more efficient. Specifically, it takes two and a half times longer to file documents in a clipped fashion. Consider using files that allow for drop filing.

Place in one section all one-time items, such as the application form, the letters of reference, and so on. In another section, include the recurring-date-related documents that need to be immediately accessible, such as state licenses, the DEA registration, and professional liability coverage documents. For these items, a tickler file is usually placed in the computer for renewal purposes. In another section of the paper file, include the staff reappointment information, usually with the most current on top. A separate section should be reserved for clinical privileges. Some hospitals use an additional separate section for peer review information (both good and bad) and related actions. The CD that accompanies this book provides a sample policy and procedure outlining the contents and organization of a credentials file.

Paper files become thicker and thicker over time as more paper is added. It is possible to purge files of nonessential information, and this practice should be addressed in the organization's policies and procedures. Essential information would include a complete record of which privileges were granted and when. Nonessential information might include outdated copies of DEA registration or certificates of insurance. Many MSSDs are reluctant to part with any paper (and purging files in a large medical staff organization may take considerable time). Additionally, many hospital attorneys advise against destruction of any paper included a credentials file. In these cases, it may sometimes be more practical to start a new file and put the old file in storage. The old file can still be retrieved if necessary. The new file is clearly marked to indicate that a previous file has been archived.

Many hospitals are interested in paperless files and are using scanning technology to achieve an electronic—rather than paper—credentials file. Documents that are scanned into the system can be printed out, if necessary. Some organizations have raised concerns about data security if electronic files are used, although use of password protection can alleviate some of these issues. It should be noted that maintaining paper files is not a foolproof method of maintaining security. Indeed, whatever method is selected, the organization should make appropriate provisions for maintaining the security of confidential information.

Verifying Information on the Application

As stated previously, a healthcare practitioner's credentials result from education, training, licensure, board certification, and other documentation that helps to demonstrate qualifications to practice in his or her specialty. This section provides details about each type of credential, as well as other items that are routinely subject to verification and collection during a credentialing and privileging process.

What to verify is included with each type of credential, as well as which methods of verification might be used. Of course, potential methods of verification have changed rapidly over the past few years because of the proliferation of databases and Web sites that may be rapidly accessed by healthcare organizations. This trend is likely to continue, so the methods of verification listed in this section should simply be a starting point for exploration of a particular organization's approved methods for verification of information.

A Web site that provides many links useful for verification purposes can be found at www.docboard.org. Administrators in Medicine—the national organization for state medical and osteopathic board executive directors—supports this site. In addition, the National Association Medical Staff Services has a link on its Web site (www.namss.org) that provides useful information about sources of verification organizations.

A chart containing verification requirements and methods can be found on the CD that accompanies the book.

Medical, Dental, and Other Professional Education (Domestic Graduates)

Premedical education is obtained at a college or university and is usually four years in duration. In some institutions, three years will qualify a student to apply for admission to a medical/professional school. Premedical education is not usually subject to verification.

Dental and podiatric schools also have four-year curricula. Upon completion, dentists are conferred the DDS (Doctor of Dental Science) or DMD (Doctor of Dental Medicine) degree. Podiatrists earn a DPM (Doctor of Podiatric Medicine) degree upon completion of podiatric school.

- What to verify: Institution (e.g., medical school, podiatric school, dental school), completion date, and degree received.
- Potential verification methods: Confirm directly with the institution in writing or orally, or use the AMA (www.ama-assn.org) or American Osteopathic Association [AOA] (www.aoa-net.org) profile services (physicians only).
- When to verify: At time of initial appointment/privileges.

Educational Commission for Foreign Medical Graduates

Through its process of certification, the Educational Commission for Foreign Medical Graduates (ECFMG) assesses the readiness of graduates of foreign medical schools to enter residency or fellowship programs in the United States. Examination is administered on knowledge of basic medical sciences and ability to understand the English language. Any graduate of a foreign medical school who wants to enter a postdoctoral training program in the United States must have an ECFMG certificate. All education that occurs after receipt of the ECFMG should be verified, but not necessarily the education that preceded receipt of the

ECFMG (unless the training received prior to receipt of the ECFMG is crucial to demonstrating competency to exercise clinical privileges).

- What to verify: ECFMG number and date issued.
- Potential verification methods: Contact the ECFMG (www.ecfmg.org) for verification instructions.
- When to verify: At time of initial appointment/privileges

Postgraduate Education (Internship, Residency, or Fellowship)

Upon graduation from medical (or other professional) school, current graduates attend training conducted in a hospital that is referred to as postgraduate year one (PGY1). PGY1 was previously referred to as an internship program. PGY1 may consist of various rotations (a short period of time spent in several services such as medicine, obstetrics, and surgery), it may be specialty oriented (e.g., solely pathology), or it may be a combination of both approaches.

PGY2 and onward is training related to the specialty selected by the practitioner (e.g. family medicine, pediatrics, general surgery). PGY2 training and beyond was previously referred to as a residency program. The length of time that it takes to complete PGY2 training and beyond depends on the specialty selected. For example, it takes three years (PGY2–4) to complete training in internal medicine and four years (PGY2–5) to complete an obstetrics/gynecology residency training program.

Training that takes place beyond completion of the specialty training (i.e., the residency) in a subspecialty (e.g., cardiology, gastroenterology, colorectal surgery) is referred to as a fellowship. A fellowship may be of one, two, or three years in duration, depending on the discipline.

- What to verify: Institution, begin/end dates, type of training/specialty, successful completion.
- Potential verification methods: Confirm directly with the institution in writing or orally, or use the AMA or AOA profile services (physicians only).
- When to verify: At time of initial appointment/privileges or whenever additional training is obtained.

Board Certification

Specialty and subspecialty medical disciplines have established boards that perform testing of practitioners who are qualified for examination in the specified area. After passing the exam and meeting certain other criteria, a practitioner may become board certified in his or her specialty. If the practitioner is a subspecialist, has completed the required training, and has achieved certification in the specialty area, he or she may also become certified in the subspecialty. For example, the subspecialty board for gastroenterology may certify a physician who is board certified in internal medicine and has completed a fellowship in gastroenterology. Certification boards

Exhibit 6-1 Sample Training Director Letter and Questionnaire

(Date)

Residency Program
(Street Address)
(City/State/ZIP)

RE: (Name of Applicant)
    (Applicant's date of birth—for identification purposes)

Dear Sir or Madam:

The above-named practitioner has applied to _____ Medical Center for medical staff appointment and/or clinical privileges. The purpose of this letter is to request verification of his or her completion of a residency program. Because this training program was recently completed, we also need to obtain information concerning the applicant's current clinical competency.

Please complete the information below and return it in the self-addressed envelope enclosed for your convenience. I have enclosed a copy of a signed waiver executed by the practitioner, which gives us permission to obtain the requested information.

If you have confidential information you would like to discuss, please call _____ at _____ .

Your prompt reply will be greatly appreciated.

Sincerely,

_____
Title

_____

Did the above-named practitioner successfully complete a residency program?
                                            ❑ Yes   ❑ No
Type of residency: _____
From: _____ to _____

_____

Evaluation

This evaluation should be based on demonstrated performance compared to that reasonably expected of a practitioner with a similar level of training, experience, and background as this one. A copy of the practitioner's request for clinical

124 CHAPTER 6 The Hospital Credentials Process

Exhibit 6-1: Sample Training Director Letter and Questionnaire (continued)

privileges at _____ Medical Center is enclosed for reference purposes. If you do not have knowledge to answer a particular question, please indicate "no information."

	Favorable	Not Favorable	No Information
Basic medical knowledge			
Professional judgment and responsibility			
Clinical competence			
Ability to exercise the privileges requested			
Ability to work with others			
Medical records			
Patient management			
Practitioner–patient relationship			
Ability to understand, speak, and write English			
Relationship with nursing and other professional staff			

Actions Taken and Conduct and Health Status

If any of the following questions are answered "yes," please give details on separate sheet.

	Yes	No	Don't Know
During the applicant's residency program has this applicant ever been subject to any type of disciplinary action, including, but not limited to, suspension, probation, or termination?			
To your knowledge, has the applicant ever been under investigation by any governmental or other legal body?			
At the time the applicant left your institution, were any investigations or actions instituted, in process, or pending against the applicant?			
Has the applicant ever shown signs of any behavior, drug, or alcohol problems?			
Has the applicant ever shown signs of any mental or physical health problems?			

Exhibit 6-1 — Sample Training Director Letter and Questionnaire (continued)

Recommendations
❏ Recommend without reservation
❏ Recommend with the following reservations
_____
_____
_____

❏ Do not recommend

What is the best time to contact you by telephone? _____
Telephone number: _____

Reference provided by:

_____   _____
Date   **Signature**

_____
Typed or Printed Name

---

exist for physicians (those recognized by the American Board of Medical Specialties [ABMS] and the American Osteopathic Association [AOA]) as well as for podiatrists and other disciplines. The World Wide Web can be used to access information about certifying boards for various disciplines and specialties.

Each healthcare organization must determine which certifying boards will be recognized for its own credentialing purposes. In recent years, a plethora of "certification" boards have emerged, some of which are not generally recognized in the healthcare industry. Most hospitals recognized the ABMS and AOA boards for physicians. Some hospitals also recognize certifying boards in Canada and the United Kingdom (Royal College of Physicians). It is best to determine which certification boards will be recognized when requirements related to board certification are established, rather than waiting until an applicant presents credentials that show board certification by an unrecognized board.

"Board qualified" refers to the practitioner's admissibility to take the specialty board certification examination and usually refers to completion of an approved residency/fellowship training program. In addition to the training programs, some boards require the practitioner to practice for a specified length of time prior to being eligible to take the examination. For example, an obstetrician/gynecologist must complete the residency program, practice obstetrics/gynecology for a period of 18 months, and submit a clinical resume of patients treated prior to being qualified to sit for the board certification examination.

Many boards administer written and oral examinations. Candidates usually have a waiting period between taking the written exam and taking the oral exam.

Depending on the specialty, practitioners are qualified to take the examination for a specified numbers of years after completion of training. If the board's time limits are exceeded, the practitioner is no longer admissible to apply for the certification examination. In some specialties, practitioners may have to complete additional training to become admissible again. These practitioners are no longer considered board qualified or board admissible.

Most specialty boards currently have requirements for recertification after a given number of years (in the past, practitioners were often board certified with no expiration date). In these cases, when the initial board certification status expires, the practitioner is no longer considered board certified. Some specialty boards do not require recertification, but encourage practitioners to accomplish recertification on a voluntary basis. For additional information about board certification, explore the Web sites of the American Board of Medical Specialties (www.abms.org) or the American Osteopathic Board (www.osteopathic.org).

For many years, the term "board eligible" was used by hospitals in the context of a physician's progress toward becoming board certified. In 1977, the ABMS issued this statement:

> *The term board eligible has been given such a variety of meaning by various agencies that it has lost usefulness as an indicator of a physician's progress towards certification by a specialty board. Furthermore, because some candidates have used the term year after year while making no perceptible progress toward certification, it has sometimes been accepted improperly as a more or less permanent alternative to certification.*
>
> *For those reasons, the American Board of Medical Specialties recommended to its member boards that the use of the term board eligible be disavowed. Instead the Boards are urged to respond to inquiries by stating the individual's precise position in the certifying process.*

Therefore, the term "board eligible" should not be used to describe a physician's qualifications.

- **What to verify** (for each board certification): Certifying board, specialty or subspecialty, date certified/recertified, and expiration date, if applicable.
- **Potential verification methods**: Confirm directly with the certifying board in writing, orally, or via an authorized Web site, or use the AMA or AOA profile services.

- **When to verify:** At the time of initial appointment/profiles and at the time of expiration of certification. In addition, some hospitals confirm current certification at the time of reappointment.

License to Practice

To practice medicine (as well as dentistry or podiatry), a practitioner must obtain a license from the appropriate state licensing agency (i.e., state medical board). A physician usually applies for a state license after completing medical school and passing an examination that establishes his or her knowledge in the basic sciences. Generally, this application occurs prior to PGY1. State licensure boards require reregistration of the license to practice on an annual or biennial basis, depending on the state.

Many practitioners hold licensure in more than one state. Some states issue a license by reciprocity, which is recognition by the state of the validity of the medical license issued by another state. Other states will not issue a license by reciprocity and require applying practitioners to pass a medical sciences examination.

- **What to verify:** License to practice in the state in which services will be provided (i.e., the location of the healthcare facility credentialing the practitioner). It is not required (although it may be good practice) that licensure in other states be verified. Verify license, expiration date, and sanctions and/or limitations.
- **Potential verification methods:** Confirm directly with the state licensing authority in writing, orally, or via an approved Web site.
- **When to verify:** At the time of initial appointment/privileges, reappointment, and at the time of license expiration. Also verify this information if new privileges are requested between reappointment periods.

Drug Enforcement Administration Registration

The U.S. Department of Justice operates the Drug Enforcement Administration (DEA). For a practitioner to prescribe medications and narcotics, he or she must have a DEA registration, which constitutes the practitioner's authorization to prescribe drugs. The drug schedules that may be prescribed are listed on the practitioner's DEA registration: 2, 2n, 3, 3n, 4, and 5. Not all practitioners apply for or are granted prescribing authority for all schedules. Some practitioners do not apply for DEA registration at all, because they do not need or intend to prescribe drugs. For example, many pathologists do not maintain a DEA registration.

In addition to the federal DEA registration, some states require practitioners to register at the state level to prescribe drugs. The state registration also expires periodically and must be verified to ensure that it remains current.

- **What to verify:** Federal and/or state DEA registration number, expiration date, and schedules. (The drug schedule information should be provided to the hospital pharmacy for monitoring purposes.)

- Potential verification methods: Obtain a copy from the practitioner or use the National Technical Information Service (NTIS).
- When to verify: At the time of initial appointment/privileges and update at expiration.

Healthcare Organization Affiliations

Each hospital should determine the extent to which the practitioner's service at current and previous healthcare organizations (e.g., hospitals, ambulatory care facilities) will be verified. Until the past few years, it was common for hospitals to query all current and all past affiliations at the time of initial appointment (referred to as "cradle-to-grave credentialing"). Today, hospitals, however, often limit the numbers of years they go back to seek this information. For example, some hospitals verify all current and previous healthcare organization affiliations for the previous seven to ten years, rather than go back to the practitioner's entire career. One of the reasons for the limitation on the number of years to go back is that many applications approved for statewide use (e.g., the California Participating Physician Application Form) ask only for a ten-year affiliation history. Some organizations believe that information going back more than ten years in the past is not particularly relevant to current clinical competency and only go back more than ten years to verify a pattern of behavior or other important issue.

Additionally, some healthcare organizations select a percentage of the past seven to ten years to verify. One reason for this practice is because of the number of locum tenens and telemedicine practitioners now being credentialed—some of these practitioners may have hundreds of previous affiliations. The Joint Commission does not require verification of hospital affiliations, so each organization should use common sense in establishing its own requirements.

It is very common for healthcare organizations to release only the "name, rank and serial number" about their current and past members. It is often necessary to contact individuals at a healthcare organization personally if a problem is suspected.

- What to verify: Current status (e.g., active, resigned), begin/end dates of affiliation, adverse actions, performance or behavior problems, and if the practitioner is or was in good standing. Ideally, the MSSP should also verify the range and scope of the practitioner's privileges.
- Potential verification methods: Write directly to the healthcare organization or contact it via telephone. Some organizations have authorized Web sites for this purpose, but provide only limited information via these sites.
- When to verify: At the time of initial appointment/privileges. Also verify this information at the time of reappointment, particularly for practitioners whose primary healthcare organization affiliation is elsewhere and clinical activity at the requesting organization is low or nonexistent.

Professional Liability Insurance

Each organization establishes its own requirements regarding whether professional liability insurance is required and, if so, which type and how much insurance. The Joint Commission requires that information about previous settlements and judgments be obtained—not simply that a practitioner has insurance. Some of the various types of professional liability insurance are profiled here:

- Claims made policies protect policyholders for alleged acts of malpractice that both occur and are reported to the insurance company while the claims made policy is in continuous force.
- Occurrence policies provide coverage for a specific dollar amount for each individual year. For example, suppose a practitioner carries a $100,000/$300,000 policy in 2008 and increases the coverage to $1 million/$3 million in 2010. The practitioner is sued in 2009 for something that occurred in 2008. The insurance company is liable for no more than $100,000 for the claim.
- Tail coverage provides coverage after cancellation of a policy (i.e., when a physician retires or changes insurance carriers).

Most hospital attorneys advocate for obtaining not only previous settlement and judgment information, but also information about currently pending claims.

- What to verify: Depending on the internal healthcare organization requirements, verify current coverage and dates of coverage (expiration date), and confirm that the type of insurance and the amount meet organization requirements. Additional items that may be verified include whether there are any current or pending claims and whether the practitioner is covered to exercise the privileges requested.
- Potential verification methods: Obtain a certificate of insurance directly from practitioner or write the insurance carrier to verify coverage and claims history. Payments made since September 1, 1990, should be covered by the National Practitioner Data Bank (NPDB) report.
- When to verify: At the time of initial appointment/privileges and update as insurance expires.

Continuing Medical Education

Participation in continuing medical education (CME) is one way to maintain current clinical competency. It is customary to require that practitioners provide information about their involvement in CME at the time they are initially appointed and at each reappointment period. This information is usually self-reported by the practitioner. The healthcare organization should assess the information submitted by the practitioner to make sure that the CME (or at least a portion of the CME) is related to the privileges requested.

- What to verify: Number and types of CME activities.
- Potential verification methods: Several options are available to healthcare organizations. First, the applicant could be required to submit a listing of CME activities for the previous 24-month period. An alternative method (and one that is approved by the Joint Commission) is to allow applicants to attest to their involvement in CME that pertains to the privileges requested. Applicants who completed residency or fellowship training within the past two-year period are commonly exempted from providing documentation of CME.
- When to verify: At the time of initial appointment/privileges and at reappointment.

Peer References and Recommendations

The Joint Commission requires that peer recommendations be obtained for initial appointment and privileging and at the time of reappointment. The number of peer recommendations is organization specific, but usually ranges from two to four recommendations for initial appointment and at least one for reappointment (the reappointment peer recommendation may be the department chair, credentials committee, or other peer within the organization). A "peer," according to the Joint Commission, means an individual in the same professional discipline (i.e., the same type of license) with essentially the same privileges.

Application forms should be clear about the organization's definition of who may be listed as a potential peer reference. For example, some organizations use the following definition:

> A peer must be someone who has had contact with the applicant during the past three to five years. If the applicant finished training during the past three years, one of the letters must be from the training program director. At least one reference must be from the colleague in the applicant's specialty. Individuals who are related by family or via financial relationships may not provide references.

It should be noted that an organization is not obligated to only seek information from the names of peers provided by the applicant. Perhaps additional individuals potentially have information about the applicant that can be queried even though their names were not provided by the applicant.

- What to verify: Relationship of the peer to the applicant; how the peer is aware of the applicant's current clinical competency; validation by the peer of the applicant's request for clinical privileges (send a copy of the requested clinical privileges to the peer so that the peer can comment directly upon whether the applicant is qualified to exercise the privileges requested).

- Potential verification methods: Send a letter, a copy of the requested privileges, and the questionnaire directly to the peer reference. Letters submitted by the applicant may not be used. Telephone inquiries may also be made but must be documented.
- When to verify: At the time of initial appointment/privileges and at reappointment. If a practitioner requests new privileges between appointments, obtaining a peer recommendation may also be advisable.

A sample letter to a peer reference is included on the CD that accompanies the book.

Background Checks

Many organizations now conduct background checks (sometimes referred to as criminal background checks) to find out if there is information in an applicant's background that should be known and evaluated before the organization considers granting membership and/or privileges. In some states, conducting a background check of some type is required. Unfortunately, some states that require background checks only require checking records in the state in which the applicant practices or plans to practice. If an organization has an application from a candidate from another state, checking the records of the state to which the candidate is moving will probably yield no information. Checking the state(s) where the candidate has been living and working is a more rational approach.

Each organization should determine the scope and content of a background check. The more extensive the search (and the more locations that must be checked for an applicant), the more expensive the background check will be. Some organizations perform a background check on all new applicants. Others check only those applicants who meet specific criteria, such as the following:

- Moved practice more than two times during professional career
- All locum tenens (i.e., traveling) practitioners
- Moved practice after five years in same area or city
- More than three state licenses during professional career
- Gap of six months in which the practitioner was not practicing or in training at any location
- Noncompletion of any professional training program

These criteria are given for illustrative purposes only. An organization that is considering using criteria to determine when to conduct a background check should consult legal counsel when establishing its policy in this area.

The first step in the background investigation process begins with obtaining a comprehensive authorization and release form from the candidate. The candidate should be aware that a background check will be conducted as part of the credentialing process. The applicant will have already provided his or her full name, any other names under which the candidate had attended schooling or practiced, a date of birth, and a Social Security number as part of the application form. These pieces of information are critical in confirming the individual's records and identity. If a candidate hesitates or refuses to sign an authorization to conduct a background check, it should be the first red flag in the screening process.

From there, a Social Security trace and validation are obtained. This report will generally provide any alternate names utilized, current and past addresses, and the date and state of issuance. This information is key in determining whether the candidate has practiced in any locations not noted on the application form. States listed on a Social Security trace that do not correspond to information on the application should immediately be contacted for licensure information and may even be considered prime locations for a search of court records.

A comprehensive background search will include a search of court records, including both criminal and civil records at the county and federal level. Criminal records are always of concern; however, when dealing with medical personnel, the civil records are just as important as—if not more important than—the criminal records. Civil records will contain suits involving medical malpractice, negligence, breach of contract, and antitrust litigation to name a few. Contact with the court systems may uncover a pattern of behavior or litigation that may not otherwise be found.

Validation of the Identity of the Applicant

The Joint Commission requires that during the credentialing process, the healthcare organization use some mechanism to ensure that the individual requesting privileges is, in fact, the same individual who is identified in the credentialing documents. A credentialing "best practice" is to obtain a current picture of the applicant, and then to ask peer references and healthcare organization affiliations to verify the applicant's identity. However, despite that fact that this practice is a good one, it does not meet the Joint Commission requirements. To confirm identity, someone at the healthcare organization must view government-issued identification (e.g., passport, driver's license, military identification). Some organizations require that the newly appointed practitioner go to the MSSD with his or her government-issued identification prior to providing any type of patient care. An alternative method might be to have hospital security view identification prior to issuing a name badge.

Additional Sources of Information on Applicants

Another potential source of information on physician applicants that may be used is the Federation of State Medical Boards (www.fsmb.org), which is a data bank containing disciplinary action information as reported by all state boards of medical examiners and other sources. The National Practitioner Data Bank must be queried as well. This data bank, which began collecting information in September 1990, should eventually contain a wealth of information, especially information concerning licensure and inadequate performance (www.npdb.org). For completeness of information sources, the American Medical Association Physician Masterfile may be obtained for physician applicants (www.ama-assn.org).

Red Flags

Some points need to be specifically considered in reviewing the completed application form and in relation to source verification. Any incomplete item that is pertinent to the application requires a letter telling the applicant that his or her application is on hold. This is particularly true regarding the critical questions section, particularly in relation to liability and health issues. Telephone calls to the applicant usually are not productive, and there is no hard copy record of the information exchange when this medium is used for communication. If a second letter to request information is needed, it should be sent by certified mail to document its arrival and ensure a signed receipt. The second letter should also indicate a final date by which the information must be received if the application is not to be placed in the "incomplete" file. The medical staff bylaws should define what constitutes a completed application and include language specifying that unresolved questions about an applicant make an application incomplete.

Look for red-flag items, such as those listed below and in TABLE 6-1:

- When the application reveals an unexplained time gap in the training or practice sequence since graduation, this gap requires serious attention. The applicant must explain why there was a long period of inactivity or the application cannot be processed. The healthcare organization should define the amount of time that constitutes a gap in time that requires explanation and follow-up. Most organizations define a gap as 30 to 90 days.
- Any indication of a voluntary or involuntary loss of one or more privileges at another hospital or a restriction or loss of a license or DEA registration certificate, past or present, is another red flag that requires clarification before further processing of the application. If both the other facility or agency and the applicant refuse to cooperate in providing the needed information, then the application should go into the incomplete file and the practitioner be so notified.
- Because it takes time to build a practice, frequent changes in location in a short span of time require investigation of the applicant. Practitioners may have a sound reason for moving from one location or state to another. Sometimes, however, a move may be related to problems with the state licensing agency, litigation problems, felony convictions, or health problems, none of which were mentioned on the application form. The health problems may relate to impaired physician status that has not been resolved.
- The practitioner who has a number of lawsuits pending or settled requires additional investigation. Professional liability claims are not necessarily an indication of a problem, but extra checking should be undertaken to determine that a

Table 6-1   Some Credentialing "Red Flags" and Recommended Responses

Lowell C. Brown, Esq.
FOLEY & LARDNER
2029 Century Park East, Suite 3500
Los Angeles, California 90067
(310) 957-7843

The Problem	Recommended Approach
1. Failure by any hospital, medical staff organization, training program, or professional society with which the applicant has been affiliated to respond completely to any written or oral reference inquiry	This is the most common indication that a problem may exist. If a complete reference response is not forthcoming from any such entity, the hospital credentialing committee should inform the applicant that the application will be deemed incomplete until a complete reference is obtained, and that failure to provide the reference within a set period of time will be considered a withdrawal of the application.
2. Equivocal or incomplete response to a written or oral reference request	The hospital credentialing committee should inform the applicant that it will be necessary for him or her to authorize the reference individual to provide a full and complete explanation of any equivocal or incomplete response and that the application will be deemed incomplete until that explanation is received. If the applicant fails to produce the full explanation required by the committee within a set period of time, the application will be filed incomplete.
3. "Off the record" (but credible) reports of problems relating in any way to an applicant's professional practice	This is the second most common form of evidence that a problem exists. Individuals may report investigations, concerns, or disciplinary actions taken at other facilities (or of other problems) of which they are aware. The reporting individuals may be known to membership committee members and may be credible, but the reporting individuals may be unwilling to provide information on the record.
	The hospital credentialing committee should never base its recommendation on unconfirmed, "off the record" information. Such information may turn out to be unreliable or may not result in any usable information at a subsequent hearing.

Table 6-1	Some Credentialing "Red Flags" and Recommended Responses (continued)
The Problem	**Recommended Approach**
	Instead, the hospital credentialing committee should get as much detail as possible about the reported problem, even if that detail is "off the record." Then, the committee should require the applicant to furnish specific documentary evidence relating to whatever problems were reported off the record. For example, the committee may require the applicant to produce all correspondence with another hospital or medical staff organization, or to authorize another medical staff organization to provide a verified statement including copies of all peer review reports and minutes reflecting an evaluation of the applicant's practice. Likewise, the committee may require the applicant to provide a verified statement transmitting copies of particular office or hospital patient records (with names expunged) or other documents that may confirm information received off the record. The application should be considered incomplete until all such information is received and should be considered to be withdrawn if the information is not *produced by a particular* date.
4. Difficulty in verifying nature and volume of recent hospital practice	The applicant should be informed that the application is incomplete until documentation of such information in whatever form the hospital credentialing committee requires is received. If the information is not received within a set period of time, the application should be deemed withdrawn.
5. Difficulty in verifying compliance with general requirements, such as professional liability insurance coverage, patient coverage arrangements, and establishment of office practice in the hospital's area	The applicant should be informed that the application is incomplete until documentation of such information in whatever form the hospital credentialing committee requires is received. If the information is not received within a set period of time, the application should be deemed withdrawn.

Table 6-1	Some Credentialing "Red Flags" and Recommended Responses (continued)
The Problem	**Recommended Approach**
6. Any resignation or withdrawal of an application for appointment or reappointment from any hospital, medical staff, or professional society at any time in an applicant's career	This is another strong sign of a potential problem. The hospital credentialing committee should require the applicant to produce a signed verification from the facility or organization involved, transmitting copies of all correspondence, committee minutes, memoranda, reports, or other documents relating in any way to the withdrawal or any pending investigations or disciplinary actions.
7. Past disciplinary actions by another hospital, medical staff, professional society, or practice arrangement	This is the type of information that the hospital credentialing committee is required to obtain and evaluate carefully. The committee should inform the applicant that it will be necessary for him or her to produce signed verification from the facility or organization transmitting all correspondence, memoranda, reports, committee minutes, transcripts, statements of charges, exhibits, and other documentation in any way relating to the disciplinary action.
	The application should be deemed incomplete until that information is provided. Failure to provide the information within a set period of time should be deemed a withdrawal of the application.
8. Pending investigation by any hospital, medical staff organization, or professional society	This is also the type of information that the hospital credentialing committee is required to obtain and evaluate carefully. As with past disciplinary actions, the committee should inform the applicant that it will be necessary for him or her to produce a signed verification from the facility or organization transmitting all correspondence, memoranda, reports, committee minutes, transcripts, statements of charges, exhibits, and other documentation in any way relating to the disciplinary action.
	The application should be deemed incomplete until that information is provided. Failure to provide the information within a set period of time should be deemed a withdrawal of the application.

Table 6-1	Some Credentialing "Red Flags" and Recommended Responses (continued)
The Problem	**Recommended Approach**
9. Pending recommendation of disciplinary action by any hospital, medical staff organization, professional society, or practice affiliation	As with items 7 and 8, the hospital credentialing committee should inform the applicant that it will be necessary for him or her to produce a signed verification from the facility or organization transmitting all correspondence, memoranda, reports, committee minutes, transcripts, statements of charges, exhibits, and other documentation in any way relating to the disciplinary action.
	The application should be deemed incomplete until that information is provided. Failure to provide the information within a set period of time should be deemed a withdrawal of the application.
10. Past or present investigation by the state medical board	The hospital credentialing committee should inform the applicant that he or she must provide a signed verification from the medical board transmitting all correspondence, memoranda, investigative reports, witness statements, expert evaluations, and other investigative material relating to the investigation. In addition, if that material discloses any disciplinary actions at other facilities, the applicant should be required to produce a signed verification from that facility transmitting all relevant documentation. If this information is not received within a set period of time, the application should be deemed withdrawn.
11. Disciplinary action by the state medical board	As with item 10, the hospital credentialing committee should inform the applicant that he or she must provide a signed verification from the medical board transmitting all correspondence, memoranda, investigative reports, witness statements, expert evaluations, and other investigative material relating to the investigation. In addition, if that material discloses any disciplinary actions at other facilities, the applicant should be required to produce a signed verification from that facility transmitting all relevant documentation. If this information is not received within a set period of time, the application should be deemed withdrawn.

Table 6-1	Some Credentialing "Red Flags" and Recommended Responses (continued)
The Problem	**Recommended Approach**
12. Pending state medical board accusation (regardless of whether an administrative hearing has been completed or whether the applicant is appealing the administrative determination in court)	The hospital credentialing committee should inform the applicant that he or she must provide a signed verification from the state medical board transmitting all correspondence, memoranda, investigative reports, witness statements, expert evaluations, and other investigative material relating to the investigation. In addition, if that material discloses any disciplinary actions at other facilities, the applicant should be required to produce a signed verification from that facility transmitting all relevant documentation. If this information is not received within a set period of time, the application should be deemed withdrawn.
13. Settlement of any professional liability claims (whether or not they resulted in litigation) within the past five years	The applicant should be asked to provide a signed verification from an individual, other than himself or herself, who is knowledgeable about the settlement, transmitting copies of all settlement agreements, documentation, court pleadings, deposition transcripts, expert opinion reports, correspondence, or other documents relating to the terms of the settlement or the charges on which the claim was based. The application should be deemed incomplete until this information is received, and if the information is not received within a set period of time, the application should be deemed withdrawn.
14. Adverse judgment in any professional liability action during the past five years	The application should be required to produce signed verifications transmitting copies of the judgment, and court papers demonstrating the specific charges upon which the claim was based. In appropriate cases, the information requested might include deposition transcripts, expert opinion reports, correspondence, and other documents relating to the claim, as well as patient records, office records, hospital investigation reports, and documents relating to disciplinary actions by any other facilities. Until all such documentation is received, the application should be deemed incomplete.

Table 6-1	Some Credentialing "Red Flags" and Recommended Responses (continued)
The Problem	**Recommended Approach**
15. Pending professional liability actions	This is one of the most important pieces of information that may come to the hospital's attention, and one which the hospital is probably legally required to review. The applicant should be required to produce signed verifications transmitting the materials generally described in item 14.
16. Other civil litigation relating to the applicant's professional practice or qualifications. (This may include, for example, claims of sexual misconduct with patients or claims of insurance fraud or investigations by a professional review organization.) Such information would probably not come to the hospital's attention as a result of the applicant's completion of the hospital's application. It would probably come to light through news reports or other unofficial means.	The applicant should be required to produce signed verifications in transmitting copies of court documents sufficient to explain the nature of charges against him or her and the status of the litigation (including any settlement thereof). In addition, the applicant should be required to produce signed verifications transmitting copies of correspondence, reports, committee minutes, and any other documents relating to the underlying charges or any investigation or disciplinary actions relating to those charges. The application should be deemed incomplete until that information is produced, and it should be deemed withdrawn if the information is not produced within a set period of time.
17. Investigations or disciplinary actions by a professional review organization, or any third-party payer (including Medicare, Medi-Cal, or private insurance)	The applicant should be required to provide a signed verification transmitting copies of all investigative reports, correspondence, related disciplinary actions, or administrative investigations relating to this matter. The application should be deemed incomplete until such information is received and should be deemed withdrawn if the information is not received within a set period of time.

Table 6-1	Some Credentialing "Red Flags" and Recommended Responses (continued)
The Problem	**Recommended Approach**
18. Participation, in the last five years in any treatment or diversion program relating to drug use, alcohol dependency, or psychiatric problems	The applicant should be required to provide signed verifications transmitting copies of all documents relating to the terms and conditions of participation, correspondence relating to such participation, and all evaluations of the applicant's physical, mental, or emotional condition. The application should be deemed incomplete until all such information is received and should be deemed withdrawn unless all such information is received within a certain period of time.
19. Evidence of any criminal charges brought against the applicant with the past five years	The applicant should be required to provide signed verifications from public authorities transmitting copies of charges and of any court documents demonstrating the resolution or status of such actions. The applicant should also be required to produce signed verifications transmitting such documents as the committee deems necessary relating to the underlying conduct reflected in the criminal accusations. The application should be deemed incomplete until such information is furnished and should be deemed withdrawn unless the information is produced within a set period of time.
20. Pending criminal charges	In many cases, the criminal charges, if proven, would disqualify the applicant from hospital membership. Accordingly, the applicant should be required to produce signed verifications of court documents as well as such related documentation as the hospital credentialing committee requires. Generally, it will be impossible for the committee to resolve the issues presented by a criminal charge relating to the applicant's professional practice or qualifications until after the criminal proceeding is completed. Accordingly, the committee, in appropriate circumstances, may consider the application incomplete until the criminal matter is fully resolved.
21. Criminal conviction during the past five years	In many cases, the criminal charges if proven would disqualify the applicant from the hospital membership. The hospital credentialing committee should require the same information from the applicant as recommended in item 20.

pattern of substandard practice was not the cause. Obtaining source information on the applicant's professional liability coverage may require the applicant's written permission unless the bylaws or the application form or the cover letters accompanying it provide otherwise. The insurer, however, can still insist on written permission to release the information.
- The practitioner who was previously impaired by alcohol or drug abuse may apply for membership and privileges. Documentation of rehabilitation and a period of monitoring will help to verify recovery and provide evidence that the problem has been corrected. Chapter 13 provides additional information about practitioner health problems.

Telephone Calls Concerning Applicants

Occasionally insight about the previously mentioned problems can be gained through an administrator-to-administrator (or physician-to-physician) phone call. Unless a dated memo detailing the conversation is created, however, there will be no hard information on which to help base a decision or provide documentation of the rationale for a decision. When phone calls are made to discuss an application problem or a negative reference letter, specific questions should be asked of the physician or administrator contacted. Included might be questions about the receipt of reports of poor medical practice, poor relationships with peers or hospital staff that have been detrimental to patient care or hospital operations, and mental or physical illness or substance abuse problems that have interfered with the ability to practice quality medicine. Names of other informants who might be contacted can be obtained at the time these phone calls are made to previous hospitals and peer references.

■ Evaluation and Decision-Making Process

The completed application form and all supporting information should be prepared for evaluation by the MSSP. "Prepared for evaluation" means that the file should be organized in a manner that facilitates evaluation, a summary of the information in the file should be prepared, and red flags (or potentially adverse information) should be clearly identified. Even though it is the medical staff organization's responsibility (through delegation to elected and/or appointed representatives) to make informed recommendations, the role played by the MSSP in properly preparing the file for evaluation cannot be overstated. Physicians are busy people, and it is in the best interest of the healthcare organization to assure that physicians are assisted in carrying out their responsibilities in the important work of credentialing.

Each file is evaluated by the following parties, who then provide an indication of approval, approval with stated exceptions (e.g., denial of certain privileges), or disapproval and the rationale for any disapprovals:

1. The medical staff clinical department chair. This individual should indicate that he or she has (a) reviewed the application and found it in satisfactory order, (b) has no knowledge of any health problem that would prevent the individual seeking appointment from exercising the privileges requested, and (c) has made a recommendation (e.g., approval). (This statement may have to be made by the chief of staff in a hospital that is still not departmentalized.)
2. The credentials committee or the body performing the credentialing function.
3. The medical staff executive committee.
4. The governing body, which has final decision-making authority.

Any person required to evaluate the request for appointment can request further relevant information before making a recommendation or decision. If the process is performed properly, however, this type of delay will rarely occur. EXHIBIT 6-2 is a sample initial appointment recommendation form that the department chair should complete upon review of the completed credentials file.

Expedited credentialing is permitted by the Joint Commission when essentially there is a complete, problem-free application (there is no current or previously successful challenge to any licensure or registration; no involuntary termination of medical staff membership; and no involuntary limitation, denial, or loss of clinical privileges; and the organization has determined that there has not been an unusual pattern of, or an excessive number of, professional liability actions that have resulted in a final judgment against the applicant). "Expedited" means that the governing body may delegate the authority to make decisions on appointment, granting of clinical privileges, and reappointment to a committee consisting of at least two voting members of the governing body. An expedited credentialing process does not include bypassing the MEC in an effort to make an earlier decision. Organizations that decide to use provisions for expedited credentialing should carefully consider the Joint Commission standards and cautiously craft policies and procedures that meet the intent of accreditation requirements, as many organizations have misinterpreted the extent to which credentialing can actually be expedited.

■ Staff Reappointment

Credentials

The credentials process also involves staff reappointment. Reappointment is required by the CMS and the Joint Commission for multiple reasons, including the updating of information relating to claims and litigation, health, and changes in outside affiliations, and additional training, education, and certification. It is also mandatory to ensure that the practitioner is currently competent to exercise the clinical privileges

Exhibit 6-2 Initial Appointment Recommendation Form

Initial Appointment Recommendation Form

Applicant: _____

Specialty: _____

1. Review of request for clinical privileges (check all that apply):
   - ❏ Privileges requested supported by residency/fellowship training
   - ❏ Privileges requested supported by CME experience
   - ❏ Privileges requested supported by practice experience

   Other comments related to request for privileges: _____
   _____
   _____
   _____

   Special training or areas of expertise: _____
   _____
   _____

2. Previous experience and reason(s) for leaving past practices (if applicable):
   _____
   _____
   _____
   _____

3. Professional liability actions (if applicable, please comment on any past or pending claims): _____
   _____
   _____
   _____

4. Health status:
   - ❏ To the best of our knowledge, the applicant is competent and physically and mentally able to perform the duties and clinical privileges.
   - ❏ Has the following health problem(s): _____
   _____
   _____

   Additional comments (address any potentially adverse information flagged by the medical staff coordinator): _____
   _____
   _____
   _____

Exhibit 6-2 — Initial Appointment Recommendation Form (continued)

Recommendation of department chair:

Appointment: ❑ Recommended
❑ Not recommended
❑ Recommended with the following conditions:

_____
_____
_____

Privileges: See privilege delineation form

_____   _____
Signature of Department Chair   Date

Recommendation of credentials committee:

_____

DATE
❑ Confirm recommendation of the department chair
❑ Recommend the following: _____
_____
_____

Recommendation of Medical Executive Committee:

_____

DATE
❑ Confirm recommendation of the credentials committee
❑ Recommend the following: _____
_____
_____

Board Action

_____
_____

DATE
❑ Confirm recommendation of the medical executive committee
❑ Recommend the following: _____
_____

Staff Reappointment   145

that he or she has been granted. Beginning in 2008, healthcare organizations accredited by the Joint Commission were required to have an "ongoing professional practice evaluation" (OPPE) process in place that provides data to be used to regularly evaluate the performance of each practitioner granted clinical privileges. At the same time, the reappointment process is still required and the same type of information used for OPPE is used at the time of reappointment.

One frequently overlooked medical staff and governing body responsibility is the obligation to ensure that the practitioner has met any requirements for privileges, the exercise of which requires evidence of continued proficiency. See Chapter 7 for additional information about clinical privileging requirements.

During the period between staff appointments, a staff member's credentials are established through the medical staff quality and peer review system. The medical staff committees and departments review performance data; they may also review specific patient care cases. Ongoing practitioner performance data are maintained, including the findings of the hospital's performance improvement program (see Chapter 11). Findings should be included from procedure evaluation, drug therapy evaluation, blood therapy evaluation, medical record documentation review, utilization review, hospital risk management, and other monitoring and evaluation programs. These numerator findings should be included on a profile that also notes denominator information (i.e., the number of admissions, procedures performed, and consultations). The denominator information is important as it helps to put into perspective any negative data generated. A practitioner who has admitted only three patients and had quality problems with the treatment of all three patients is in a different category from a practitioner who has admitted dozens of patients but experienced quality problems with only three. Additionally, each practitioner's data should be compared to data for other practitioners within the same specialty as well as to data from an external source.

It is important, especially for a large medical staff, to have a staggered system of reappointment. That is, the entire staff should not be reappointed at the same time but rather have their reappointment dates divided by department, by birth date, by appointment date, or alphabetically, so that large numbers are not reappointed at the same time. This permits a more in-depth evaluation of each candidate for reappointment and of the related clinical privilege delineation.

The Reappointment Form

A reappointment form should be provided to each staff member for completion along with a record of his or her current privileges. The reappointment form should require the following evidence:

1. Confirmation of all required demographic information.
2. Confirmation of current licenses, DEA registration, and professional liability coverage (this information should be updated at the time of expiration;

therefore, it may not be necessary to query the applicant regarding current information that is already on file). Because states vary with respect to licensure date requirements and hospital medical staffs vary with respect to reappointment dates, it may be necessary to verify the state licensure twice—once at expiration date and once at time of reappointment. This issue has become more important in recent years as medical staffs have wisely shifted to staggered reappointment systems.

3. Confirmation of the attainment of specialty board certification since appointment or last reappointment.
4. An indication as to whether a privilege change is being requested and, if so, whether specific additional privileges are the issue. (If additional privileges are requested, the staff member must state, in terms of training and so on, why he or she is qualified to exercise the additional privileges.) A practitioner may also wish to drop privileges due to a change in the pattern of practice. For example, an obstetrician/gynecologist may want to discontinue practicing obstetrics and limit his or her practice to gynecology. It is important that this change be noted on the clinical privilege form.
5. The answers to critical questions relating to status since the previous appointment, including the following:
    - Has your membership in another healthcare facility been denied, revoked, or otherwise acted against, or been subjected to disciplinary action?
    - Have any privileges been voluntarily or involuntarily withdrawn in another healthcare facility?
    - Are you currently under charges that, if upheld, could lead to conviction for a felony or misdemeanor (other than minor traffic offenses)?
    - Have any judgments been made against or settlements been obtained from you in professional liability cases?
    - Are any professional liability cases pending against you?
    - Have you been under treatment for drug addiction or alcoholism?
    - Have you been under psychiatric treatment or care?
    - Are you currently under care for a continuing health problem? (Note: If the answer to any of the previous items is "yes," please include details.)
    - Do you feel that your health status is adequate enough to permit you to provide the patient care services for which you are requesting clinical privileges? (Note: If the answer is no, please include details.)
6. Description of continuing education since last appointment.
7. Any other requirements of the medical staff bylaws, rules, and regulations.
8. The signature of the individual seeking reappointment.
9. The reappointment fee (if any).

The completed application will be routed through the evaluation process, accompanied by the profile information supplied through the quality improvement program and the MSSD. This information usually includes both information on administrative aspects of staff membership (e.g., meeting attendance statistics—if attendance is required, medical record delinquency status, committee appointments, and hospital practice statistics) and clinical performance data (e.g., clinical outcome statistics, committee and department citations, governing board sanctions, and peer review and quality improvement reviews and actions). All hospitals are required to check with the National Practitioner Data Bank to determine whether any adverse information has been reported during the past period of appointment. This step would be omitted if the healthcare organization used the NPDB's Proactive Disclosure Service. The use of this service provides subscribers with information about credentialed practitioners at the time reports are made to the NPDB.

Reappointment of Practitioners with Low Activity

Some hospitals have large numbers of staff members whose primary practices are centered at other area facilities. It is difficult to obtain adequate performance data for these practitioners at the time of reappointment. In each such case, the facilities at which the practitioner most actively practices must be contacted to obtain the information needed for reappointment. As with the reference letters used to obtain information for the initial appointment, these requests should be carefully worded to elicit the precise information needed. The value of the information obtained also depends on the quality and scope of the quality and peer review programs at the other facilities. Even so, some attempt should be made to determine whether the practitioner has experienced professional problems at these facilities. Some hospitals are attempting to reduce the number of staff members who mainly practice elsewhere by requiring (as provided in the bylaws) a minimum number of admissions, procedures, or consultations for maintenance of staff membership and privileges.

Routing Reappointments Through Channels

The completed reappointment form and profile information should be evaluated by the following parties, who should provide an indication of approval, approval with stated exceptions (e.g., denial of certain privileges), or disapproval and the rationale for any disapprovals:

1. The medical staff clinical department chair. This individual should indicate that he or she has (a) reviewed the application and profile information and found it in satisfactory order, (b) has no knowledge of any health problem that would prevent the individual seeking reappointment from exercising the privileges requested, and (c) has made a recommendation (e.g., approval).

(This statement may have to be made by the chief of staff in a hospital that is not departmentalized.)
2. The credentials committee or the body performing the credentialing function.
3. The medical staff executive committee.
4. The governing body, which has final decision-making authority.

Any person required to evaluate the reappointment request can request further relevant information before making a recommendation or decision. However, if the process is performed properly, this type of delay will rarely occur.

If a medical staff member voluntarily relinquishes certain privileges (e.g., because of age, a desire to cut back practice, or poor results), it is critical that the change be formalized through the medical staff and governing body system. Otherwise, the staff member may decide after several years of inactivity to exercise the same privileges again. This could be catastrophic. Before formalizing the voluntary relinquishment of privileges, check state or federal reporting requirements relating to privilege changes.

Conclusion

Whereas it is the responsibility of the medical staff organization to evaluate the information on applicants for medical staff membership and privileges, it is the responsibility of the MSSP to actually gather the information. Credentialing policies and procedures in place in the hospital must be applied objectively and equally by the MSSP to each applicant. The MSSP must be alert to potential problems and initiate further investigation whenever there is questionable, equivocal, or negative information on an applicant.

The vast majority of applicants for medical staff membership and/or clinical privileges will be well-trained, well-qualified practitioners. It is the unqualified or substandard few for whom the MSSP needs to keep a watch. When verifying information returned to the hospital is incomplete, vague, or negative, the MSSP must take the initiative to start the process of further checking. Medical staff leaders are frequently inexperienced in these matters and will look to the MSSP for guidance.

As mentioned earlier, medical staff leaders should be asked by the MSSP in these cases to make telephone calls to peer references, training program directors, or past hospital affiliations in an effort to clarify vague or incomplete information or confirm (or disconfirm) negative information. Respondents will frequently be willing to discuss on a physician-to-physician or administrator-to-administrator basis sensitive information they do not want to put in writing. An effort should be made to obtain names of additional references for the purpose of checking further into reports of professional problems. All persons contacted should be encouraged to put the information in writing to the hospital. Should they be unwilling to do so, the person making the call should prepare a memo to the file that contains a summary of the conversation.

For each applicant, the information gathered should be sufficient to dispel any discomfort in recommending appointment and clinical privileges or be sufficient to demonstrate the unreasonableness in doing so (in which case the appointment should be denied).

When the credentials file is completed, the MSSP is responsible for routing it through the appropriate medical staff channels to the governing body (see Figure 6-1). Supporting the credentials process is one of the most critical responsibilities of the MSSP. In providing this support, medical staff bylaws and credentialing policies should be followed to the letter. Accurate, thorough, and complete documentation should be obtained on each applicant. Legal counsel should be consulted when a question arises as to whether the hospital is carrying out the process appropriately. Medical staff and hospital leaders will look to the MSSP to guide this process.

■ Notes

1. *Merriam-Webster Online Dictionary.* Springfield, MA: Merriam Webster; 2005. Available at: www.m-w.com. Accessed August 17, 2009.
2. "The Joint Commission Glossary." In: *Comprehensive Accreditation Manual for Hospitals, 2009.* Oakbrook Terrace, IL: The Joint Commission; 2009.

CHAPTER 7

Hospital Privileging

Christina W. Giles, CPMSM, MS

■ Delineation of Privileges

Delineation is the process of organizing the procedures offered by an organization into a workable privilege system. By delineating privileges, the organization is authorizing a practitioner to perform certain procedures, provide certain services, or care for or treat specific types of patients. Privilege delineation, when properly performed and monitored, continues to be the most important patient safety function performed by the medical staff and governing body. If the delineation process is unclear or inappropriately defined, or if it does not include specific criteria for each privilege or group of privileges, then the chances of incompetent or poorly trained practitioners providing services or performing procedures increase, as does the opportunity for medical errors and bad outcomes.

Traditionally, privilege delineation has not been very sophisticated, but it is evolving to be the most important part of the credentialing process and will only continue to become more important. Professional specialty groups, certifying and accrediting bodies, licensure boards, and healthcare organizations all tie privilege delineation to assessment of competency—a process that is continually being developed.

Methods for Delineating Privileges

Privilege delineation forms are critical documents because they collectively describe the scope of services provided by a hospital, the services that can be provided individually by a particular practitioner, or the services that can be provided by a specific specialty. Current methods used to describe or delineate clinical privileges include the following:

- A detailed laundry list
- Categories or levels
- Core and special privileges

The laundry list is a lengthy list that attempts to include any and all procedures or treatments performed by a specific specialty. Some people prefer this approach because it appears to be all-inclusive, and it is quite clear which privileges an individual has been granted. The disadvantages are that it is cumbersome and difficult to maintain. If a specific procedure is not included in the list, the implication is that the practitioner is not privileged to perform the procedure. Laundry lists also work best with surgical or procedural types of practice; they are more difficult to use for internal medicine or family practice, which are specialties that rely more heavily on cognitive abilities (i.e., treatment of conditions and illnesses).

A category or levels approach to privileging describes the practice in terms of a hierarchy of levels based either on treatment groupings, acuity of patient disease, or the level of training and experience. An example of categories based on treatment levels follows:

Category I: Privileges for the treatment of uncomplicated illnesses, injuries, or conditions that have lower risk for the patient and represent no apparent serious threat to life

Category II: Privileges for the treatment of major illnesses, injuries, or conditions that pose no significant risk to life and require skills usually acquired upon completion of residency training sufficient to qualify the applicant for board certification

Category III: Privileges for the treatment of severe, life-threatening or potentially life-threatening illnesses, injuries, or conditions usually requiring skills acquired upon completion of fellowship training sufficient to qualify the applicant for subspecialty board certification

The core privileging approach has been many hospitals' preferred method of delineating privileges. The core privileges for a specialty are usually described in a simple, straightforward paragraph. The privileges, which comprise a combination of medical assessment and management as well as procedures, are those medical conditions and procedures that a practitioner would almost always be qualified to perform upon completion of residency training in a particular specialty. Practitioners who have not recently completed a residency training program would be qualified based on continual practice experience in their specialty. Often, a set of special procedures or medical management of conditions are not part of the core because they are either new, are associated with high risk, or require additional training and experience. Privileges to perform these special procedures must be requested separately, and specific criteria must be fulfilled before the privileges are granted. For example, privileges for the management of patients in a critical care unit may be included in the core privilege for a pulmonologist or a physician trained in critical care medicine but would be a special privilege with special criteria for a general internist or family practitioner. The specific criteria for critical care management as a special privilege might be related to clinical activity such as treatment of 20 critically ill patients during a two-year period with acceptable outcomes, along with documentation of recent continuing medical education in critical care medicine or specific recent training, such as successful completion of a one-year fellowship in critical care medicine.

Because the core approach is so very different from the laundry list approach, and because some accrediting bodies have recently spoken out about the inadequacies of the core approach, many hospitals are also including within the core description a list of procedures or treatments. In this way, the core description becomes more specific and complete. This approach also helps define the majority of procedures or treatments that *are* included. EXHIBIT 7-1 is an example of a core privilege form for General Surgery.

In addition, sometimes combinations of these methods are used. When the category approach to clinical privilege delineation is used, care must be taken to ensure that the privileges are actually classified in a way that makes the limits of practice very clear. Some specialty organizations have published sample categories. When these examples are read carefully, however, it becomes obvious that within each category level, the practitioner actually delineates what his or her practice will be. This is inappropriate: There should never be a situation where the practitioner delineates his or her own privileges. The delineation process must include a mechanism for a practitioner to request a new privilege or procedure or to not request something that is included, such as removing a procedure or service from a core description. The practitioner should never be allowed to "write in a new privilege or service on the delineation form." The governing body must authorize, based on medical staff recommendation, any treatment, procedure, or service that is to be added to the delineation form.

Although determination of staff membership and the delineation of clinical privileges are two separate processes, they are interrelated and typically culminate simultaneously in a governing board decision. Nevertheless, a practitioner may request privileges without membership or request membership without privileges. There will be times when a staff member requests a change in privileges or a reduction in or additional or new privileges outside of the reappointment process. The processing of a privilege request mirrors that of an application for membership. Whatever process the medical staff has identified in its medical staff bylaws or related documents for reviewing this request must be followed. Typically that process includes receipt of a departmental recommendation, presentation of credentials, receipt of medical executive committee recommendations, and presentation to the governing body for final approval. The individual should receive a letter after the governing body has met informing him or her of acceptance, modification, or denial of the privilege request. A copy of the privileges granted should always be provided to the practitioner. If there is a modification of the original request, a written explanation should also be supplied. If there is a denial, then the practitioner must be informed of his or her rights to an appeal according to the fair hearing plan laid out in the bylaws.

Exhibit 7-1 Sample Core Privilege Form

Criteria and Privilege Request Form: General and Vascular Surgery

Applicant's Name: _____ **Date:** _____

Background: The American Board of Surgery states that general surgery is a "discipline having a central core of knowledge embracing anatomy, physiology, metabolism, immunology, nutrition, pathology, wound healing, shock and resuscitation, and intensive care and neoplasia, which are common to all surgical specialties." Furthermore, the ABS holds that the general surgeon is an individual who has specialized knowledge and skills relating to the diagnosis, preoperative, operative, and postoperative management in the following areas: alimentary tract; abdomen and its contents; breasts, skin, and soft tissue; head and neck (including trauma, vascular, endocrine, congenital and oncologic disorders—particularly tumors of the skin, salivary glands, thyroid, parathyroid, and the oral cavity); vascular system (excluding the intracranial vessels, the heart, and those vessels intrinsic and immediately adjacent thereto); endocrine system; surgical oncology (including coordinated multimodality management of the cancer patient by screening, surveillance, surgical adjunctive therapy, rehabilitation, and follow-up); management of trauma, including musculoskeletal, hand, and head injuries (the responsibility for all phases of care of the injured patient is an essential component of general surgery); and complete care of critically ill patients with underlying surgical conditions in emergency departments, intensive care units, and the trauma/burn units.

To be eligible to use this form to request clinical privileges, the following minimum threshold criteria must be met:

Basic Education: MD or DO

Minimal Formal Training: Successful completion of a postgraduate residency program in general surgery approved by the Accreditation Council for Graduate Medical Education or its equivalent.

Board Certification: Certification by the American Board of Surgery or the American Osteopathic Board of Surgery.

Required The successful applicant must be able to demonstrate that he or she has performed at least

Previous Experience: 100 general surgical procedures during the past 24 months.

Exhibit 7-1 Sample Core Privilege Form (continued)

Indicate Privileges Requested by Checking Those Privileges You Are Requesting and for Which Documentation Is Submitted.

If you meet the criteria above, you may request privileges as specified below. Any special requests you make will be considered only if you meet the threshold criteria for each request.

_____ I hereby request <u>core general surgical privileges as follows:</u> The performance of surgical procedures on patients of all ages (including related admission, consultation, work-up, preoperative and postoperative care) to correct or treat various conditions, illnesses, and injuries of the:

_____ Alimentary tract
_____ Abdomen and its contents
_____ Breasts, skin, and soft tissue
_____ Head and neck
_____ Vascular system, excluding the intracranial vessels, the heart, and those vessels intrinsic and immediately adjacent thereto (15 cases per year are required to maintain privileges)
_____ Endocrine system
_____ Minor extremity surgery (biopsy, I&D, varicose veins, foreign body removal, and skin grafts)

Also included within this core of privileges is the comprehensive management of trauma, including musculoskeletal, hand, and head injuries, and the complete care of critically ill patients with underlying surgical conditions in the Emergency Department.

Privilege Request Form: General and Vascular Surgery Special Procedures

For each special request, the applicant must meet minimum threshold criteria. Special requests in general surgery include:

_____ Laser Surgery _____ CO_2 _____ YAG

<u>**Criteria:**</u> *Documentation of completion of an approved 8- to 10-hour CME course inclusive of laser principles and safety, basic laser physics, laser tissue interaction, discussions of the clinical specialty field and hands-on experience, OR letter from residency or fellowship director attesting to laser education as part of the training curriculum AND successful completion of eye exam.*

<u>**Required Clinical Activity:**</u> *At least 4 procedures during the last 24 months.*

 Tumor Resection

Exhibit 7-1 Sample Core Privilege Form (continued)

Criteria: No fewer than 3 procedures per wavelength must be performed under the direct supervision of preceptor who has already been granted laser privileges. A preceptor checklist shall be completed for each procedure.

- **Administration of Moderate Sedation**

Criteria: Current ACLS certification; evidence of successful completion of 5 or more moderate sedation/analgesia cases performed in the last 12 months and compliance with _____ hospital's administrative policy and procedures.

- **Laparoscopic Surgery**

Criteria: Documentation of training and performance of at least 12 procedures in the past 12 months with acceptable outcomes.

- **Gastroscopy**

Criteria: Documentation of training and performance of at least 15 procedures in the past 12 months with acceptable outcomes.

- **Swan-Ganz Catheter**

Criteria: Documentation of training and performance of at least 20 procedures in the past 12 months with acceptable outcomes.

- **Bronchoscopy**

Criteria: Documentation of training and performance of at least 15 procedures in the past 12 months with acceptable outcomes.

- **Endoscopy**

Criteria: Documentation of training and performance of at least 12 procedures in the past 12 months with acceptable outcomes.

- **Hand-Assisted Laparoscopy**

Criteria: Documentation of training and performance of at least 12 procedures in the past 12 months with acceptable outcomes.

Minimal Formal Training: Evidence of training from residency program (including a letter of support from the training director) Completion of an acceptable course in hand-assisted laparoscopy, or an acceptable course is defined as a course that includes both didactic and hands-on training.

Required Previous Experience: Present evidence of experience from residency training (including a letter of support from the training director) or documentation of 5 cases in another facility.

Exhibit 7-1 Sample Core Privilege Form (continued)

I understand that in making this request I am bound by the applicable medical staff bylaws, rules and regulations, and any and all policies of the medical staff, hospital, and surgical services, and hereby stipulate that I meet the threshold criteria for each request.

I am capable of caring for patients in age ranges expected to be part of the usual and customary training in my specialty.

_____   _____
Signature of Applicant   Date

_____   _____
Approval of Department Chair   Date

The goal of the privileging process is to identify the practitioner's competency level and then recommend and authorize him or her to practice within that competency level (i.e., to match capability with authorization to practice). Privileges need to be renewed or reviewed at the time of the practitioner's reappointment (every two years). It is recommended that an applicant for reappointment should complete a new delineation form at each reappointment. If a new delineation form is not used, the applicant must update the current form and sign and date it to confirm that he or she wishes to continue with the current privileges or to note any modifications requested.

Traditionally, privilege forms contained all specialties on one form, but this approach is not acceptable today. Specialty-specific forms should be developed and the practitioner provided with the appropriate form based on his or her training, experience, and practice. In addition, the privilege forms sent out to applicants or used for practitioners seeking reappointment should contain only hospital-specific privileges. For example, privileges for obstetrics, radiation therapy, or cardiac surgery should not be listed if these services are not offered by the hospital.

■ The Joint Commission Requirements

The Joint Commission has multiple standards relevant to privileging. According to its 2009 standards, "the decision to grant or deny a privilege(s), and/or to renew an existing privilege(s), is an objective, evidence based process."[1] The standards language references the development of criteria for privileging and states that the criteria must be, at the minimum, based on current competence and peer recommendations. When developing privilege forms, the medical staff services professional (MSSP) should always review the current standards in place at the time to ensure compliance.

The Joint Commission has adopted recommendations concerning core competencies made by the Accreditation Council on Graduate Education (ACGME) and the American Board of Medical Specialties (ABMS). These recommendations are designed to transition the privileging process from a subjective exercise to a more objective, evidence-based activity. The ACGME, ABMS, and Joint Commission have suggested that six areas of general competencies are key to assessing healthcare practitioners: patient care, medical knowledge, practice-based learning and improvement, interpersonal and communication skills, professionalism and systems-based practice. (The Joint Commission actually references a slightly revised version of those competencies—medical/clinical knowledge, technical and clinical skills, clinical judgment, interpersonal skills, communication skills and professionalism—in the standards that requires peer recommendations within the privileging process.[2]) These competencies are expectations adopted by the ACGME for physicians in training and residency programs and by the ABMS for individuals who have been certified and who are looking to maintain their certification.

■ Centers for Medicare and Medicaid Services Requirements

The Conditions for Participation of Hospitals published by the Centers for Medicare and Medicaid Services (CMS) also contain requirements concerning privileging in hospitals. In November 2004, the CMS disseminated a statement clarifying its requirements and reiterating that the agency does not support any one particular type of privileging process. Instead, it has the following expectations:

- All medical staffs must ensure that their privileging process and privileging criteria are authorized by the governing body.
- The medical staff bylaws must describe the privileging process.
- All privileging criteria must be applied to individual practitioners.
- Specific privileges must reflect activities that the majority of practitioners in that category can do and that the hospital can support.
- The individual practitioner's ability to perform each task, activity, and privilege is assessed and not assumed.[3]

When developing a privileging process, CMS' Conditions of Participation, the accrediting body standards, and any relevant state regulations must be used as the basis for the particular institution's process.

■ Developing and Revising Privileges

Once a decision is made in terms of which privileging approach will be used (laundry list, category, core, or a combination of these), development of a new privileging approach must be handled as a special project. The following discussion refers to the use of a paper-based form and process; a later discussion will address a paperless privileging process.

Revision of or development of a new type of privilege format and content is a major undertaking. The first requirement is that there must be a physician "champion" who will help spearhead the project—he or she must be the medical staff spokesperson and support the MSSP during all steps of the process. Privilege development or revision has to be a project that the medical staff supports. If they see it as an administrative project or just another "new idea," they will not support or participate in the creation of the new format and criteria development, and the project will not be successful.

The MSSP's role in this project should be as project manager or coordinator and major researcher. It is best if the forms and content are developed and presented to the specialty representatives of the medical staff for their input rather than expecting them to develop the format and content. The MSSP has many sources available for researching specialty specific requirements. For example, the ACGME's Web site (www.acgme.org/review committees) provides information about the content of all accredited residency and fellowship training programs.[4] It is an excellent source for developing a better understanding of what a physician is expected to learn in each residency program. In addition, the ABMS and American Osteopathic Association (AOA) are the boards that oversee all of the specialty-specific certification boards. Their Web sites (www.abms.org and www.do-online.org/index.cfm?PageID=crt_speclist, respectively) contain links to their individual boards, which in turn provide a description of the qualifications for board admissibility/qualification that is helpful in establishing privileging criteria. Almost every specialty has a professional group that develops position papers on privileging in that specialty. The availability of information through the Internet is almost endless.

Internal sources of information are also helpful in developing new privilege forms. For example, asking for a listing of the top five diagnosis-related groups (DRGs) for internists and family practitioners and a listing of procedures performed in the operating room and day surgery for the past year will provide a good idea of actual practice at the hospital. A discussion with department chiefs about new technologies and new procedures they are anticipating within their specialty will help you begin the research for identifying criteria or for benchmarking with other local hospitals about the development of criteria.

Once the draft forms are prepared, a medical staff specialty representative should be identified for each specialty who will review the forms and privileging content and provide feedback to the MSSP, who will then prepare second drafts of these documents. Although many department chiefs would like to include all members of the department or specialty in the review of the new content, that practice can wreak havoc on the process and make it unbearably unwieldy. Almost everyone who reviews the content will have recommendations for changes. The more input that is requested, the more information that will be received. The review and recommendation process needs to be defined *before* the project is begun; the specific individuals who will be involved in the process should be identified and oriented to the process and procedures prior to beginning the project.

Once the designated specialty representatives have accepted the new form and content, each form should be reviewed and recommended by the credentials committee (if there is one) or a special task force specifically charged with review of all new privilege forms/content. Next, the forms should be reviewed and approved by the medical executive committee. Only then are the new form and content eligible to be authorized by the governing body.

The forms should contain no blank spaces that would allow practitioners to write in additional privilege requests—the only privileges a practitioner may request are those that are listed or described. If a new procedure or technology comes along, then the hospital should have a process for authorizing its use by the governing body prior to actually granting privileges to any one practitioner.

Privilege forms are expected to change over time as practice changes. The MSSP should maintain historical changes to each specialty form. The forms should always be dated so that the most current version is readily recognizable. No matter which format is used, each form should contain the same type of header that indicates the name of the organization, the specialty, the name of the practitioner, and the time period of the privileges being granted. It should also contain a clear mechanism for noting which privileges the practitioner is requesting and which privileges are being recommended and ultimately authorized. There should also be a way to document any privileges that are being modified or that may require a consultation, assistant, or proctor.

■ Implementation of New Forms

Typically, three approaches to implementation of new forms are used:

- Implement all new forms at once.
- Implement new forms by department or specialty.
- Implement new forms at the time of next reappointment.

There is no single right way to handle this process. It really depends on the size of the medical staff and the workload and capabilities of the personnel in the medical staff services department (MSSD). If the staff is large, sending new privilege forms to everyone at once is a difficult task.

Once the new forms have been approved by the governing body, it would be best to plan an educational or orientation session for practitioners with privileges. This can be done in various ways—for example, at department meetings, via a memorandum, in a newsletter, through a posting on the medical staff affairs Web site. Use whatever works best to get the word out that the organization will be moving to a new privileging process. (In actuality, this could be the end result of a complete educational plan that would have been initiated early on so that the members of the medical staff were well aware that these changes were coming.) The goal is to have all licensed independent practitioners with privileges complete the new form and submit it back to the MSSD within a specified time frame. You may consider providing them with the old form; however, it is critical that any new criteria for privileges that practitioners have had in the past be highlighted. Often, new criteria are written with a "grandfather clause" that allows anyone who held the privileges prior to the initiation of the criteria being developed to continue to practice as long as they have acceptable outcomes.

The most difficult part of this process is reviewing the new forms once they have been returned to note whether there are any changes in privilege requests. Most of the time, practitioners will ask for the same privileges as they had before. When you are moving from a laundry list to a core privilege approach, however, questions will undoubtedly be raised and many clarifications will be required concerning which procedures are included in the core. If the practitioner does not make any changes in his or her privileges, but merely transfers his or her request to the new form, then no further processing is required. In contrast, if additions or deletions are noted, then this form must be processed through the department chair, the credentials and medical executive committees, and the governing body (or whatever process is defined in the medical staff bylaws) to be finalized. At this point in the process, a great deal of attention needs to be given to assessing the privileges requested on the new form—many privileging issues have been discovered at a later time when a particular privilege was left off a new form or when a new privilege was requested and submission of qualifications was not provided.

Another aspect of implementation is to identify all of the internal end users of privilege information—those individuals in the hospital who have previously received copies of privilege forms or who have lookup capability to view the privileges of a particular practitioner—and to provide an educational session for them. It is very important for those individuals (typically nurse managers in the various areas, such as the emergency department, intensive care units, labor and delivery, or operating room) to understand the new privileging approach, including what the new definitions of privileges are and how they will affect their work. If this step is omitted, there will be many telephone calls to medical staff services and much misunderstanding concerning privilege changes.

■ Criteria for Granting Privileges

The medical staff is required by the Joint Commission to establish an objective framework for determining which privileges will be granted to an applicant. Criteria must be established that describe minimum training or direct experience that must be documented or demonstrated before privileges are granted.

The medical staff bylaws usually describe broad membership criteria, which include licensure, training, experience, current competence, and health status. More specific criteria must also be developed to determine precisely which training or experience an applicant must have obtained to be approved for specific procedures or treatment of a particular diagnosis. These criteria must also be developed for new procedures that evolve as a result of new or improved technology.

Criteria for granting privileges may include the following:

1. Minimal formal training, such as an approved residency training program
2. Required previous experience, such as performance of 50 major surgical procedures within the last two years or treatment of a minimum of 50 patients within the last two years
3. Certificates of attendance for approved formal training course(s), accompanied by the course outline(s)
4. Completion of a specified number of proctored cases
5. Documentation of a certain number of hours of continuing medical education, accompanied by course outline(s)
6. Successful completion of a specific number of procedures with less than a specific percentage of complication

Exhibit 7-1 provides an example of core and special privileges for the specialty of general surgery, which includes the criteria for granting privileges. TABLE 7-1 is an example of criteria for granting privileges for neuroradiology procedures. These privileges usually cross specialty lines, which means that the criteria must be broad enough to allow for multiple types of specialists to qualify for the privileges. The Joint Commission also requires that prior to any privilege being granted within an institution, the institution must make an assessment to determine whether the necessary resources (i.e., equipment, types of personnel, space that is available or will be available within a specified time frame).[5]

When an applicant applies for specific clinical privileges, his or her training and experience are compared to the required criteria established previously by the medical staff and authorized by the governing body. The applicant should always be provided with the criteria prior to submitting a request for privileges. It is best if the criteria can be included on the actual delineation of privilege form. If criteria are printed on a separate document, then that document should always be provided to an applicant along with the delineation form. If the applicant does not meet established criteria, he or she cannot request the privileges. If he or she submits a

Table 7-1	Criteria for Granting Privileges
ABC Hospital	
Criteria for Granting Neuroradiology Privileges	
Information Required	**Information Submitted**
Specialties Involved	Neurological surgery Diagnostic radiology Neuroradiology
Procedure/Condition/ Privilege/Service Requested	Endovascular surgical neuroradiology
GENERAL Requirements	1. Must be a member in good standing of the ABC Medical Center Medical Staff 2. Staff category requirement: N/A 3. Current licensure in the state of: MA with no sanctions 4. Current state and federal DEA certificate with no sanctions 5. Concurrent privileges with no disciplinary action in the specialty(ies) of radiology, neuroradiology, or neurosurgery
Required Education and Training	1. Successful completion of an accredited medical/ professional school 2. Successful completion of an ACGME or AOA accredited residency/fellowship in: • Diagnostic radiology + one year of neuroradiology training + at least 3 months of clinical experience in neurological surgery OR • Neurosurgery + course in basic radiology skills OR • Neurology + 1 year in vascular neurology + 3 months of clinical skills in diagnostic radiology + 3 months of clinical experience in an ACGME-accredited neurological surgery program
Specialty Board Status XX ABMS XX AOA ❐ ABPS ❐ ABPOPPM ❐ ADA ❐ Other: _____	Board certified in diagnostic radiology, neurosurgery, or neuroradiology

Table 7-1	Criteria for Granting Privileges (continued)
ABC Hospital	
Criteria for Granting Neuroradiology Privileges	
Information Required	**Information Submitted**
Peer References and/or Evaluations	XX Letter from chairman of the relevant clinical department or residency training program director attesting to the applicant's competence in this privilege/procedure/service. XX Written confirmation of 12 cases/procedures within the past 12 months/years. (Documentation should indicate satisfactory performance with acceptable outcomes.) XX Peer recommendations from at least 2 persons who have had extensive experience and knowledge of the applicant and can attest to the applicant's health status and current clinical competence for the privilege(s) being requested. ❐ Other: _____
Monitoring/Proctoring	XX Concurrent observation of first 5 cases/procedures with documentation from proctor on appropriate form. XX Retrospective review of medical records of 10 cases/procedures ❐ Other: _____
CME Requirements	❐ Documentation confirming 10 hours of category 1 CME activity during the previous 12 months/years on the specific procedure/service ❐ Attendance at specific CME program(s) Specifications: _____
Reappointment/ Reprivileging Requirements	XX 1. Confirmation of successful completion of 10 procedures/services with acceptable outcomes within the past 24 months as determined by medical staff peer review activities 2. Confirmation of _____ patients treated with a specific condition/service required with acceptable outcomes within the past 2 months as determined by medical staff peer review activities XX Documentation from an accredited healthcare facility of 1 or 2 above for practitioners who have not met the numeric requirements at this institution XX Peer recommendations (2) ❐ Other: _____

Table 7-1   Criteria for Granting Privileges (continued)

ABC Hospital

Criteria for Granting Neuroradiology Privileges

Information Required	Information Submitted
Hospital Assessment Hospital CEO/Designee Signature Date Hospital CFO/Designee Signature Date Hospital CNO/Designee Signature Date	Hospital CEO, CNO, and CFO or designees have reviewed the request to perform this procedure or to provide this service and the suggested criteria and agree that: ❐ Hospital has sufficient space ❐ Hospital has sufficient resource personnel appropriately trained ❐ Financial/reimbursement issues have been clarified ❐ Hospital can accommodate this new procedure, treatment, or service ❐ Issues/problems have been identified concerning the following: _____ _____ _____ _____
Approval	Division Chief Date Department Chair Date Second Department Chair Date Credentials Committee Chair Date MEC Chair Date Board of Trustees Chair Date
This Form Reviewed and Approved: Credentials Committee: MEC: Board of Trustees Revisions:	

request for which criteria are not met, the request for privileges will not be considered. This is not considered a denial of privileges but rather a failure to fulfill criteria; therefore, this action is not a reportable action to the National Practitioner Data Bank (NPDB).

Sometimes practitioners attempt to keep otherwise qualified practitioners from performing certain procedures based on economic considerations. When developing criteria for granting privileges, care should be taken to ensure that all qualified groups have input into the criteria and that requirements are reasonable, defensible, and, ideally, backed up by literature and community standards.

■ Process for Adding New Privileges

As noted earlier, a policy and procedure should be established to address the method for adding new privileges to a specialty form. The same process can be used for adding new privileges as is used for granting cross-over or multispecialty privileges (when two or more specialties want to perform the same procedure). In case of a new procedure, service, treatment, or therapy, the question is not only relevant to the individual requesting the privilege and the medical staff, but also has to consider issues related to many other departments of the hospital. The policy and procedure should include a mechanism for this request to be considered by nursing, hospital administration, and finance. Questions that should be answered include these:

- Will there be a need for new equipment?
- Will there be a need for additional personnel or specialized training for support personnel?
- Is this a service that the hospital wants to offer or that the community needs?
- Will the hospital be able to be reimbursed for this service?

Basically, the governing body, the medical staff, nursing, finance, and hospital administration must all authorize the initiation of this new procedure, technology, or treatment. Once the hospital, through its governing body, has authorized the new privilege, treatment, or service and its recommended criteria, then the individual who requested the privilege can submit his or her request and be considered. Often the practitioner requesting the privilege will be a good source of information and can assist the MSSP in collecting the necessary information concerning the background and need for the privilege or treatment and any criteria that may already have been established by a professional society or training programs. The CD that accompanies this book includes a sample tool that can be used to consider adding new privileges for procedures or treatments by ensuring all relevant medical staff and hospital departments are included in the assessment process.

Focused Professional Practice Evaluation

In the past, any new privileges granted were considered "provisional" for a period of time to allow the medical staff to assess the competency of the practitioner in performing the new privilege, procedure, or service. The Joint Commission no longer uses the term "provisional" in the standards but does include the requirement of a process called focused professional practice evaluation (FPPE). This type of evaluation must be performed in two circumstances: (1) when a practitioner does not have documented evidence of competently performing the requested privilege at the organization (i.e., a new practitioner or a practitioner requesting a new privilege) and (2) when a question arises regarding a currently privileged practitioner's ability to provide safe, high-quality patient care.[6]

Although the terminology is new, the idea behind the first application of FPPE is not. Any practitioner new to the organization or anyone requesting a new privilege has traditionally been observed or assessed by the medical staff to ensure that the individual is competent to perform the privileges requested. Although each organization may decide how it will perform this evaluation, it is imperative that each specialty have input into the development of criteria that will be used to assess and evaluate the performance of the practitioners practicing in that specialty. An important component to this evaluation is consistency: Whatever criteria are established must be applied consistently to each applicable practitioner. Each specialty is also responsible for identifying the triggers (a single incident or evidence of a clinical practice trend)[7] that indicate the need for performance monitoring.

The second application of FPPE occurs when a practice problem has been identified with a particular practitioner. It is very important that each specialty identify those situations prior to them occurring, so that evaluation is a known outcome of that trigger. This approach ensures that no one can charge the medical staff with discrimination or favoritism in terms of which incidents or situations are targeted for FPPE.

The information that is collected during the FPPE period needs to have a specific time frame for collection, and a direct action needs to take place at the conclusion of the evaluation. FPPE can be individualized for each practitioner. Be aware that the more practitioners being evaluated, the more difficult it will be to collect data and define competency. The process should be defined in a policy and procedure that should address the following issues:

- What will be evaluated (i.e., outcomes, complications, techniques, or clinical management)
- Which method of evaluation will be used (i.e., retrospective review, proctoring, or statistical review)
- How long the evaluation will take place
- How the information will be communicated to the practitioner

- How the information will be integrated into the ongoing monitoring evaluation[8]

Further discussion of this issue appears in Chapter 11. EXHIBIT 7-2 shows a sample FPPE policy.

Exhibit 7-2 Policy and Procedure Manual

Focused Professional Practice Evaluation

Purpose

To establish a systematic process to assure there is sufficient information available to confirm the current competency of practitioners initially granted privileges at facilities that are part of "XX" Health System (XXHS). This process, termed focused professional practice evaluation (FPPE) by the Joint Commission, will provide the basis for obtaining organization-specific information that substantiates current competence for those practitioners.

For purposes of this policy, the term "practitioner" means any medical staff member or allied health professional granted clinical privileges. When the title "Department Chair" is used, it means the Department Chair or the Department Chair's designee (for example, a Service Chief may serve as the Department Chair's designee).

Medical Staff Oversight

The Credentials/Privileging Committee is charged with the responsibility of monitoring compliance with this policy and procedure. It accomplishes this oversight through receiving regular status reports related to the progress of all practitioners undergoing FPPE as well as any issues or problems involved in implementing this policy and procedure. Department Chairs shall be responsible for overseeing the FPPE process for all applicants assigned to their Departments.

The medical staff committees involved with ongoing professional practice evaluation (OPPE) will provide the Credentials/Privileging Committee with data systematically collected for OPPE that is appropriate to confirm current competence for these practitioners during the FPPE period.

Scope of the FPPE Program

Proctoring is the primary mechanism used to confirm competency of granted privileges during the FPPE period of time.

Definition of Proctoring

For purposes of this policy, proctoring is an FPPE to confirm an individual practitioner's current competence at the time new privileges are granted, either at initial appointment or as a current member of the medical or AHP staff. In addition to

Exhibit 7-2 Policy and Procedure Manual (continued)

specialty specific issues, proctoring will address the six general competencies of practitioner performance:

- Patient care
- Medical knowledge
- Practice-based learning and improvement
- Interpersonal and communication skills
- Professionalism
- Systems-based practice

Practitioners requesting membership but not requesting specific privileges are not subject to the provisions of this policy. They are not proctored and may not act as proctors. The decision and process to perform FPPE for current practitioners with existing privileges based on trends or patterns of performance identified by OPPE are outside the scope of this policy.

Selection of Methods for Each Specialty

The appropriate proctoring methods to determine current competency for an individual practitioner will be part of the recommendation for granting of privileges by the Department Chair/designee and will be reviewed and approved by the Credentials/Privileging Committee and Medical Executive Committee and recommended to the Board for final approval. Each specialty will define the appropriate methods on the approved privilege delineation form and will include the types of proctoring to be used, and the number of cases to be proctored, depending on the privileges requested by an applicant. It should be noted that these are general guidelines and that the Department Chair is expected to customize proctoring requirements based on the practitioner's background, training, and reputation, and the Department Chair's first-hand knowledge of a practitioner's current competency (all of which must be documented when the Department Chair makes his or her recommendation related to clinical privileges and FPPE).

Proctoring Methods

Proctoring may utilize any combination of the following methods to obtain the best understanding of the care provider by the practitioner:

- **Prospective Proctoring:** Presentation of cases with planned treatment outlined for treatment concurrence, review of case documentation for treatment concurrence, or completion of a written or oral examination or case simulation.
- **Concurrent Proctoring:** Direct observation of the procedure being performed or medical management either through observation of practitioner interactions with patients and staff or review of clinical history and physical and review of treatment orders during the hospital stay of a patient.

Exhibit 7-2 Policy and Procedure Manual (continued)

- **Retrospective Evaluation:** Review of case record after care has been completed. May also involve interviews of personnel directly involved in the care of a patient.

Sources of Data

FPPE data may include:

- Personal interaction with the practitioner by the proctor
- Detailed medical record review by the proctor
- Interviews of hospital staff interacting with the practitioner
- Surveys of hospital staff interacting with the practitioner
- Chart audits by nonmedical staff personnel based on medical staff–defined criteria for initial appointees

The data obtained by the proctor will be recorded on the approved proctoring form for consistency and inter-rater reliability.

Proctoring Data Analysis

The Department Chair will review both the case-specific and aggregate data and provide the Credentials/Privileging Committee with an interpretation as to whether a practitioner's performance was acceptable, in need of further data to complete the evaluation, or unacceptable. For aggregate rate data, the acceptable targets will be determined by the medical staff.

Proctoring Period

Proctoring shall begin when a practitioner is informed of appointment to the medical or AHP staff and the granting of clinical privileges or upon being granted a new privilege. Based on the specialty of the practitioner, newly granted privileges shall be considered under FPPE for 6 months or for a specific number of patients or procedures. The FPPE period may be extended for a period not to exceed a total of 12 months from the granting of the privilege(s) that require proctoring if either initial concerns are raised that require further evaluation or if there is insufficient activity during the initial 6-month period.

The medical staff may take into account the practitioner's previous experience in determining the approach and extent of proctoring needed to confirm current competency.

Results and Recommendations

At the end of the 6-month FPPE period, the Department Chair shall provide a summary report to the Credentials/Privileging Committee that shall include one or more of the following:

Exhibit 7-2 Policy and Procedure Manual (continued)

- Whether a sufficient number of cases done at XXHS have been presented for review to properly evaluate the clinical privileges requested.
- If a sufficient number of cases have not been presented for review, whether in the Department Chair's opinion, the FPPE period should be extended for an additional 6-month period.
- If sufficient treatment of patients has occurred to properly evaluate the clinical privileges requested, the Department Chair shall make his or her report concerning the appointee's qualifications and competence to exercise these privileges.
- Make a recommendation related to the appropriate medical staff category (if applicable) and clinical privileges as requested or recommend an additional period of proctoring or *not* membership and clinical privileges as requested.
- If there is a recommendation by the MEC to terminate the practitioner's appointment or additional clinical privileges due to questions about qualifications, behavior, or clinical competence, the medical staff member shall be entitled to the hearing and appeal process outlined in the medical staff bylaws. AHPs shall be entitled to rights as defined in AHP policies and procedures.

Responsibilities

Responsibilities of the Proctor

Proctor(s) must be members in good standing of the medical staff (or AHP staff) of XXHS and must have privileges in the specialty area relative to the privileges(s) to be evaluated. Proctors must not be in the FPPE process or undergoing any type of focus review by XXHS. The proctor shall:

1. Use appropriate methods and tools approved by the Credentials/Privileging Committee.
2. Assure the confidentiality of the proctoring results and forms and deliver the completed proctoring forms to the Medical Staff Services Department (MSSD).
3. Submit any summary reports or additional information requested by the Department Chair.
4. If the practitioner being proctored is not sufficiently available or lacks sufficient cases to complete the proctoring process in the prescribed time frame, the Department Chair may recommend to the Credentials/Privileging Committee an extension of the proctoring period to complete the report.
5. If at any time during the FPPE period, the proctor has concerns about the practitioner's competency to perform specific clinical privileges or care related to a specific patient(s), the proctor shall promptly notify the Department Chair.

Exhibit 7-2 Policy and Procedure Manual (continued)

Responsibilities of the Practitioner Undergoing FPPE

The practitioner undergoing FPPE shall:

1. For concurrent proctoring, make every reasonable effort to be available to the proctor, including notifying the proctor of each patient where care is to be evaluated in sufficient time to allow the proctor to concurrently observe or review the care provided. For elective surgical or invasive procedures where direct observation is required, and the department requires proctoring be completed before the practitioner can perform the procedure without a proctor present, the practitioner must secure agreement from the proctor to attend the procedure. In an emergency, the practitioner may admit and treat the patient and must notify the proctor as soon as reasonably possible.
2. Provide the proctor with information about the patient's clinical history, pertinent physical findings, pertinent lab and radiology results, and the planned course of treatment or management, and direct delivery to the proctor of a copy of all histories and physicals, operative reports, consultation reports, and discharge summaries documented by the proctored practitioner.
3. Shall have the prerogative of requesting from the Department Chair a change of proctor if disagreements with the current proctor may adversely affect his or her ability to satisfactorily complete the proctorship. The Department Chair will keep the Credentials/Privileging Committee and MEC informed about changes in proctors.
4. Inform the proctor of any unusual incident(s) associated with his or her patients.

Responsibilities of Department Chairs

In accordance with the Credentials Procedure Manual, the Department Chair of each practitioner's anticipated primary facility will take the lead in confirmation of competency for granted privileges. The Department Chair shall be responsible for:

1. Assignment of proctors as noted above.
2. Assist in establishing a minimum number of cases or procedures to be proctored and determining when the proctor must be present. The minimum number of cases to be proctored and type of proctoring required shall be made at the time privileges are recommended. When there are interdepartmental privileges, the Credentials/Privileging Committee shall determine the minimum number of cases or procedures to be reviewed.
3. Identifying the names of practitioners eligible to serve as proctors as noted above.
4. If at any time during the proctoring period, the proctor notifies the Department Chair that he or she has concerns about the practitioner's competency to perform specific clinical privileges or care related to a specific patient(s), based

Exhibit 7-2 Policy and Procedure Manual (continued)

on the recommendations of the proctor, the Department Chair shall then review the medical records of the patient(s) treated by the practitioner being proctoring and shall:
a. Intervene and adjudicate the conflict if the proctor and the practitioner disagree as to what constitutes appropriate care for a patient.
b. Review the case for possible referral to the peer review committee.
c. Recommend to the Medical Executive Committee that:
   1) Additional or revised proctoring requirements be imposed upon the practitioner.
   2) Corrective action be undertaken pursuant to applicable corrective action procedures.

Responsibilities of the Medical Staff Services Department

The MSSD shall assure that the following steps are taken:

1. Send a letter to the practitioner being proctored and to the assigned proctor containing the following information:
   a. A copy of the privilege form of the practitioner being proctored
   b. A copy of the FPPE policy and procedure
   c. Proctoring forms to be completed by the proctor
2. Provide information to appropriate hospital departments about practitioners being proctored, including the name of the proctor and a supply of proctoring forms as needed.
3. Contact both the proctor and the practitioner being proctored on a monthly basis to ensure that proctoring and chart reviews are being conducted as required.
4. Periodically submit a report to Credentials/Privileging Committee related to proctorship activity for all practitioners being proctored.

Responsibilities of the Credentials/Privileging Committee

The Credentials/Privileging Committee shall:

1. Have the responsibility of monitoring compliance with this policy and procedure.
2. Receive regular status reports related to the progress of all practitioners required to complete FPPE as well as any issues or problems involved in implementation of this policy and procedure.
3. Make recommendations to the MEC regarding clinical privileges based on information obtained from the FPPE process.

Exhibit 7-2 Policy and Procedure Manual (continued)

Medical Staff Ethical Position on Proctoring

The proctor's role is typically that of an evaluator, not a consultant or a mentor. A practitioner serving as a proctor for the purpose of assessing and reporting on the competence of another practitioner is an agent of XXHS. The proctor shall receive no compensation directly or indirectly from any patient for this service, and shall have no duty to the patient to intervene if the care provided by the proctored practitioner appears to be deficient. However, the proctor is expected to report immediately to the appropriate Department Chair or XXHS authority (i.e., President of the applicable Medical Staff organization, the Chief Medical Officer) any concerns regarding the care being rendered by the proctored practitioner that has the potential for imminent patient harm. The proctor, or any other practitioner, may render emergency medical care to a patient for medical complications arising from the care provided by a proctored practitioner. XXHS will defend and indemnify any practitioner who is subjected to a claim or suit arising out of his or her acts or omissions in the role of proctor.

Note: The preceding paragraph is controversial and should be discussed by medical staff organization representatives as well as legal counsel.

■ Proctoring

One mechanism used to observe and assess newly granted privileges is called proctoring. Not every medical staff has a proctoring program, however. It is not a required function by accrediting bodies but may be required by state statute.

It makes good sense that a practitioner recently granted privileges or granted a new privilege should be observed. The period of observation is needed to confirm that the decision of granting one or more privileges was justified. Nevertheless, establishing a proctoring program has both pros and cons. The reality is that very few such programs are successful because they are difficult to administer, volunteer physicians are few and far between, and inconsistency in practice often makes physicians uncomfortable with assessing their colleagues' work.

If a decision is made to initiate a proctoring program, it is very important to ensure that the process is clearly defined in a policy and procedure or in the bylaws and that whatever is documented will be followed consistently by all practitioners. It should be decided whether the program will consist of a retrospective review of records (after the fact) or a concurrent review (direct observation of work), or a combination of the two. Although each specialty may define the proctoring requirements for that specialty, the requirements then need to be consistently applied to everyone.

Advantages of having a proctoring program include the following:

- Concurrent, direct observation of the practitioner's practice is a good way to assess skills.
- Direct observation will provide for better protection of the patient if the policy states that the proctor will "take over" if the proctored practitioner is having difficulty.
- The proctor is to observe if any health problems are present.

Disadvantages of a proctoring program include the following:

- Liability for the proctor and hospital. Many practitioners do not want to volunteer to be proctors; they are concerned about the liability issues if something goes wrong, and they are uncomfortable with assessing another practitioner. The hospital and medical staff are liable if there is a proctoring program in place, but it is not consistently applied.
- Difficulty in persuading physicians to participate. Physicians often see very little advantage for this type of program and many disadvantages, including the fact that when they are acting as proctors, they are usually not earning money. Many are also uncomfortable with performing the role of proctor.
- Information systems. Such systems are often not available or lack the capability to maintain the required data for tracking, especially which cases or procedures must be proctored and what the time frames for completion of proctoring requirements are.

The word "proctoring" is typically not well received by the medical staff; other terms may be used in an attempt to alleviate their concerns, such as "observing," "monitoring," or "sponsoring." Whatever it is called, several rules apply when proctoring is undertaken, and the whole process itself should be defined in the medical staff bylaws or in a policy approved by the executive committee of the medical staff.

The written document, whether it is the bylaws or a policy and procedure, should define the following:

- How proctors are selected. The selection is ordinarily done by the department chair in a departmentalized medical staff and by the chief of staff in a nondepartmentalized medical staff.
- The relationship of the proctor to the practitioner being proctored. The proctor should not be a relative or a practice partner or associate of the person being observed.
- The mechanism for how the proctoring will take place (i.e., concurrent or retrospective review) and the documentation that will be maintained (including by whom and how).

- Department- and specialty-specific requirements that cover the full scope of privileges granted. Proctoring should include the most sophisticated type of procedures that have been granted and cover the full scope of privileges granted. For instance, performing varicose vein surgery, varicocelectomies, and hemorrhoidectomies does not equate with surgery for aortic aneurysm or femoropopliteal bypass surgery when proctoring a physician granted vascular surgery privileges. Similarly, an inguinal hernioplasty and appendectomy do not equate with surgery of the common bile duct for general surgery proctoring purposes.
- The process for interceding in the care being provided, if that is required to protect the patient.
- The process for assisting in remediation of the practitioner, should that be a determination.
- The mechanism for the practitioner to submit cases performed and proctored at another institution if he or she has not had sufficient cases at the present institution.
- The method of documenting recommendations, the location where the documentation will be maintained, and possible outcomes of the process.
- What will happen if the practitioner does not fulfill the minimum requirements for activity.

A sample proctoring policy and procedure, as well as an evaluation form and its attachments, can be found on the CD accompanying this book.

■ Ongoing Professional Practice Evaluation

Ongoing professional practice evaluation (OPPE) is a continual evaluation intended to ensure that any practitioner granted privileges is assessed for competency in those privileges and to collect data as the basis for deciding whether a practitioner should be allowed to maintain the existing privileges or have the privileges revised or revoked. This standard, which was implemented in 2008 by the Joint Commission, allows each organization to identify the practice trends taking place in that facility and track the impact of that practice on the quality of care and patient safety. (See Chapter 11 for a full discussion of types of criteria that may be used in this evaluation.)

The information used in this process may be obtained from periodic chart review, direct observation, monitoring of diagnostic and treatment techniques, or discussion with other individuals involved in the care of each patient. Each organization may designate which information will be collected and assessed for each specialty and how that information will be collected. The data collected are key because medical staff leaders and the governing body need to be able to quantify which privileges each practitioner should be allowed to maintain by assessing the collected data and noting positive outcomes EXHIBIT 7-3 shows a sample OPPE policy.

Exhibit 7-3 Sample Ongoing Professional Practice Evaluation (OPPE) Policy

Purpose

The purpose of this policy is to identify the process used to perform the ongoing professional practice evaluation of the medical staff members.

Policy

It will be the policy of the Medical Center to conduct ongoing professional practice evaluation (OPPE) of its medical staff on a continuous basis. This is done through a variety of processes, including medical staff peer review, monitoring of performance metrics in key or prioritized areas, the profiling of the physician at the time of initial and reappointment, and formal OPPE reports that identify practitioner-specific performance with aggregated and/or comparison information.

Formal OPPE reports are to be presented to the medical staff leadership no less than twice each calendar year. The formal OPPE reports or a summary of the findings will be presented to various committees within the medical staff committee structure, including the Performance Improvement Committee, the Credentials Committee, the Medical Executive Committee, and the Health System Board.

In the event that issues are identified during the OPPE process that may lead to a focused professional practice evaluation (FPPE) of a practitioner's performance and could result in action to limit, suspend, or revoke privileges, the appropriate mechanism described in the medical staff bylaws will guide this process.

Procedure

1. The medical staff peer review process will be conducted as described in the Medical Staff Peer Review Policy as part of the medical staff and hospital leadership's efforts to evaluate the professional practice of the medical staff on a continuous basis.
2. Another key mechanism used to evaluate the ongoing professional practice of the medical staff is the review and assessment of the formal OPPE reports that are presented to the medical staff committee structure no less than twice each calendar year.
   a. The OPPE reports will provide practitioner-specific performance information, with comparative or target performance expectations when possible, in areas not limited to the following:
      i. Core measures
      ii. Medical record documentation
      iii. Medical record suspensions

Exhibit 7-3   Sample Ongoing Professional Practice Evaluation (OPPE) Policy (continued)

  iv. Peer review findings
   v. Patient satisfaction
  vi. Infection control
 vii. Physician health referrals
viii. Medical Executive Committee investigations regarding practitioner performance
b. With the OPPE reports, information will be provided to medical staff and hospital leadership regarding trends in performance that may require additional review or assessment.
c. The following performance triggers and interventions may be initiated based on the information provided on the OPPE reports:

Topic	Target	Number of Occurrences with Performance Below Stated Target	Action	Report
Core measures	Performance is expected to be at 100%.	All core measures that do not have 100% performance will trigger an intervention.	The physician will be sent a letter asking for his or her response regarding the failure to meet the core measure indicator. If no response is received, the Department Chair will be sent the letter asking for a response. An FPPE is triggered on the fourth letter to a physician regarding his or her performance. The Performance Improvement Committee and/or the Medical Executive Committee will identify the structure of the FPPE process for the physician.	Report of the letter being sent to the physician will be placed in the provider's quality file. (Record of correspondence is maintained in the medical record documentation report.) The results of the FPPE activity will be reported to the appropriate committees.

Exhibit 7-3 Sample Ongoing Professional Practice Evaluation (OPPE) Policy (continued)

Topic	Target	Number of Occurrences with Performance Below Stated Target	Action	Report
Medical record documentation	All medical staff members are subject to be included in the review of medical record documentation. A letter will be sent to inform the physician of legibility issues, the use of unacceptable abbreviations, and/or missing signature/contact information.	Fourth letter.	The Medical Director, PI will send a letter to the practitioner stating the performance expectation and that the fourth occurrence has triggered a FPPE. An FPPE is triggered on the fourth letter to a physician regarding his or her performance. The Performance Improvement Committee and/or the Medical Executive Committee will identify the structure of the FPPE process for the physician. **In the event that the documentation FPPE process does not demonstrate improved performance, the Medical Executive Committee has the option of requiring the physician to participate in mandatory documentation training that may be followed by an additional evaluation to determine if improved performance has been noted.**	Report of the letter being sent to the physician will be placed in the provider's quality file. (record of correspondence is maintained in the medical record documentation report.) The results of the FPPE activity will be reported to the appropriate committees.

Exhibit 7-3 Sample Ongoing Professional Practice Evaluation (OPPE) Policy (continued)

Topic	Target	Number of Occurrences with Performance Below Stated Target	Action	Report
Medical record suspensions	No more than three in a calendar year.	Fourth occurrence in a calendar year.	The Medical Executive Committee (MEC) will send a letter to the practitioner to inform him or her of the need to address the performance issue at a MEC meeting. Fines may be considered for additional suspensions. (See Medical Record Suspension Policy.)	Medical record suspensions will be noted in the physician's quality file.
Peer review findings	Fewer than three occurrences of a "3" or "4" rating during a reappointment period.	The third occurrence of a "3" or "4" rating will trigger a review of the cases/issues by the Best Practice Oversight Committee.	The Best Practice Oversight Committee (BPOC) reviews each "3" or "4" rating from the medical staff peer review process. The BPOC has the authority to intervene and recommend further action to provide for the safe care of the patients when a quality issue is identified. This may include requesting an investigation or referring the matter to the Credentials Committee and to the MEC if actions regarding privileges are suggested.	Peer review information will be maintained in the physician's quality file.

Exhibit 7-3 Sample Ongoing Professional Practice Evaluation (OPPE) Policy (continued)

Topic	Target	Number of Occurrences with Performance Below Stated Target	Action	Report
Patient satisfaction	Overall performance rating is < 50th percentile of the system comparison.	First occurrence starting with the 2007 annual Press Ganey Report.	Informational letter regarding ranking and score will be mailed to the physician.	
Infection control/surgical site infections	To be determined.	To be determined.	To be determined.	
Physician health referrals	N/A	The number of referrals is provided on the OPPE report.	The referral is tracked to identify other patterns/trends with the practitioner's performance. Performance issues may be shared with Physician Health.	The referral to Physician Health will be maintained in the physician's quality file.
MEC investigations	N/A	All issues resulting in a MEC investigation will be noted on the OPPE report.	The MEC will determine the appropriate response/action on a case-specific basis.	The results and summary of the MEC investigation will be maintained in the provider's quality file.

3. Medical staff leadership and the medical staff committees reserve the right to revise the performance triggers and the intervention based on information known at the time of the review of the OPPE report.
4. Additional items, not included in the table above, will have interventions defined at the time a pattern or trend with performance is identified.

■ Temporary Privileges

In the absence of a rule prohibiting the use of temporary privileges, the medical staff should be quite strict in recommending or approving such privileges. Temporary privileges are considered a high-risk activity because often the practitioner is not a known quantity to the institution and is being granted temporary privileges for an important patient care need. The institution may not have as much information about the practitioner being granted temporary privileges. Given that the practitioner who is applying for membership and/or clinical privileges, there are some inherent risks in the temporary privilege situation.

The Joint Commission standards allow for granting of temporary privileges in specific situations:

- To fulfill an important patient care, treatment, and service need
- When a new applicant with a complete application that raises no concerns is awaiting review and approval of the medical staff executive committee and the governing body[9]

In addition, the elements of performance of this standard are very specific about which information must be collected and verified in both instances. From a patient safety and risk management point of view, the institution would be wise to collect and verify as much information as possible. Even though there is often a "pressured" or "rush" situation presented when requiring temporary privileges, the institution's first responsibility is to the patient. The MSSP must ensure that whatever the policy requires is obtained and that the medical staff leaders entrusted with the responsibility of recommending these privileges feel sufficiently satisfied that the necessary information has been collected and verified prior to making a recommendation.

Temporary privileges should be granted for only a limited period of time. Some state statutes and the Joint Commission require that temporary privileges never be granted for more than 120 days; a more cautious approach would be to grant them for 30 days at a time and renew them, if necessary.

Another important aspect of this process is the need to record and track who has temporary privileges and for how long to ensure that no one goes beyond the time limit established by the bylaws or policies and procedures or 120 days. This information should be maintained in a computerized database; if that is not available, then a manual tracking process should be developed. According to the Healthcare Quality Improvement Act, the NPDB must be queried whenever privileges are requested, so every temporary privilege request must include a NPDB query and report.[10]

Temporary privileges should never be granted solely for patient desire or convenience. When temporary privileges are granted to a new medical staff applicant awaiting review and approval by the organized medical staff, the following information must have been collected and verified:

- Current licensure
- Relevant training or experience
- Current competence
- Ability to perform the privileges requested
- Other criteria required by the organized medical staff bylaws
- A query and evaluation of the NPDB information
- A complete application
- No current or previously successful challenge to licensure or registration
- No subjection to involuntary termination of medical staff membership at another organization
- No subjection to involuntary limitation, reduction, denial, or loss of clinical privileges

The Joint Commission requires that temporary privileges be granted on the recommendation of the medical staff president or authorized designee and be formally granted by the CEO or authorized designee.[11] Many departmentalized hospitals also involve and require the department chief and/or the credentials committee chair to review and provide recommendations for requests for temporary privileges. In any event, the procedure should not be unduly complicated because often the request for temporary privileges comes at the end of the day or the week, and it is much more difficult to have to reach four individuals rather than two individuals.

The CD that accompanies this book includes a sample application for temporary privileges that could be used for those instances when the request comes from an individual who has not submitted an application for privileges or medical staff membership.

■ *Locum Tenens* Privileges

Locum tenens means "one practitioner taking the place of another." Typically hospitals become involved in this situation when there are insufficient individuals to cover an individual's practice, the emergency department, or the radiology department. Some placement firms and staffing firms provide temporary medical staff who will contract with either the institution or a physician group to provide this coverage. Such a contract should contain some language concerning what the staffing company will do to credential its practitioners, although this may mean different things to different people.

It is very important that the MSSP obtain a copy of the contract made with the staffing company. If at all possible, it is most advantageous if the MSSP can actually be involved in the negotiation prior to contract finalization. Unfortunately, often the contract is handled in hospital administration or finance and the MSSD is not notified until the contract is finalized. The MSSP's input would be essential to outline what sort of information the staffing company should provide to the hospital prior to sending a *locum tenens* practitioner to work at the hospital.

The difficulty in processing requests for privileges from *locum tenens* practitioners arises because these individuals have often worked at multiple locations for many years, which makes it more challenging to obtain references from all of their previous healthcare affiliations. The important thing to remember is that this type of practitioner, even though he or she will be on-site for a short period of time, must be reviewed and assessed in the same manner and in the same depth as any other practitioner.

The *locum tenens* practitioner should complete an application and provide all of the same type of information that would be collected from any other applicant seeking privileges at the institution. You may want to retitle the application "Application for *Locum Tenens* Privileges," rather than using the more traditional "Application for Medical Staff Appointment." Chances are the individual will not want to become a medical staff member, but he or she will be applying for privileges and should complete an application and a delineation of privileges form for the appropriate specialty or specialties.

Often this situation seems to occur with a "Rush" label—the hospital needs coverage in radiology or the emergency department this weekend or a medical staff member will be away and needs someone to cover his or her practice tomorrow. There should be a long-term plan for these situations. If people planned ahead, then the "Rush" label wouldn't have to be applied.

The privileging process should not be any different for a *locum tenens* practitioner than for any other practitioner. The major problem in processing these individuals, however, is that they often have 20 to 40 (or more) previous healthcare affiliations. The medical staff could recommend a change in policy in this instance and require a certain number of references be obtained from the most recent references (e.g., going back five years), thereby eliminating the nearly impossible task of obtaining references from all the facilities where the *locum tenens* practitioner has worked. The reality is that often these practitioners are in and out so quickly that the other healthcare organizations will not be able to provide much meaningful information. If the *locum tenens* practitioner will be returning multiple times, consideration should be given to granting him or her privileges for a two-year period, and then at the time of reprivileging determine whether he or she will be returning. This is one way to avoid having to process a request for privileges every time the individual's name appears on the call schedule.

The Joint Commission has initiated a Health Care Staffing Services Certification program that evaluates staffing organizations, which may prove helpful when staffing companies provide practitioners to the MSSP's institution. Those companies that have achieved certification are listed on the Joint Commission's Web site. The certification program provides a comprehensive evaluation of key processes, such as verifying the credentials and competencies of healthcare staff. Standards address the following areas:

- Leadership
- Human resources management
- Performance measurement and improvement
- Information management

A Certificate of Distinction is awarded to healthcare staffing firms that meet the requirements for certification.[12]

■ Disaster Privileges

The Joint Commission differentiates between disaster privileges and emergency privileges. Emergency privileges are used in an emergent situation, and basically any licensed independent practitioner is authorized to do whatever he or she can to the patient to prevent death or to save a patient from serious harm to the degree permitted by the practitioner's license, regardless of department affiliation, medical staff status, or clinical privileges granted. Once the patient has been stabilized, then a practitioner with the appropriate privileges must take over the care.

Disaster privileges are something different. The Joint Commission standards outline these requirements in the "Emergency Management" chapter. These privileges may be initiated only when the hospital's emergency operations plan has been activated, and the hospital is unable to handle the immediate patient needs. These privileges allow nonstaff practitioners to come to the aid of the hospital at the time of a disaster. The CEO, the medical staff president, or their designees have the option of granting these privileges, but certain requirements must be fulfilled according to the Joint Commission standards. There should be a policy and procedure concerning disaster privileges, and this document should address all current Joint Commission requirements. Those current at the time of this publication include the following:

- As described in the bylaws, the individual(s) responsible for granting disaster privileges to volunteer licensed independent practitioners must be identified.
- The hospital determines how it will distinguish volunteer licensed independent practitioners from other licensed independent practitioners.
- The medical staff describes, in writing, a mechanism to oversee the professional performance of volunteer licensed independent practitioners who are granted disaster privileges.
- The organization has a mechanism to readily identify volunteer practitioners who have been granted disaster privileges.

- While disaster privileges are granted on a case-by-case basis, volunteers considered eligible to act as licensed independent practitioners in the organization must, at a minimum, present a valid government-issued photo identification issued by a state or federal agency and at least one of the following:
  - A current picture ID card from a healthcare organization that clearly identifies his or her professional designation
  - A current license to practice
- Primary source verification of licensure:
  - Identification indicating that the individual is a member of a Disaster Medical Assistance Team (DMAT), the Medical Reserve Corps (MRC), the Emergency System for Advance Registration of Volunteer Health Professionals (ESAR-VHP), or another recognized state or federal response organization or group
  - Identification indicating that the individual has been granted authority to render patient care, treatment, and services in disaster circumstances (such authority having been granted by a federal, state, or municipal entity)
  - Confirmation by a licensed independent practitioner currently privileged by the hospital or by a staff member with personal knowledge of the volunteer's ability to act as a licensed independent practitioner during a disaster[13]

The medical staff oversees the professional practice of volunteer licensed independent practitioners.

■ Telemedicine Privileges

With the changes in world communication and the ability to send information in various modes, the possible uses of telemedicine are endless. Telemedicine (also known as e-health) can take advantage of multiple technologies such as videoconferencing between providers and patients in real time, radio links to emergency medicine personnel, teleradiology, interactive computing, e-ICUs, computer-based patient records, and many other audio, video, and data transmission technologies.

The Joint Commission's 2009 standards address this situation; however, the standards will continue to evolve over time as the situation becomes more and more common and technology continues to change. The original standards concerning telemedicine can be found in the "Medical Staff" chapter and also are covered in the "Leadership" chapter in terms of dealing with contracted services. There are also some relevant standards in the "Environment of Care" chapter. The medical staff standard clearly states that:

> The services covered under these standards are narrowly defined, focused solely on licensed independent practitioners who have either total or shared responsibility for patient care, treatment, and services (as evidenced as having the authority to write orders and direct care, treatment,

and services) through a telemedicine link. Licensed independent practitioners who provide official readings of images, tracings, or specimens through a telemedicine link are credentialed and privileged under the contracted services standards.[14]

These standards have raised many questions about how telemedicine is defined. The important language to note in the preceding quotation is "practitioners who have either total or shared responsibility." If the telemedicine practitioner is not providing the final interpretation or not authorizing the treatment, then he or she is considered a consultant.

The telemedicine standards previously allowed hospitals to credential by proxy; that is, the standards allowed a hospital to utilize the credentialing and privileging information and decision of another Joint Commission–accredited organization. Because CMS was not in agreement with the Joint Commission's concept of credentialing by proxy. The Joint Commission has now changed these standards to require hospitals that use the Joint Commission accreditation for deemed status to credential telemedicine practitioners in the same manner as any other practitioner. This means that hospitals will have to do their own credentialing of telemedicine practitioners and can no longer rely on the distant site's credentials process. If a hospital has previously approved large numbers of telemedicine practitioners by proxy, they may want to limit the number of telemedicine practitioners via the contract to allow for the need to fully verify all credentials and process through the medical staff route. Many MSSPs have complained that there are often a large number of practitioners providing care via telemedicine, such as in the teleradiology example, to the point that it becomes an almost impossible task to credential and privilege all of them. Consideration of using the leadership standards that allow organizations some alternatives when dealing with contracted services should be strongly pursued.

There is no federal law regulating telemedicine, nor is there any uniformity among state laws related to telemedicine. Physician licensure is the key issue when medicine is practiced across state lines.

Some states have statutes specifically permitting limited telemedicine physician consultations in their states by physicians licensed only in another state. Other states specifically prohibit such consultations, and still other states have no statutes on the subject. Consultants licensed in the patient's home state do not face this obstacle.

If the practice of medicine is taking place, a license is required. Therefore, healthcare facilities must first examine the interaction between all the physicians and patients involved to determine whether acts have occurred or will occur that constitute the practice of medicine. Then the licensure status of the consulting physician must be determined.

Before embarking on out-of-state telemedicine consultations, it is prudent that an organization do the following:

- Develop policies and procedures that define the credentialing and privileging process that will take place, including who is responsible for performance improvement activities and peer review and how those findings will be shared with the practitioners.
- Verify that all the physicians involved have specific professional liability insurance coverage for telemedicine consultations.
- Make sure the out-of-state physicians providing telemedicine consultations are licensed to practice in the state in which the healthcare facility is located, unless licensure is not required in that state by statute.
- Create patient consent forms specific to telemedicine and ensuring compliance with the Health Insurance Portability and Accountability Act (HIPAA). A telemedicine consent form should inform the patient that there might be problems with telemedicine transmission, so he or she is assuming risks in relying on connection with signal transmission and linkups to the satellite or cable. The patient should also consent to have another person, such as a camera operator, present during a consultation to take photos or videos of the patient.
- Maintain an accurate medical record.

■ Privileges That Cross Specialty Lines

Periodically, new procedures or services will emerge that more than one specialty will want to perform. In some instances, the hospital may have a contract with a specific group or type of specialist to perform a procedure. In that case, the contract controls the situation. If it is a new procedure and more than one specialty wishes to pursue its practice, however, the institution should establish a mechanism to deal with the situation. The MSSP will be asked to research the situation and identify whether all of the specialties requesting the privilege are, in fact, trained to provide the procedure or treatment.

For example, within the past few years, a new subspecialty has evolved called endovascular surgical neuroradiology. This subspecialty uses catheter technology, radiologic imaging, and clinical expertise to diagnose and treat diseases of the central nervous system. The training program must be administered by representatives from neurological surgery, diagnostic radiology, and neuroradiology programs. Applicants wishing to enter this program may come from various training backgrounds:

- Completion of an ACGME-accredited training program in radiology, plus one year of neuroradiology training, plus at least three months of clinical experience in neurological surgery, **or**
- Completion of an ACGME-accredited training program in neurological surgery plus a course in basic radiology skills, **or**
- Completion of an ACGME-accredited training program in neurology, plus completion of a one-year accredited program in vascular neurology, plus three

months of clinical skills in diagnostic radiology, plus three months of clinical experience in an ACGME-accredited neurological surgery program.[15]

This type of training criteria would need to be established for a procedure that more than one specialty could perform. ACGME is a good place to start the research to find out which specialties receive training in the procedure. Sometimes the procedure is new, and research will involve calling other hospitals where they are performing it already to see if they will share their criteria.

There may be economic initiatives involved in such ventures that will cause one specialty to oppose another, but the hospital must always maintain a fair and consistent approach to privileging. If there is no contract with a particular group or specialty, then all those who have sufficient training should be allowed the privilege once the hospital has decided to offer the privilege or procedure and defined the criteria. A sample policy and procedure for privileges that cross specialty lines is found on the CD that accompanies this book.

The same type of form that was shown for criteria development could also be used when establishing criteria for multispecialty privileges.

■ Turf Battles

"Turf battles" may arise when specialties are in disagreement about which one should perform certain procedures or treatments, or when there is opposition to a new procedure being done by another specialty. This term has a negative connotation and should really be eliminated from the MSSP's vocabulary. The goal is to achieve a win-win situation. This outcome may not always be possible, but the best approach to this problem is communication, communication, and more communication. Education of all sides needs to take place, and sometimes the medical director, medical staff president, or vice president of medical affairs may need to get involved.

There are multiple reasons why turf battles erupt. Many times the discord stems from issues related to finances, power, or control. The MSSP should strive to avoid being placed in the middle of any such situation. The MSSP's role is to obtain the facts, do the research, prepare documents for review, coordinate the process, try to avoid being dragged into the nitty-gritty of any argument, or avoid being persuaded to "side" with one of the representative groups.

■ Documentation of Privileges

The majority of hospitals today are still using a paper format for the privilege process. New paper forms are mailed to the applicants, and copies of authorized privileges are mailed back to the member at the end of the process. The various areas of the hospital that require this information—the emergency department, operating room, ambulatory surgery, labor and delivery, endoscopy suite, and so on—should always receive copies of the most recent privileges granted. Traditionally, these documents have been stored in notebooks in those areas. It has been the MSSP's job to distribute the revised forms. Unfortunately, some of those other areas have not maintained these documents as well as they should. The Joint Commission surveyors may ask hospital staff how they know that a particular practitioner had the privileges to do what he or she was doing. If the answer is that the information is available via notebooks, the surveyor will probably ask to see the notebooks. Obviously, it would be important for the staff to be able to locate the notebooks and, once located, for the notebooks to be current.

Today's answer to this problem is to computerize this information. Many of the credentialing software products include a privileging module that allows for computerization of privileges. In turn, this information needs to be networked, via either the hospital's main information system or another system, to those areas that require the information. Computerization of the information, once the software is defined, makes this job so much easier. The MSSP needs to update the information only once, and then everyone can look up the new privileges. If changes occur in someone's privileges, it would no longer be necessary to send that information all over the hospital in paper format. An e-mail announcing the changes and a revision to the computerized privileges for that practitioner would be sufficient.

If the medical staff services department does have computerized credentialing software but the privileges are not currently computerized, doing so should become a priority project. It will take a bit of time and effort, but information sharing will be so much easier after it is accomplished.

■ House Staff, Medical Students, and Other Trainees

Academic centers and many community hospitals have residents, medical students, or other types of students rotating through the facility as part of their training. Questions are often raised concerning whether these individuals need to be privileged.

The answer is actually quite simple: If these individuals are rotating through as part of their training, there should be a written agreement with the institution that is sending them to your facility. That written agreement should include a description of what these individuals are expected to do and what they are responsible for. In addition, there should always be a physician supervisor denoted in the agreement. The physician supervisors are the responsible individuals for any and all care provided by those in training. These supervisory personnel serve as the physician of record and are responsible for what the students are doing. No privileges need to be granted to these students as long as they are covered under a written agreement.

The Joint Commission does have a standard that requires the medical staff to have a defined process for supervision by a licensed independent practitioner with appropriate clinical privileges of each student.[16] If residents or students will be rotating through your facility, check this standard and see if you can locate the contract or documents that authorize the students and residents to be there and that it includes a definition of roles and responsibilities of the students as well as the supervising physician(s).

Sometimes hospitals use residents or fellows (physicians who have completed an accredited residency and are in an advanced program) as "moonlighters." This term refers to someone who still is in training but who is filling in nights, weekends, or extra shifts for house coverage or possibly emergency department coverage. In this case, the resident or fellow must have a full license to practice in the state, should have his or her own Drug Enforcement Administration certificate, and should obtain professional liability insurance for working outside of the training program. Moonlighting is not considered part of these individuals' formal training; they are functioning as licensed independent practitioners. The ACGME has a "moonlighting" policy on its Web site because this has become a popular practice but could be a dangerous one. The policy states:

> *The circumstance of working as a physician outside of one's authorized training program is called moonlighting. Moonlighting has been discouraged in the past for several reasons. First, it clearly competes with the opportunity to achieve the full measure of the educational objectives of the residency. Not only does the added time burden take away from study; it reduces rest and the ability for a more balanced lifestyle. Nevertheless, many residents find the need for money to be compelling and wish to use their time away from their training program to meet financial obligations.*
>
> *First and foremost, the moonlighting workload must not interfere with the ability of the resident to achieve the goals and objectives of their graduate medical education program. The program director should monitor resident performance to assure that factors such as resident fatigue are not contributing to diminished learning or performance, or detracting from patient safety. The program director may also choose to monitor the number of hours and the nature of the workload of residents engaging in moonlighting experiences.*
>
> *Residents must not be required to engage in moonlighting.*
>
> *All residents engaged in moonlighting must be licensed for unsupervised medical practice in the state where the moonlighting occurs. It is the responsibility of the institution hiring the resident to moonlight to determine whether such licensure is in place, [whether] adequate liability coverage is provided, and whether the resident has the appropriate training and skills to carry out assigned duties.*

> *The program director should acknowledge in writing that he or she is aware that the resident is moonlighting, and this information should be part of the resident's folder.*[17]

As this statement makes clear, it is incumbent upon the hospital that employs these individuals to ensure that they are not working beyond their allowable work hours.

■ Practitioners with Low Volume of Activity

As noted in the discussion in Chapter 6 concerning this same topic in relation to reappointment, practitioners with little or no activity at your institution need to provide some documentation of a hospital-based practice in another facility, and then references need to be obtained from that other facility to ensure that granting privileges to the provider is appropriate. Each hospital has an obligation to show knowledge of current competence prior to reappointing and reprivileging any practitioner. Privileges of practitioners who have low activity based on the fact that they primarily have an office-based practice should reflect their anticipated use of the hospital. It is not unusual for office-based practitioners to have admitting privileges, but no privileges for patient management. It would be difficult (if not impossible) to be able to demonstrate competency for management of acutely ill patients for practitioners who are solely office based. Some hospitals have considered asking for blinded medical records from the office practice to be reviewed and assessed to determine capability in diagnostic skills and treatment protocols. This type of care still does not qualify as working in an acute care setting, however, and privileges for hospital-based care are different. Often these practitioners can be offered a membership status that provides them with the relationship they require with a hospital without any clinical privileges.

■ Reprivileging and Profiling

At time of reappointment and reprivileging, hospitals are required to collect as much information as is available concerning the practitioner and his or her practice in the hospital. The Joint Commission requires that "the organized medical staff reviews and analyzes all relevant information regarding each requesting practitioner's current licensure status, training, experience, current competence and ability to perform the requested privilege. . . . The standard goes on to state that decisions on membership and granting of privileges include criteria that are directly related to the quality of health care, treatment, and services."[18]

The Joint Commission provides suggestions for ways to evaluate individuals with privileges:

> When renewing privileges, review of the practitioner's performance within the hospital should take place. [Items to be reviewed may include] procedures performed and outcomes based on reviews of operative and other procedures, medication usage, blood usage, medical records, and other performance improvement activities; additional criteria may include morbidity and mortality rates when available, utilization management, meeting and committee attendance, risk management data, peer recommendations, continuing medical education activities, patient safety, and sentinel event data.[19]

Each medical staff is responsible for identifying meaningful indicators and criteria for the ongoing professional practice evaluation for privileging that will provide them with practitioner-specific data as compared to aggregate data, when available, so that individuals practicing in the same specialty can be compared to similar practices. There is an expectation that an individual's privileges will change over time; new privileges may be added, privileges that are no longer used will be removed, and changes due to the evolution of technology will be reflected.

The profile should not be developed with a negative approach. Although it is a "report card," it should present the basis for renewal from a positive practice, not necessarily capturing only those cases that "fall out" of review. The profile should provide an overall view of the practice of each licensed independent practitioner. If there are problems, they will be reflected in the documentation that is collected. Nevertheless, the overall picture, if continued privileges are to be recommended, should be that of acceptable practice patterns. EXHIBIT 7-4 shows a sample practice profile.

Use of outcomes information has been part of the privileging/reprivileging process for a long time. In the past, medical staffs have atypically examined the bad outcomes, the problem outcomes, the complications, or mortalities. More recently, use of positive outcome information—that is, looking at the good results from a particular procedure, treatment, or service—has become the norm. Ideas such as "pay for performance" have been introduced by the CMS and the National Committee for Quality Assurance (NCQA), with more reimbursement being awarded for better outcomes. MSSPs would do well to begin researching the pay-for-performance idea to better understand what it means and what payers are striving to achieve. The Joint Commission has a policy statement entitled "Principles for the Construct of Pay-for-Performance Programs" that provides basic principles for future pay-for-performance programs.[20] The Medical Group Management Association has also posted a position paper on the same topic on its Web site.[21] NCQA provides a link to the Bridges to Excellence program on its Web site that explains programs already under way to help physicians measure themselves in their office practices, collect data, and submit those data for consideration of increased payment.[22] NCQA has also reached an agreement with the American Board of

Exhibit 7-4 Performance Profile

St. Elsewhere Medical Center Performance Profile

Performance Profile Goals

- To positively influence practice patterns while maintaining or improving outcomes
- To provide data that support competency of practitioners
- To meet credentialing-related requirements of the Joint Commission
- To provide data to privileging decision makers in a format that makes it difficult to ignore significant variations

Practitioner: _____

Specialty: _____

Time Period: From ___/___/___ To ___/___/___

Performance Parameter	Period Ending 6/30/10	Period Ending 12/31/10	Period Ending 6/30/11	Period Ending 12/31/11	Internal Comparative Data	Target	Flag for Further Review
Activity							
• Inpatient discharges							
• Total patient-days							
• Outpatient encounters							
• Consultations performed							
• Total procedures performed							
• Top 5 DRGs							
Litigation History							
• Number of settlements							
Staff Requirements							
• Number of medical record suspensions							
• ED call compliance measure							

Exhibit 7-4 Performance Profile (continued)

Performance Parameter	Period Ending 6/30/10	Period Ending 12/31/10	Period Ending 6/30/11	Period Ending 12/31/11	Internal Comparative Data	Target	Flag for Further Review
Indicators for Medical Staff Who Admit/Manage Patients							
• Readmission rate (unplanned for same diagnosis)							
• Unexpected mortality rate							
• Unplanned returns to intensive care unit							
• Blood order intervention rate							
• Pharmacy intervention rate							
• Indicator related to patient/family satisfaction							
Medical Record Review							
• Indicator(s) related to documentation quality							
• Indicator(s) related to documentation timeliness							
• Indicator(s) related to documentation completeness							

Exhibit 7-4 Performance Profile (continued)

Performance Parameter	Period Ending 6/30/10	Period Ending 12/31/10	Period Ending 6/30/11	Period Ending 12/31/11	Internal Comparative Data	Target	Flag for Further Review
Utilization Management							
• Indicator(s) related to resource utilization							
Specialty-Specific Indicators							
• Related to privileges and/or specialty							
Case-Specific Review							
• Total number of cases reviewed							
• Number of cases receiving scores of "X" or "Y"							

Evidence of Department Chair Evaluation and Any Required Follow-Up

Analysis of Performance Profile

☐ Sufficient data. No significant variations.
☐ Insufficient data for analysis.
☐ Sufficient data. Significant variations, or potential issues, as follows, with recommended action:

_____

_____

_____

Signature _____ Date _____
Chair, Department of _____

Internal Medicine (ABIM) so that a portion of the data submitted by a physician from his or her practice can also be used in the ABIM's maintenance of certification process.

All of these activities may very well have some components that can be used in the hospital or healthcare system privileging process. For this reason, MSSPs should broaden their education to include learning about these types of programs and look for ways to apply them to the organization's privileging program.

■ Clinical Activity Requirements Related to Competency

Some specialty professional organizations, such as the American College of Cardiology (www.acc.org), the American Society of Bariatric Physicians (www.asbp.org), and the American College of Gastroenterology (www.acg-gi.org), have developed guidelines stating the minimal acceptable numbers of procedures to be performed to maintain competency. The majority of specialties, however, have not accepted the theory that a minimal number of procedures performed necessarily equals competency. The American Academy of Family Practice (AAFP) has actually come out against using numbers in privileging:

> *The AAFP believes that privileging should be based on documented training and/or experience, demonstrated abilities, and current competence. Therefore, a policy recommending a minimum quota (or number) of procedures as a requirement for privileging should be formulated scientifically from data derived from physicians within a given specialty, rather than on arbitrary or consensus based quotas (or numbers) of procedures. This data derived privileging policy is only applicable to physicians in the specialty group from which it was derived. (1995) (2001)*
>
> Quota Privileging
>
> *The AAFP believes that each specialty society should maintain responsibility for recommending, implementing, maintaining, and evaluating privileging policies for its members. The AAFP also believes that privileging should be based on documented training and/or experience, demonstrated abilities and current competence, and, whenever possible, be evidence based.*
>
> *Recognizing that on rare occasions minimum quotas (or numbers) may be required in specific privileging instances where insufficient data exists, the AAFP believes that a consensus opinion of experts from within the specialty may be necessary until such time as an evidence-based recommendation is available. (1995) (2007)*[23]

Medical staffs are sometimes hesitant to include a required number of procedures in their privileging criteria because they are fearful that, if the minimum numbers are not achieved, practitioners will lose the privilege. In some instances, studies have proved that performing a higher number of procedures or caring for a specific number of patients leads to better outcomes. In fact, some studies have shown that positive outcomes are often influenced by the fact that not only is the individual practitioner more competent, but the whole team involved in the patients' care—nurses, assistants, and other professionals—influence the positive outcomes.

Medicare will not reimburse hospitals for some procedures if the volume is too low. In addition, this federal program has established criteria for Centers of Excellence. The Centers of Excellence idea originated as a demonstration project in the early 1990s to evaluate the effect of volume on quality and mortality for coronary artery bypass graft (CABG) surgery. The Department of Health and Human Services selected facilities on the basis of their outstanding experience, outcomes, and efficiency in performing these procedures. The agency found that hospitals that perform large volumes of a certain type of procedure tend to have better outcomes and quality. The demonstration resulted in an 8% average annual decline in mortality, and saved Medicare an average of 14% on CABG procedures. In 1999, the Congressional Budget Office scored the Centers of Excellence proposal as saving $300 million over five years and $600 million over ten years.[24]

Since the early 1990s, numerous reports have been published documenting higher-quality care and lower mortality in facilities that perform a large volume of cancer treatments, cardiac surgeries, and transplants, among others. These conditions often require highly specialized care that should be provided only by the highest-rated facilities. The Centers of Excellence designation is also currently being used in the private sector to improve quality and decrease costs in such areas as knee and hip replacement surgery.

The ideas underlying the Centers of Excellence proposal could be cited as a rationale for medical staffs to require minimum numbers for certain types of procedures where they believe that repetition (with good outcomes) equates to competency. Numbers plus outcome are what really matter and what should be considered when assessing for future privileges.

■ Privileging Questions

Questions are often raised about situations when the organization is unsure whether it must grant privileges to an individual. For example, what about transplant or organ procurement surgeons? The Joint Commission provides a FAQ section on its Web site for each accreditation product. Under the "Hospital" section, it states that the hospital does not have to credential or privilege these individuals if the arrangement or contract with their originating organization indicates that the originating organization is accredited by the Joint Commission and the original organization has credentialed and privileged those individuals.

Most of the time, common sense should prevail. If no other organization is responsible for authorizing what an individual will be doing in your organization, then it would make sense that your organization needs to be responsible for the practitioner's activities. There may be ways to check on the practitioner other than the medical staff credentialing and privileging process—for example, through human resources or through a contract. But the bottom line is clear: If a practitioner is touching a patient, the organization controlling the environment where the patient care is taking place is responsible.

■ An Innovative and Creative Solution

Here is an idea to consider: A group of hospitals in Jacksonville, Florida, got together in 1989 to explore the development of a centralized credentialing program through the local medical society. The original idea did not come to fruition; however, the advisory committee that had initiated the meetings challenged the local MSSPs to develop an alternative method to streamline the credentialing process. The result was a cooperative credentialing process. The group of MSSPs and legal counsels representing each organization were able to develop common initial appointment and reappointment applications and obtain agreement on a common reappointment cycle, a common evaluation form, a common statement of authorization and release, and delineation of privilege forms that are used by 12 hospitals. The goal—and eventually achievement—of this group was to have all applicants to any of the 12 hospitals complete only one application and one privilege form, and to do the same at time of reappointment. Through a cooperative agreement signed by all institutions, the hospitals agreed that whichever medical staff office received the first application for a new applicant would perform primary source verification and copy and send the application and all verification documents to the other hospitals where the applicant was applying. Today, each institution participating in this coalition is responsible for appraising and reappraising the applicants to that institution and for processing the application through its own approval process. The information collection and verification data are what is shared.

The Joint Commission has surveyed most of the Jacksonville institutions two to three times since this project was initiated and has been supportive of the program. The participating hospitals indicate that this cooperative credentialing venture has yielded the following benefits:

- Elimination of work duplication through the creation of a credentialing process that is less cumbersome and easier for the practitioners
- Creation of quality credentialing tools (forms and documents) through collaborative efforts

- Establishment and maintenance of a standard process
- Improvement of communication among participating healthcare institutions

All the forms developed by this cooperative, including the applications and evaluation forms as well as the delineation of privilege forms, can be found on the Florida Association of Medical Staff Services' Web site (www.famss.org/FAMSSTODAY/NECooperative Credentialing forms). EXHIBITS 7-5 AND 7-6 are examples of the privilege forms used by the cooperative credentialing group.

The cooperative credentialing group concept was developed and implemented through the collective efforts of medical staff services professionals at the following Northeast Florida healthcare institutions: Baptist Medical Center, Baptist Medical Center-Beaches, Baptist Medical Center-Nassau, Methodist Medical Center, St. Luke's Hospital, St. Vincent's Medical Center, University Medical Center, and Wolfson Children's Hospital.

■ Acknowledgment

Thanks to Betsy Miller, the head of the NE Florida Cooperative, for sharing the history and a written monograph detailing the development of this creative solution. She is the contact person if you desire further information about this initiative.

■ Notes

1. The Joint Commission. *2009 Hospital Accreditation Standards.* Oakbrook Terrace, IL: Author; 2009:,MS.06.01.05, p. 204.
2. The Joint Commission, note 1, MS.06.01.01, p. 205.
3. Department of Health and Human Services, Centers for Medicare and Medicaid Services. "Center for Medicaid and State Operations/Survey and Certification Group Memorandum." November 12, 2004: Ref:S&C-05-04.
4. Accreditation Council for Graduate Medical Education. "Review Committees/ Program Requirements." Available at: http://www.acgme.org/review committees. Accessed July 2009.
5. The Joint Commission, note 1, MS.08.01.01, p. 210.
6. The Joint Commission, note 1, MS.08.01.01, p. 210.
7. The Joint Commission, note 1, MS.08.01.01, p. 212.
8. Prichard B. "Still Struggling with OPPE and FPPE? You've Come to the Right Place." Presentation at the NAMSS Annual Meeting, Milwaukee, WI, October 13, 2008.
9. The Joint Commission, note 1, MS.06.01.13, p. 208.
10. National Practitioner Data Bank. "Guidebook," Chapter D. Available at: http://www.npdb-hipdb.hrsa.gov/query.html. Accessed July 27, 2009.
11. The Joint Commission, note 1, MS.06.01.13, p. 208.
12. Joint Commission on Accreditation of Healthcare Organizations. Available at: http://www.jcaho.org/dscc/hcss/index.htm. Accessed August 18, 2009.
13. The Joint Commission, note 1, EM .02.02.13.

Exhibit 7-5 Advanced Registered Nurse Practitioner Privilege Form

Name: _____ Effective Date: _____ to _____

Legend: 1–Baptist 2–Beaches 3–Memorial 4–Nassau 5–Orange Park 6–St. Luke's
7–St. Vincent's 8–Shands/Jax 9–Specialty 10–Wolfson 11–Brooks 12–South

The minimum education, training, and experience qualifications for core privileges are as delineated in each hospital's medical staff bylaws, rules and regulations, or policies. Please consult these documents to determine your eligibility to request these privileges.

To request core privileges, please place an "X" in the appropriate hospital column.

1	2	3	4	5	6	7	8	9	10	11	12	Core Privileges	Approval
												Initial and ongoing assessment of patient's medical, physical, and psychosocial status, including conduct, history and physical; develop treatment plan; provide patient education, perform rounds; record progress notes; order tests, examinations, medications, and therapies; and write discharge summary. **All privileges are conducted in accordance with an approved written protocol between the nurse practitioner and the supervising physician, and do not take the place of timely physician visits.**	

Exhibit 7-5 Advanced Registered Nurse Practitioner Privilege Form (continued)

To request special procedures, please place an "X" in the appropriate hospital column. If the condition/privilege you desire in is not included on this form, please submit a separate written request for the privilege along with documentation of training and/or experience.

Special Procedures (Procedures that are not routinely part of training, and may require proof of training or experience)	1	2	3	4	5	6	7	8	9	10	11	12	Approval
Apply/remove orthopedic splints/casts for closed fractures and severe sprains [++Hospitals 9]									■				
Arterial line placement [++Hospitals 2]		■											
Bone marrow biopsies [++Hospitals 2, 6]		■				■							
Cardiac stress testing [++Hospitals 3, 7]			■				■						
Central venous catheters—insertion [++Hospitals 7, 9]							■		■				
Central venous catheters—removal [++Hospitals 9]									■				
Cerebrospinal fluid (CSF) shunt puncture [++Hospitals 10]										■			
Chest tubes—insertion [++Hospitals 7]							■						
Chest tubes—removal [++Hospitals 9]									■				
Emergency Department—may manage illness of minimal severity with no serious threat to life													
Emergency Department—may perform initial evaluation of illness of moderate or major severity and manage in conjunction with supervising physician [++Hospitals 2]		■											
Emergency Department—perform medical screening exams													

202   CHAPTER 7 Hospital Privileging

Exhibit 7-5 Advanced Registered Nurse Practitioner Privilege Form (continued)

Special Procedures (Procedures that are not routinely part of training, and may require proof of training or experience)	1	2	3	4	5	6	7	8	9	10	11	12	Approval
Endotracheal intubation [++Hospitals 9]									X				
Exchange transfusions													
First/second surgical assistant [++Hospitals 2, 5]		X			X								
Implantation of temporary cardiac pacemakers [++Hospitals 1, 3]	X		X										
Insertion pulmonary artery catheter (Swan-Ganz) [++Hospitals 3, 5, 7, 8]			X		X		X	X					
Intra-aortic balloon pump (IABP)—insertion [++Hospitals 1, 6, 7, 10]	X					X	X			X			
Intra-aortic balloon pump (IABP)—removal [++Hospitals 1, 6, 7, 10]	X					X	X			X			
Limited fiberoptic-bronchoscopy [++Hospitals 8]								X					
Local infiltrative anesthesia administration [++Hospitals 9]									X				
Long-term ventilator management [++Hospitals 9]									X				
Lumbar puncture [++Hospitals 6, 9]						X			X				
Moderate sedation/analgesia [++Hospitals 6, 8, 12]						X		X				X	
Open, close, harvest, and prepare saphenous vein for bypass graft [++Hospitals 6, 7]						X	X						
Peripheral indwelling central venous catheter (PICC) insertion [++Hospitals 7, 8, 9]							X	X	X				

Exhibit 7-5 Advanced Registered Nurse Practitioner Privilege Form (continued)

Special Procedures (Procedures that are not routinely part of training, and may require proof of training or experience)	1	2	3	4	5	6	7	8	9	10	11	12	Approval
Pre- and post-operative surgical care [++Hospitals 9]									■				
Puncture and aspiration of subcutaneous abscess or cyst [++Hospitals 10]										■			
Resuscitative measures (ACLS, NCLS, PALS) [++Hospitals 1, 2, 3, 4, 6, 7, 9, 10, 12]	■	■	■	■		■	■		■	■		■	
Reprogramming of programmable shunt system [++Hospitals 10]										■			
Skin biopsy or excise lesions [++Hospitals 2, 6, 7, 9]		■				■	■		■				
Sternal closure [++Hospitals 7]							■						
Subdural puncture [++Hospitals 10]										■			
Suture lacerations and provide wound care [++Hospitals 9]									■				
Temporary pacer wires—removal													
Venous cut-down [++Hospitals 7]							■						
Ventricular tap [++Hospitals 10]										■			
Umbilical vessel catheterization													

Exhibit 7-5 Advanced Registered Nurse Practitioner Privilege Form (continued)

Privilege not available in this specialty at this hospital.
++ Please refer to this hospital's bylaws or rules and regulations regarding specific criteria to be met before this privilege may be granted.

Acknowledgment of Practitioner: I understand that (a) in exercising clinical privileges granted, I am constrained by each hospital's medical staff policies, rules and regulations, and (b) any restriction on the clinical privileges granted to me is waived in an emergency situation and in such situation my actions are governed by the applicable section of each hospital's medical staff bylaws.

Applicant Signature: _____ *Date:* _____

Acknowledgment of Supervising Physician: The above named practitioner shall be under my supervision in the exercise of clinical privileges. I acknowledge that above named practitioner is competent and qualified to perform the requested privileges.

Supervising Physician Signature: _____ *Date:* _____
Supervising Physician Signature: _____ *Date:* _____
Supervising Physician Signature: _____ *Date:* _____
Supervising Physician Signature: _____ *Date:* _____

Source: Courtesy of Florida's North Eastern Cooperative

Exhibit 7-6 Cardiology Privilege Form

Name: _____ Effective Date: _____ to _____

Legend: 1–Baptist 2–Beaches 3–Memorial 4–Nassau 5–Orange Park 6–St. Luke's
7–St. Vincent's 8–Shands/Jax 9–Specialty 10–Wolfson 11–Brooks 12–South

The minimum education, training, and experience qualifications for core privileges are as delineated in each hospital's medical staff bylaws, rules and regulations, or policies. Please consult these documents to determine your eligibility to request these privileges.

To request core privileges, please place an "X" in the appropriate hospital column.

1	2	3	4	5	6	7	8	9	10	11	12	Internal Medicine Core Privileges	Approval
												Work-up, admission, evaluation, performance of any laboratory procedure classified under CLIA 88 rules and regulations as provider-performed microscopy or any waived procedure approved by the director designated on the hospital waived testing certificate, diagnosis, consultation, and/or provision of nonsurgical treatment to patients from adolescence through old age during times of health and through all stages of acute and chronic illness. Core privileges include CVP line placement.	

To request core privileges, please place an "X" in the appropriate hospital column.

1	2	3	4	5	6	7	8	9	10	11	12	Cardiology Core Privileges	Approval
												Work-up, admission, evaluation, diagnosis, consultation, and/or provision of treatment to patients presenting with cardiovascular disease or disorders. Privileges include Advanced Cardiac Life Support (ACLS), CVP line placement, and cardioversion.	

Exhibit 7-6 Cardiology Privilege Form (continued)

To request special procedures, please place an "X" in the appropriate hospital column. If the condition or privilege you desire is not included on this form, please submit a separate written request for the privilege along with appropriate documentation of training and/or experience.

1	2	3	4	5	6	7	8	9	10	11	12	Special Procedures (Procedures that may not be part of residency/fellowship training and/or may require proof of additional training or experience)	Approval
							■					Arterial Dopplers [++Hospital 8]	
■		■			■	■	■					AICD implantation [++Hospitals 1, 3, 6, 7, 8]	
■						■	■		■		■	Atrial fibrillation ablation [++Hospitals 1, 7, 8, 10, 12]	
					■	■	■					Echocardiography (2D, m-mode) [++Hospitals 6, 7, 8]	
					■	■	■					Echocardiography (Doppler) [++Hospitals 6, 7, 8]	
	■	■				■						Echocardiography (stress) [++Hospitals 2, 3, 7]	
■	■	■		■	■	■	■				■	Echocardiography (transesophageal) [++Hospitals 1, 2, 3, 5, 6, 7, 8, 12]	
■	■	■		■	■	■	■	■	■		■	EKG reading list [++Hospitals 1, 2, 3, 5, 6, 7, 8, 9, 10, 12]	
■		■			■	■	■					Electrophysiological studies [++Hospitals 1, 3, 6, 7, 8]	
	■					■	■	■				Holter monitor interpretation [++Hospitals 2, 7, 8, 9]	
	■	■		■		■						Implantation of temporary cardiac pacemakers [++Hospitals 2, 3, 5, 7]	
■	■	■		■	■	■	■					Implantation of permanent pacemakers [++Hospitals 1, 2, 3, 5, 6, 7, 8]	
				■	■	■						Insertion pulmonary artery catheters (Swan-Ganz) [++Hospitals 5, 6, 7]	

Notes

Exhibit 7-6 Cardiology Privilege Form (continued)

1	2	3	4	5	6	7	8	9	10	11	12		Approval
												Special Procedures (Procedures that may not be part of residency/fellowship training and/or may require proof of additional training or experience)	
												Moderate sedation [++Hospitals 1, 2, 3, 4, 5, 6, 7, 8, 9, 10, 12]	
												Nuclear cardiology [++Hospitals 1, 2, 3, 5, 6, 7, 8, 12]	
												Treadmill stress testing [++Hospitals 2, 6, 7]	
												Cardiac-Vascular Laboratory Procedures	
												Angiography; coronary [++Hospitals 3, 5, 6, 7]	
												Angiography; extracranial (head and neck) [++Hospitals 3, 5, 6, 7, 8]	
												Angiography; extremity [++Hospitals 1, 2, 3, 5, 6, 7, 8]	
												Angiography; intracranial [++Hospitals 6, 7, 8]	
												Angiography; pulmonary [++Hospitals 5, 6, 7, 8]	
												Angiography; renal/mesenteric [++Hospitals 1, 3, 5, 6, 7, 8]	
												Angioplasty/stent; coronary [++Hospitals 1, 3, 6, 7, 8]	
												Angioplasty/stent; extracranial (head and neck) [++Hospitals 1, 3, 5, 6, 7, 8]	
												Angioplasty/stent; extremity (including thrombolysis/thrombectomy) [++Hospitals 1, 3, 5, 6, 7, 8]	
												Angioplasty/stent; intracranial [++Hospitals 1, 6, 7, 8]	

Exhibit 7-6 Cardiology Privilege Form (continued)

1	2	3	4	5	6	7	8	9	10	11	12	Special Procedures (Procedures that may not be part of residency/fellowship training and/or may require proof of additional training or experience)	Approval
												Angioplasty/stent; pulmonary [++Hospitals 3, 6, 7, 8]	
												Angioplasty/stent; renal/mesenteric [++Hospitals 1, 3, 5, 6, 7, 8]	
												Aortography [++Hospitals 3, 6, 7]	
												Coronary rotablator [++ Hospitals 1, 3, 6, 7, 8]	
												Coronary flow wire/pressure wire insertion [++Hospitals 3, 7]	
												Endovascular abdominal aortic stent graft [++Hospital 3, 7]	
												Intra-aortic balloon pump [++Hospital 5, 6, 7]	
												Intracoronary thrombectomy devices (AngioJet, X-sizer, others) [++Hospitals 3, 8]	
												Intracoronary thrombolysis [++Hospital 8]	
												Intracoronary ultrasound [++Hospital 3, 8]	
												Intravascular brachytherapy [++Hospital 7, 8]	
												Laser: excimer [++Hospital 3, 8]	
												Thrombolysis/thrombectomy procedures—pulmonary [++Hospitals 6, 7, 8]	
												Valvuloplasty [++Hospitals 3, 6, 7]	

Notes

Exhibit 7-6 Cardiology Privilege Form (continued)

Acknowledgement of Practitioner: I understand that (a) in exercising clinical privileges granted, I am constrained by each hospital's medical staff policies, rules and regulations, and (b) any restriction on the clinical privileges granted to me is waived in an emergency situation and in such situation my actions are governed by the applicable section of each hospital's medical staff bylaws.

Applicant Signature: _____ *Date:* _____

■ Privilege not available in this specialty at this hospital.
++ Please refer to this hospital's bylaws or rules and regulations regarding specific criteria to be met before this privilege may be granted.

Source: Courtesy of Florida's North Eastern Cooperative

14. The Joint Commission, note 1, MS.06.01.03–.06.01.07, excluding MS.06.01.03, EP2; MS.13.01.01, EP1, LD.04.03.09.
15. Accreditation Council for Graduate Medical Education. "Residency Review Committees/Program Requirements." Available at: http://www.acgme.org/. Accessed September 2009.
16. The Joint Commission, note 1, MS.04.01.01.
17. Accreditation Council for Graduate Medical Education. "Resident Information—Moonlighting Policy—ACGME Approved." June 27, 2000. Available at: http://www.acgme.org/acWebsite/navPages/commonpr_documents/VIFG_DutyHours_MoonlightingandExceptions_Documentation.pdf. Accessed September 2009.
18. The Joint Commission, note 1, MS.06.01.07.
19. The Joint Commission, note 1, MS.06.01.07, .06.01.05.
20. The Joint Commission. "Pay for Performance." Available at: http://www.jointcommission.org/PublicPolicy/pay.htm. Accessed September 2009.
21. Medical Group Management Association. "Pay for Performance." Available at: http://www.mgma.com/workarea/downloadasset.aspx?id=17518. Accessed September 2009.
22. National Committee on Quality Assurance. "Communications/News: Bridges to Excellence." Available at: http://www.ncqa.org/tabid/431/Default.aspx. Accessed September 2009.
23. American Academy of Family Practice. "Policies on Health Issues: Privileges, Pay for Performance, and Physician Profiling." Available at: http://www.aafp.org. Accessed September 2009.
24. U.S. House of Representatives, Pete Stark. April 1999. Available at: http://www.house.gov/stark/webarchives/Stark%20Web%20Page/documents/centerexpress.html. Accessed August 29, 2005.

CHAPTER 8

Credentialing Allied Health Professionals

Cindy A. Gassiot, CPMSM, CPCS

■ What Is an Allied Health Professional?

There is no universally accepted definition of an allied health professional (AHP), if only because the types of practitioners who might be considered to be AHPs differ from state to state. Put simply, allied health professionals are individuals other than the licensed physicians and other practitioners who are members of a medical staff organization, who provide patient care services in a healthcare organization. Some AHPs may be accorded "licensed independent practitioner" status (which means that they function without supervision or direction). Most AHPs, however, function under a defined degree of supervision by a medical staff member who has been granted clinical privileges. AHPs exercise judgment within the areas of documented professional competence and consistent with their applicable state practice act.

The board of the healthcare organization should periodically determine the categories of healthcare professionals who are eligible to apply for privileges as an AHP.

■ Historical Perspective

Managing credentialing of AHPs has been a challenge to medical staff services professionals. Early on, resources and guidance for credentialing and privileging AHPs were scarce. Over the years, resources have been developed to assist with this demanding responsibility, and the information now available in print and online concerning the many AHP disciplines has proved very beneficial. Some of these helpful Web sites are listed at the end of this chapter. Despite these resources, credentialing AHPs can still be a headache, and many medical staff services professionals have expressed some degree of frustration about how to facilitate this sometimes onerous chore.

Historically, AHPs were brought into a hospital because they were employed by a physician member of the medical staff organization who wished to use the services of his or her employee while attending to patients. These AHPs were often nurses from physician offices who assisted as scrub nurses in the operating room or accompanied the physician on patient rounds, providing patient teaching, and so on. Not knowing what else to do, medical staff services professionals simply treated AHPs the same as physicians when it came to credentialing. An application form similar to that used for a medical practitioner was developed, a laundry list of "privileges" was devised, and AHP applications were processed in the same manner as those of physicians and dentists. Many have since come to believe that this process is not necessarily the most appropriate for many categories of AHPs.

■ The Current Picture

AHPs are entering healthcare organizations in greater numbers than ever before. Today, a wide array of AHPs provide services in hospitals and related ambulatory care settings. In addition, AHPs are being used to extend the services of the physician. These individuals may be hospital or physician employees, or they may have a contract with the organization to provide services. They may be granted privileges or the authority to provide designated patient services. There appears to be no limit to the number of possible titles, such as physician assistant (PA), advanced practice nurse (APRN), speech pathologist, and acupuncturist and other alternative care provider. Advanced practice nurses include members of the following four categories: (1) nurse practitioners, some of whom specialize in one area of medicine such as family practice or pediatrics; (2) certified registered nurse anesthetists; (3) clinical nurse specialists; and (4) nurse-midwives. The governing board determines which types of AHPs will be permitted to provide patient care services within the organization, and the procedure for appointment and the scope of practice should be defined in the organization-wide documents, not the medical staff bylaws.

Common Factors

Factors common to allied health professionals include the following:

- The source of employment has absolutely no bearing on their need to be authorized to provide services or credentialed. In other words, a hospital-employed nurse anesthetist, a physician assistant employed by a medical staff member, or a speech pathologist under contract with the hospital must be credentialed through the regular medical staff channels or authorized to perform by an alternative method, such as through human resources.
- AHPs usually provide direct care to patients; that is, they "lay hands on" or are in close verbal contact with patients.
- Some exercise a great deal of independent judgment.
- Some practice independently with no physician supervision. If this is the case, it should be noted that Joint Commission requires that all licensed independent practitioners be credentialed and privileged through the medical staff process.

- Although some AHPs are granted privileges, they are not necessarily granted medical staff membership. In fact, they are usually not permitted to be members of the medical staff. In some states, however, certain categories of licensed independent practice AHPs (e.g., psychologists) are eligible for medical staff membership.

Members of many AHP disciplines must have a license, certification, or registration and are regulated or guided by state requirements. Medical staff services professionals should read the practice acts or statutes regulating their activities in their states to obtain this information. In some states, physician assistants and advanced practice nurses have prescriptive authority and may write orders for medications and prescriptions for take-home medications. However, the hospital has the final say as to the extent of services the individual may provide within the hospital's jurisdiction. These limitations are defined in a job description or privilege list of allowable services.

More recently, forward-thinking individuals have realized that the majority of allied health disciplines practice in a totally dependent manner (with physician supervision) and do not need to be "credentialed" in the same manner as one would credential a physician, nor is a physician-equivalent credentialing process for AHPs required by accreditation organizations other than for PAs and APRNs. Also, AHPs other than PAs and APRNs certainly do not need to be granted clinical privileges as one would grant privileges to a physician. Many of these disciplines, such as surgical technologists, surgical assistants, cardiovascular perfusionists, and dental assistants—to name a few—can be authorized to function under a scope of practice or a job description. Additionally, there is no good reason why the paperwork for AHPs other than PAs and APRNs cannot be handled by a hospital department other than medical staff services.

Because medical staff services departments are typically overwhelmed with work, some of them have been successful in transferring the responsibility for processing the applications of AHP disciplines other than PAs and APRNs to another hospital department, usually human resources. In such cases, the AHP application is processed and handled in the same manner as that of a hospital employee and is not forwarded through medical staff channels to the governing board. For AHP disciplines other than PAs and APRNs (whose credentialing will be discussed later), the review process may entail primary source verification of licensure, certification, or registration; a check of education and experience references; a criminal background check; applicable health screening; professional references; and other verifications that human resources personnel may perform; the AHP is then authorized to function in the hospital under a job description or scope of practice. The organization must meet the Joint Commission's human resources (HR) standards when using this process. The organization must also determine that nonemployed AHPs have the same qualifications and competencies as employed individuals who provide the same services. The HR standards have requirements for assessing competency at orientation as well as periodically—at least once every three years.[1] A competency validation or skills checklist can be used for this purpose.

Many hospitals have defined core competencies or devised skills checklists for each category of AHP. If the same category of AHP is already employed by the hospital, the core competencies or skills checklists should exist in the human resources or home department of the employee. The department head in the hospital where the nonemployed AHP functions most frequently must be asked to validate competencies in compliance with this standard.

In 2004, the Joint Commission revised its standards to state that PAs and APRNs who are not licensed independent practitioners may be privileged through the medical staff process or an equivalent process that was developed and approved by the governing body. The Centers for Medicare and Medicaid Services' (CMS's) Conditions of Participation do not recognize an equivalent process for privileging practitioners, however, and organizations that are using an alternative process for PAs and APRNs should credential and privilege these disciplines through the regular medical staff channels.

■ Who Must Be Credentialed and Privileged

Numerous physician assistants and advanced practice registered nurses practice in today's healthcare organizations. Some perform high-risk procedures and provide complex care. Although laws in none of the 50 states allow PAs to practice without supervision, and few APRNs practice in hospitals without some physician supervision (although some states allow APRNs to function as licensed independent practitioners), healthcare organizations must credential and privilege these AHPs to assure that they are qualified, that they practice within the scope of their approved privileges, and that their performance is evaluated.

■ Multidisciplinary AHP Committees

Some organizations have formed a committee to perform the authorization process for AHPs—a task that was previously handled by the credentials committee. Such a committee is usually composed of representative AHPs, nursing administration, medical staff services, and one or more physicians. In California, a state regulation requires establishment of an interdisciplinary practice committee that is responsible for recommending policies and procedures for the granting of expanded role privileges to advanced practice nurses, whether or not they are employed by the facility. The policies and procedures are required to be administered by the committee on interdisciplinary practice, which is responsible for reviewing credentials and making recommendations for granting and/or rescinding privileges. The same regulation requires that a physician approved by the California medical licensing board supervise PAs who practice in a licensed facility, and that PAs apply to and be approved by the executive committee of the medical staff of the facility in which they wish to practice.[2]

■ AHP Policy

As with any process performed by the medical staff services department (MSSD), credentialing AHPs should be guided by a policy that has been approved by the medical staff and governing body. This policy serves as the medical staff services professional's (MSSP's) guide for handling requests for applications, the credentials verification process, the approvals process, and other questions or issues that may arise with an AHP. A sample AHP policy can be found on the CD that accompanies this book.

■ The Application Form

An application form for an allied health professional should obtain the following information:

- Name, home and office addresses, telephone numbers, citizenship, marital status, and professional affiliations
- Licensure, certification, and registration, with expiration dates
- Education and training (college, allied health school, other graduate education or training)
- Current hospital affiliations
- Military service and any specialized training
- Previous experience in hospitals or other healthcare facilities
- References (three individuals with personal knowledge of the applicant's professional ability, ethics, and character)
- Evidence of professional liability insurance (carrier, policy number, dates, and limits)
- Type of practice anticipated if granted privileges:
  - Self-employed (freelance)
  - Employed by medical staff member part-time
  - Employed by medical staff member full-time
  - Member of, or affiliated with, a group practicing this specialty
  - Other (specify)
- Distance from office or home to hospital (in miles)
- Answers to the following questions:
  - Has your license to practice in any jurisdiction ever been voluntarily or involuntarily limited, suspended, placed on probation, or revoked?

- Has your certification or registration status ever been voluntarily or involuntarily revoked?
- Have your privileges at any hospital or other healthcare facility ever been voluntarily or involuntarily revoked, suspended, reduced, subject to observation (beyond what is normal), or not renewed?
- Have you ever been denied membership (or renewal thereof) or been subject to disciplinary action in any professional organization?
- Have you ever been a defendant in a professional liability or negligence case?
- Is there any professional liability claim pending against you?
- Has a settlement of any professional liability claim involving you ever been made?
- Is there any health status problem that could prevent you from safely performing the privileges requested?

If the answer to any of these questions is yes, the applicant should be asked to give full details on a separate sheet of paper. All questions must be answered. (One possible answer is "not applicable.")

- Continuing education information (all continuing education courses attended and for which the applicant received credit in the past two years).
- Duties that the applicant desires to perform in the hospital (a specific list—if the hospital is to employ the AHP and a current job description covers all areas of the AHP's practice, then the applicant should state that information).
- Liability coverage information. If the applicant is the employee of a member of the hospital's medical staff, his or her employer should answer the following two questions:
  - Is this applicant covered by your liability carrier? List carrier name, amount of coverage, and expiration date.
  - Is this applicant covered by his or her own liability insurance? List carrier name, amount of coverage, and expiration date.

The applicant should sign a statement authorizing the inspection of records and documents that may be pertinent to the evaluation of professional, moral, and ethical qualifications and competence to carry out the clinical privileges or duties requested. The AHP applicant should also sign a statement agreeing to the following:

- Never engage in the practice of medicine as defined by the state medical practice act, the State Board of Medical Examiners, or other statutory or regulatory provisions
- Adhere to the medical staff bylaws, rules, and regulations and hospital or facility policies as they apply to actions or duties
- Comply with all relevant requirements of the Joint Commission (or other accrediting organization) as interpreted by the hospital

- Wear proper identification indicating name and title whenever in the hospital
- Maintain adequate liability insurance coverage at all times

The supervising or sponsoring physician should sign a statement attesting that all duties performed by the AHP must be done by his or her authority and under his or her supervision.

The application form is accompanied by a request for privileges form for licensed independent practitioners (for PAs and APRNs) or a scope of practice or job description (for AHP disciplines other than PAs or APRNs).

■ Delineation of Privileges

PAs and APRNs must be granted clinical privileges, and delineation of privilege forms must be developed for them. A sample request for privileges form for a PA that includes a generic PA privilege request form as well as one for a PA who specializes in emergency medicine can be found on the CD that accompanies this book.

■ Scope of Practice

A scope of practice may be designed for an AHP other than a PA or APRN with the help of the state practice act and/or the professional association for the particular discipline. The scope of practice should contain a description of the allied health discipline's permissible tasks; specify the education and training required commensurate with those required for hospital employees in the discipline; note whether licensure, certification, or registration is required; and identify any other specific qualifications. A list of tasks or procedures that would require additional training or education would then follow. The scope of practice decision should be based on what the organization has decided that the particular AHP discipline will be allowed to do within the facility. The scope of practice can also be used as a basis for competency validation. There is an example of a scope of practice on the CD that accompanies this book.

■ Processing the Application

The AHP application for the licensed independent practitioner or the APRN or PA is processed in the same manner as an application from a physician. That is, licensure, education, training, certification, peer references, previous hospital affiliations, previous employment (if relevant), and professional liability insurance coverage are verified. The AMA's Profile can be used as an approved primary source to verify education and training for PAs. In some states, PAs and APRNs have prescriptive authority and have either a Drug Enforcement Administration certificate or a state-issued narcotics registration (and sometimes both). Some organizations also verify these items online, although this step is not required. Most organizations check for Medicare sanctions through the Office of the Inspector General and perform a criminal history background check and a National Practitioner Data Bank (NPDB) query, although this usually does not produce any information. (Healthcare facilities are not required by the Health Care Quality Improvement Act to report adverse events concerning AHPs to the NPDB.)

Many organizations require that all applicants provide the names of three peers for the purpose of obtaining references about the applicant's competence. Because AHPs sometimes have difficulty listing three peers who can provide a professional reference, some organizations require only one true peer reference (e.g., PA for a PA; APRN for an APRN) and accept references from physicians for the other two.

When all verifications are received, the credentials file of the AHP is assembled, along with an evaluation tool for the department chair's signature, and the department chair reviews the file. In most hospitals, the file is forwarded with the department chair's recommendation to the credentials committee and then to the medical executive committee. An alternative process is to have an individual (for example, a designee of an AHP committee) review the file prior to the department chair's review. If the file raises concerns related to supervision, privileges, or other issues, these potential problems can be addressed by someone with expertise in this specialty area. The regular review and evaluation process is then followed. The final step is review of the application by the governing body, which approves appointment and clinical privileges.

■ Reappointment of AHPs

PAs and APRNs should be reprivileged every two years in the same manner as medical staff members. For other categories of nonemployed AHPs, the same competency validation or skills checklist used at time of initial authorization can be used for the periodic performance appraisal.

The reappointment application form should obtain the following information:

- Confirmation of current license, registration, or certification
- Confirmation of the current liability carrier, address, policy number, and amount of coverage
- A list of any liability litigation, claims, or settlements since the previous reappraisal or now pending
- Any change in employment status
- Any change desired in privileges or patient services allowed in the hospital (if additional privileges are requested, supporting information on education and training should be included)

- Any health status problems that would keep the professional from performing the privileges or tasks requested
- Relevant continuing education programs completed since the previous appraisal

■ Competency Assessment

The reappointment form should be accompanied by an evaluation of the AHP's professional performance. Performance reports used for ongoing professional practice evaluation are ideal resources to be used at the time of reappointment to confirm competency of requested or granted privileges.

It is difficult to collect clinical performance data on most AHP disciplines. The medical records of patients for whom they provide services are typically coded to the admitting physician and not to the AHP, making it difficult to retrieve the records. Nevertheless, a PA or APRN who routinely takes patient histories, conducts physical examinations, and assists in treating patients of a physician or group of physicians can be required to maintain a log of those patients for assessment purposes. Additionally, as more organizations transition to computerized patient records, information related to clinical activity will become more readily available, as these systems can identify all practitioners who access and document in the patient record. The routine screening of AHPs' performance through the regular performance improvement process can also be used for this purpose. The certified registered nurse anesthetist (CRNA) and nurse-midwife (NM) are good examples of the types of personnel who are candidates for this kind of review. Several examples of screening tools that can be used for this purpose can be found on the CD that accompanies the book.

Information from screening clinical performance should be compiled with any other available information such as incident reports, patient or staff complaints, and the information displayed on a reappointment profile. This reappointment information should be routed through the department—first to the credentials and executive committees for recommendations, and then to the governing body for final action in the same manner as a medical staff reappointment. Performance data with regard to the practitioner in question must be included.

■ Maintaining Expirables

The MSSD or human resources department, whichever is applicable, will also be responsible for maintaining current documents for AHPs. These documents, which expire periodically, may include those related to licensure, certification, registration, narcotics registration(s), and professional liability insurance.

■ Due Process for AHPs

All licensed independent practitioners who have clinical privileges have the same rights to a hearing and appeal of an adverse recommendation regarding membership or privileges that are available to medical staff members. Because the majority of AHPs are not licensed independent practitioners and are not members of the medical staff, they do not have the same rights to due process that medical staff members do. Nevertheless, some form of due process should be available to an AHP whose privileges have been reduced, terminated, or otherwise negatively affected. This process can be different from that available to medical staff members. For example, the process could be a grievance process similar to that available to employees of a hospital. Steps in the process might include the following measures:

- Notice to the AHP of adverse recommendation, with the right to request an interview
- An interview before a committee in which the AHP can present information relevant to the specifics of the adverse recommendation
- A record of the interview, which is forwarded to the medical executive committee for a recommendation
- A recommendation that is forwarded to the governing body, whose action is final

AHPs who are employed by the organization will have access to the HR grievance process.

■ Conclusion

Simplification of the process of credentialing AHPs (other than PAs and APRNs) can eliminate many of the headaches associated with this sometimes onerous process. Significant consideration should be given to discontinuing the practice of credentialing and privileging AHPs other than PAs and APRNs. It is a much less complicated process to authorize these professionals to perform in the organization through a job description or scope of practice. And the hospital will not be required to perform focused professional practice evaluation and ongoing professional practice evaluation for AHPs who have not been granted privileges, but function under a job description or scope of practice. Physicians will probably welcome this change, as they generally don't understand why they have been giving privileges to a dental assistant who has completed only on-the-job training and whose previous employment was at a pizza parlor. If you have not already done so, consider approaching organization leadership (administrative and medical staff) to see whether this change would be entertained.

■ Web Sites

American Academy of Nurse Practitioners: www.aanp.org
Advanced Nursing Credentialing Center: www.nursingworld.org/ancc
American Academy of Physician Assistants: www.aapa.org
National Commission on Certification of Physician Assistants: www.nccpa.org
American Association of Nurse Anesthetists: www.aana.com/crna
American Academy of Audiology: www.audiology.com
American Board of Cardiology Perfusion: www.abcp.org
American Academy of Cardiovascular Perfusion: http://theaacp.addr.com/
National Association of Clinical Nurse Specialists: www.nacns.org
American Psychological Association: www.apa.org
American Dental Assistants Association: www.dentalassistant.org
Association of Social Work Boards: www.aswb.org
National Association of Social Workers: www.naswcd.org
American College of Nurse Midwives: www.midwife.org
AACNM Certification Council: www.accmidwife.org
American Physical Therapy Association: www.apta.org
American Board of Physical Therapy Specialists: www.apta.org/Education/specialist/ABPTSCert
Association of Operating Room Nurses: www.aorn.org
Association of Surgical Technologists: www.ast.org
Certification Board of Perioperative Nursing: www.cc-institute.org/

■ Notes

1. The Joint Commission. "Human Resources Standards," in *2009 Accreditation Manual for Hospitals*. Oakbrook Terrace, IL: Author: 2009.
2. California Code of Regulations, Title 22, Division 5, Chapter 1, Article 7, §70706.

CHAPTER 9

The Managed Care Credentials Process

Christina W. Giles, CPMSM, MS

■ Background on the Managed Care Credentials Process

The National Committee for Quality Assurance (NCQA) issued its first credentialing standards for health maintenance organizations (HMOs) in 1991, prompting organizations across the United States to examine their credentialing systems to decide the most cost-effective and efficient method of meeting the tough new NCQA standards. This section summarizes the basic credentialing requirements in managed care organizations (MCOs) and addresses the current NCQA standards and methods of compliance.

Prior to 1991, when NCQA issued its first accreditation standards, many HMOs and MCOs relied on contracted hospitals to furnish credentialing information about their networks of physicians. The common assumption was that if a hospital performed its credentialing activities in accordance with Joint Commission standards, its staff physicians were qualified and competent to practice medicine and, therefore, competent to treat HMO/MCO patients.

The legal climate permitting this practice was soon to change. Prior to 1989, under corporate liability doctrine, an HMO was not held liable for the actions of its providers. Two landmark cases that year changed this practice. In a Pennsylvania case, *Boyd v. Einstein Medical Center*, the practitioner was judged to be an "ostensible agent" of the HMO, and the HMO was held liable for Boyd's actions. In another 1989 lawsuit, *Harrell v. Total Health Care, Inc.*, a Missouri court ruled that the HMO was liable for failure to credential a practitioner. Coupled with reporting requirements under the 1986 Health Care Quality Improvement Act, HMOs began to fall under the scrutiny of outside agencies.

Additionally, HMOs publish provider directories that list individual practitioners and organizations providing care and treatment to HMO members, and restricting access to practitioners not contracted by the HMO.

Taken in combination, these forces placed a burden on MCOs to establish credentialing systems that would thoroughly scrutinize the quality of practitioners

With thanks to Joyce Gardner, who wrote the previous edition of this chapter.

providing care to their members. The credentialing system in an MCO should be thorough and sufficiently inclusive to avoid potential liability exposure, as well as to assure that practitioners presented to MCO members in the provider directory are competent and qualified in the specialty they practice, and work well within the managed care system.

■ Types of Managed Care Organizations

A managed care organization is an organization (company) that is placed between the patient (member) and the physician, and may dictate which medical services the patient receives and from whom. These organizations generally fall into three main categories: health maintenance organization (HMO), preferred provider organization (PPO), and physician–hospital organization (PHO).

Health Maintenance Organization

An HMO is a group of facilities, physicians, and other healthcare personnel organized in a single system that provides comprehensive medical services to a specifically enrolled population for a fixed fee. The fixed fee (premium), paid in advance by employers to the MCO, is then paid to practitioners as a fixed monthly fee (called capitation) to provide the entire spectrum of care to the member (patient). Practitioners (usually primary care physicians) assume financial risk in this arrangement and act as gatekeepers for access to all other care the patient receives.

There are several models of HMOs, all designed to deliver a full range of medical care to members.

Preferred Provider Organization

A PPO is composed of healthcare providers who contract with a payer to provide health care at predetermined fixed rates. Usually working under a fee-for-service arrangement, the physician or hospital does not assume any financial risk. In a PPO arrangement, the fees are usually discounted from "usual and customary" charges.

Physician–Hospital Organization

A PHO is composed of healthcare providers who have formed an organization with one or more hospitals; the PHO contracts with various payers (on behalf of the providers and the hospitals) to provide care. PHOs may provide administrative services to an HMO's members as well. Some of these services include credentialing of the PHO's own network of healthcare practitioners, utilization review, practice management, and a wide array of other services.

The NCQA Accreditation Process

In 2004, NCQA transitioned from a paper-based, labor-intensive accreditation process to an interactive survey system (ISS). The ISS is an automated desktop review system, wherein the organization seeking accreditation submits documentation of its compliance with NCQA's standards over a secure electronic line. Through a sophisticated interactive process, NCQA's staff then works with the organization to determine its compliance with each standard. Everything is completed prior to the site review except actual hands-on file audits and review of documents not able to be transmitted electronically. As a result of the adoption of the ISS, the on-site portion of accreditation surveys has been reduced substantially. For most MCOs, the on-site portion of the survey now lasts just one to three days. For credentials verification organizations (CVOs), the on-site portion is usually one day.

Credentialing Standards

Numerous organizations—NCQA, the Joint Commission, Centers for Medicare and Medicaid Services (CMS), and URAC, among others—have issued standards for credentialing. Not surprisingly, their requirements are not all identical. Some differences are very subtle, whereas others are more readily apparent. Generally, a good rule of thumb is to select the highest standards and comply with them.

NCQA's standards for accreditation are comprehensive and detailed and cover the entire scope of an MCO's operations. They contain specific requirements for credentialing and cover policies and procedures, elements requiring primary source verification and accepted sources for the verification, timelines for processing applications, application content, and other specific details. At the time of an NCQA survey, organizations must achieve a high percentage of compliance with the standards for primary source verification to garner full certification or accreditation for the credentialing function.

Many functions, including credentialing, may be delegated to another entity that performs the services on behalf of the MCO. NCQA has very specific requirements for the contractual arrangement between these entities, and the delegated entity (doing the work on behalf of the MCO) must comply with all of NCQA's standards for the MCO to achieve accreditation.

NCQA's credentialing requirements do not include clinical privileging, but rather state only that a practitioner must be fully trained in his or her specialty, as represented in the MCO's publications. The Joint Commission requires the necessary resources (equipment and personnel) to support the requested privilege and practitioner-specific clinical privileges. MCOs may establish any requirement that exceeds NCQA's standards—such as requiring a copy of a professional liability certificate or board certification, but those requirements are not surveyed or accredited elements under NCQA's credentialing standards. Standards should be viewed as a performance measure to obtain accreditation, not the highest level of performance to aspire to. Many MCOs exceed NCQA's standards—not just in credentialing, but other areas as well. The same holds true for healthcare organizations seeking Joint Commission, URAC, or CMS accreditation.

NCQA does not require practitioners to be board certified in their specialty. Instead, it requires only that the highest level of training be verified, and that a practitioner's training match his or her specialty listed in the MCO's publications. If a practitioner is board certified, the MCO is required to verify that certification; verification of education and training leading to the board certification does not require verification. The Joint Commission requires that all relevant training be verified. Additionally, NCQA requires that practitioners attest that they do or do not have professional liability coverage and hospital privileges; the Joint Commission requires evidence of an unusual pattern or an excessive number of professional liability actions resulting in a final judgment against the applicant.[1]

■ Practitioner Credentialing

There is no uniform national definition of which types of healthcare professionals are classified as allied health professionals (AHPs). In the managed care setting, a practitioner who is not a physician may be referenced as an AHP.

NCQA began to require credentialing of certain nonphysician healthcare professionals in 1997. Its official interpretation is that under the MCO standards, NCQA does not specifically review files of practitioners other than physicians (MDs and DOs), dentists, chiropractors, and podiatrists. It does have a managed behavioral healthcare organization accreditation program that requires credentialing of the following types of providers:

- Psychiatrists and physicians certified in addiction medicine
- Doctoral and/or master's-level psychologists who are state certified or state licensed
- Master's-level clinical social workers who are state certified or stated licensed
- Master's-level clinical nurse specialists or psychiatric nurse practitioners who are nationally or state certified or state licensed
- Other behavioral healthcare specialists who are licensed, certified to, or registered by the state to practice independently [2]

The 2009 NCQA managed care standards refer to practitioners who must be credentialed as nonphysician practitioners, who have an independent relationship with the MCO or who provide care under the MCO's medical benefits. Many organizations use the directory listing as the definitive issue for contracting. Also, URAC requires all providers listed in directories, whether practitioners or facilities, to undergo credentialing and recredentialing. In addition, MCOs need to review state statutes and any other applicable standards to determine what needs to be done and where.

NCQA does not require the MCO to credential practitioners who have any of the following characteristics:

- Individuals who practice exclusively in the inpatient hospital setting or ambulatory free-standing facilities and who provide care for MCO members only as a result of the members being directed to the hospital or facility.
- Hospital-based practitioners who see members only because of their independent relationship with the MCO.
- Dentists who provide primary dental care only under a dental plan or rider.
- Covering practitioners (e.g., *locum tenens* practitioners) who are hired specifically to provide out-of-area care, and there are no incentives communicated. MCO members have no obligation to seek care from rental network practitioners and may see any out-of-area practitioner.
- Individuals who do not provide care for members in a treatment setting (e.g., board-certified consultants).[3]

The MCO's documentation (policies) must address the scope of practitioners covered, criteria and primary source verification of information used to meet the criteria, the process used to make decisions, and the extent of any delegated credentialing or recredentialing arrangements.

If a healthcare organization chooses to use a CVO to verify the credentials of its healthcare practitioners, there should be confirmation that the CVO selected understands how to perform verifications for all types of healthcare professionals whom the organization must credential.

Credentialing Committee

NCQA standards require each MCO to designate a credentialing committee to make recommendations about professional qualifications of its practitioners. The MCO may decide to delegate the responsibility to "credential" to another entity. If it takes this step, this responsibility must be clearly defined in the delegation agreement. NCQA requirements govern the composition of the credentialing committee, with the goal being to ensure that the network's primary care and specialty composition is represented appropriately on the credentialing committee.

Application

Each MCO develops a credentialing application, tailored to its individual needs and requirements. Many states have developed mandated, uniform application forms. Information gathered on the application includes demographics, work history, practice information, and any other information deemed necessary by the credentialing organization. NCQA has added specific requirements to its standards for applications, and those must be present and met for an organization to receive "credit" for its application content. MCOs may design their own application and may gather far more information than required by NCQA, but the application must always contain information that is current and complete to receive "credit" from NCQA.

Standardized Credentialing Applications

The Council for Affordable Quality Healthcare (CAQH) is a not-for-profit alliance of health plans and networks that promotes collaborative initiatives to help make health care more affordable, share knowledge to improve the quality of care, and make administration easier for physicians and their patients. CAQH has initiated the use of the universal credentialing data source, which is intended to "streamline the credentialing process by eliminating the need for multiple credentialing applications."[4] This free, online service enables providers to complete one standardized application to meet the credentialing needs of participating health plans and other healthcare organizations.

CAQH does not verify the information submitted through its online form, and no data that have been provided by the practitioner are checked for accuracy. Further, there is no guarantee of periodic updates being performed, except for the client reviewing the dates on the attestations provided by the practitioner during the data updates. This highly sophisticated technology can be electronically downloaded and, with proper interfaces, the data can be uploaded into client systems.

Primary Source Verification

Organizations providing credentialing services must adopt sources to be used for primary verification and include them in their credentialing policies and procedures. Primary sources are initiating sources—that is, the verification comes directly from the source issuing the credential and not via another party unless the third party is deemed to be a primary source. For example, board certification may be verified directly from the board issuing the certificate. At the same time, the American Board of Medical Specialties (ABMS) is an organization that obtains board certification from all boards and is considered to be primary source for board certifications. A copy of a board certificate, presented by a practitioner with his or her application, is not primary source verification because it did not come from the issuing source, but rather from the practitioner who copied the document.

Verification in a credentials file may be electronic, written, or verbal; verbal verifications must be documented in the credentials file with the date the verification was received, the name of the person from whom the verification was received, and the credentialing professional who received the verification. Internet verifications may be used provided they meet the criteria for primary source.

A caveat of the NCQA's primary source verification requirement is that certain credentialing elements are current at the time of the credentialing committee's decision and verified within the 180 days prior to the decision. Static credentials, such as medical school graduation and residency completion, are not included in this requirement; the rationale is that once these elements are verified, they do not change. (Board certifications generally last for a time-limited period; if the certification expires during the credentialing activity, it must be verified.) The Joint Commission requires only that applications be processed within a reasonable period of time; medical staff bylaws may establish a time limit for processing an application, in which case an organization would be required to complete processing within that time period. As with all standards, an MCO may elect to require its application processing to be completed in fewer than 180 days.

The elements required by NCQA for primary source verification are a valid license to practice, a valid Drug Enforcement Agency (DEA) or Controlled Dangerous Substance (CDS) certificate (as applicable), and the highest level of education. Board certification must be verified if the practitioner states that he or she is board certified on the application. (Despite occasional rumors to the contrary, NCQA does not require board certification of physicians; each MCO establishes its own criteria for participation in its network of practitioners, and board certification may or may not be one.)

Not all verifications need be obtained by letter from the credentialing entity to the verifying source. More information on this topic is located in the section of this chapter entitled "Managing Credentialing Operations."

Work History

Primary source verification of work history is not required by NCQA. NCQA does require that work history be documented and that gaps in the applicant's work history (generally gaps of six months or longer) be investigated and documented in the credentials file.

NCQA's 180-Day Rule

NCQA standards require that information presented to the credentials committee be no more than 180 days old at the time of committee review. NCQA calculates the 180 days from the date of the credentialing committee's decision backward; therefore, nothing in the file can be more than 180 days old at the time of committee decision. If an application is presented to the credentialing committee in one month, is deferred for further information, and comes back in two months, the 180 days is calculated from the date of the decision, not the date on which the application was presented the first time. If the application was signed 30, 60, or 90 days prior to its being forwarded to the credentialing department, the 180-day "clock" has been ticking for that amount of time.

While verifications must be no more than 180 days old at the time of committee review, the attestation statement is valid for 365 calendar days up to the time of the credentialing committee's decision. For a CVO, this element is valid to within 305 calendar days prior to submission of the credentials file to the client. The only exception is for MCO/PPO Medicare Advantage (MA), for which the time period remains 180 days. In such cases, CVOs must negotiate a time frame for submission of the credentials file for credentials committee review.

To see how this works, consider the following example: Dr. Doe has been contacted and has indicated an interest in affiliation with the health plan. The provider relations department sends a request to the credentialing department to check whether there are any disciplinary actions against Dr. Doe's license The credentialing department verifies the license and maintains a record of the verification. Three weeks later, Dr. Doe's completed application is received. The verification of the license was done just three weeks prior, and the attestation statement on the application was signed just a week prior and is valid for 180 days; therefore, the license verification is the "oldest" element in the application.

Credentialing professionals must be alert to any circumstance that might cause an element of the application to "fall out" of the 180-day cycle—NCQA reviews each credentialing element in a file separately for compliance with the 180-day requirement. Documents with an expiration date, such as licenses, are also reviewed for currency at the time of the credentialing decision.

Office Site Reviews

Unlike hospitals and other Joint Commission–accredited facilities, most care delivered on behalf of an MCO is done within practitioner offices. For this reason, NCQA requires MCOs to ensure that the offices of all practitioners meet requirements for physical accessibility, physical appearance, adequacy of waiting and examining room space, availability of appointments, and adequacy of treatment record keeping. The MCO must also have mechanisms to ensure that any deficiencies in the office environment are identified and corrected on an ongoing basis.

Recredentialing

MCOs are required to have an ongoing and up-to-date recredentialing process that is completed at least every three years. Hospitals and other Joint Commission–accredited organizations are required to complete recredentialing every two years. Hence, if an organization performs credentialing for both NCQA and the Joint Commission, it would, in all probability, complete recredentialing every two years and thus be compliant with both accreditors.

Performance Monitoring

The purpose of recredentialing is to evaluate a practitioner's professional performance and competence during the previous three years. Development of a practitioner profile to carry out objective evaluation of performance is helpful in making this determination. For primary care practitioners, MCOs must review data from member complaints and information from quality improvement activities.

The manner in which MCOs gather member complaints and information from quality improvement activities varies from plan to plan. Whatever process is chosen, the plan must be able to demonstrate that the information was available to the credentialing committee and was considered when the committee members made their recommendation regarding the applicant's continued participation with the plan.

Once the recredentialing information is gathered and primary verification of the file is complete, the entire file is subjected to the peer review process. Each MCO develops criteria for review of the recredentialing information. NCQA requires that this review be performed by a credentialing committee, whose recommendation is the final decision.

Ongoing Monitoring of Sanctions and Complaints

With recredentialing occurring every three years (rather than every two years), it is incumbent upon MCOs to review the appropriate data bases for sanctions and complaints between recredentialing cycles. NCQA requires MCOs to review, at a minimum, Medicare/Medicaid sanctions, sanctions or limitations on licensure, and member complaints. To do so, MCOs must collect and review information from identified adverse events received by the organization. These sources must be reviewed regularly (within 30 days of their publication), and the MCO must take corrective action when instances of poor quality are identified.

Organizational Providers

In addition to the policies and procedures described for practitioners, MCOs maintain policies and procedures covering organizational providers with whom it contracts. Such organizations include, but are not limited to, hospitals, home health agencies, skilled nursing facilities, nursing homes, behavioral health facilities, and other entities that the MCO uses to provide services to its members.

■ Contracting Versus Credentialing

Contracting and credentialing are not the same thing, and the processes used to complete these tasks may be completely separate. *Credentialing* is the verification and evaluation of professional competence by the MCO. *Contracting* is a business decision to enter into a legal arrangement with a practitioner (or group of practitioners) to supply certain services to the MCO's members. Although contracting with the provider may be desirable, the practitioner may not be able to pass a rigid credentialing evaluation process. Therefore, decisions to contract should be contingent upon the applicant's approval by the credentialing committee.

■ Managing Credentialing Operations

Even when an MCO has clearly defined policies for credentialing and recredentialing that have been approved by the governing body, the challenge of managing the credentialing department must still be met. The organization's policies provide a framework to design a system of operation; the procedures fill in this framework with actual operational processes to successfully complete credentialing and recredentialing of applicants.

A credentialing or medical staff services professional must understand operational issues to successfully manage credentialing systems. When presented with the challenge of assuming responsibility for credentialing in a managed care entity, the credentialing professional is immediately faced with several major decisions—compliance with the NCQA standards, including the 180-day rule; health plan reporting requirements; and the decision of whether to perform credentialing internally or externally. The issue of staffing a credentialing department cannot be adequately addressed until the decision is made to provide services either internally (by MCO staff members) or externally (through delegation to an outside agency).

Internal Versus External Credentialing Operations

Managed care credentialing presents numerous challenges to the credentialing professional at all levels—manager, coordinator, specialist, assistant, or any other position that is related to the credentials process. First and foremost, the decision of whether to manage the network's credentialing internally or to delegate this responsibility to external entities must be made. The credentialing department often does not make this decision alone. Factors that influence this decision may include economic issues, political issues, or simply business decisions not related to credentialing functions.

If the decision is made to delegate credentialing to an external entity, the operational challenges within the MCO's credentialing department focus on areas quite different from those that arise when the credentialing functions are managed internally. It is important for the credentialing coordinator or specialist to understand both of these processes completely so that he or she can manage either scenario effectively. It is common in a managed care credentialing department both to assign internal credentialing responsibilities and to establish external, delegated

234   CHAPTER 9   The Managed Care Credentials Process

contracts. A single provider may be internal and external, may delegate responsibilities to more than one entity, and may participate with one or more network product lines; likewise, his or her credentialing may be handled internally for one entity and externally for another. We will examine the operational aspects of these situations, one at a time.

Internal Credentialing

The term *internal credentialing* refers to credentialing operations that are carried out in a managed care credentialing department. Unfortunately, there are no clear, unified definitions of internal credentialing, external credentialing, and centralized credentialing. For now, we will consider internal credentialing to entail credentialing of a network of practitioners performed by the MCO's credentialing department.

Credentialing of a practitioner begins either simultaneously or immediately following the decision to contract with that specific practitioner to deliver services to the enrolled members of the MCO. Communication between the individuals responsible for contracting and those responsible for credentialing is absolutely essential if the two processes are to coexist and perform each of their respective functions.

Centralized Credentialing

Centralized credentialing may be a somewhat confusing term that describes credentialing done by one entity for several other entities. An in-depth discussion on centralized credentialing is found in Chapter 10.

■ Automation

Managed care organizations tend to have thousands of providers in their networks. It is virtually impossible to credential (and recredential) such large numbers of providers without an automated system. Primary source verification is very easily automated using computer databases or "Web crawlers." Web crawlers are able to perform the verification function without initiation by a human being. These databases may be purchased from one of the many software companies that have developed excellent programs designed to generate letters, track receipt of responses, query the National Practitioner Data Bank (NPDB) and the Healthcare Integrity and Protection Data Bank (HIPDB), generate profiles used for credentials committee consideration. and perform all other functions related to the credentialing process. Many credentialing departments and CVOs with thousands of providers are moving to completely electronic credentials files because storing and saving many years of credentialing history on thousands of practitioners demands storage space that is simply too expensive and too large to be efficient.

Credentialing and recredentialing can generate literally thousands of documents to be tracked, recorded, and evaluated. The software system should be capable of not only generating the necessary correspondence, but also tracking and generating reports to identify missing elements in a given credentials file. It is possible to eliminate paper documents altogether—the credentials file can be completely electronic. Thanks to modern technology's scanning capabilities, and with tracking and recording done electronically, the cumbersome, expensive, and less efficient paper file can be replaced by an electronic file. Many verifications are available online, and fax verifications are as frequent as mailed documents. Given these tremendous enhancements to the verification process, credentialing has become mainstream high tech. It is up to each individual credentialing department to decide whether it is more cost-efficient to develop the credentialing database in-house or to purchase a commercial product.

Documenting Verification

NCQA, the Joint Commission, and URAC all permit written, electronic, and verbal verification of credentialing elements. To expedite processing of an application, credentialing managers must make decisions regarding the most expeditious method to verify these elements; once verified, they must be tracked and continuously monitored against NCQA's 180-day requirement.

Written Verification (Letters)

Letter writing for verification of credentialing elements is probably the most time-consuming of the various methods for verification. "Snail mail" may take from two weeks to three months to complete a request/response exchange. Credentialing professionals whose credentialing process consists of writing letters face the challenge of constantly monitoring replies from letters written, sending second requests, and waiting for a response to the second request, while keeping a watchful eye on NCQA's 180-day requirement. The fax machine and desktop faxing are valuable tools that can expedite the written verification process. Faxed documents are generally acceptable, although specific standards governing the credentialing process should be reviewed for specific interpretation regarding faxes.

Electronic Verification

A far more efficient method of verifying credentials is through electronic queries sent to the many data sources that are acceptable to accrediting agencies. All that is needed to verify credentialing elements electronically is Internet access and agreements with various entities that allow direct communication to the database. For example, electronic verification is supported by most state licensing boards. In such a case, the state allows access to its licensing information through an electronic interface that the MCO uses to access the board's data. An agreement may be necessary before the MCO can obtain the data, because the licensing board databases may not available to the general public through electronic interface. Some state licensing boards allow public access to their databases, but the information available in those resources is limited to the general public; more comprehensive data may be available to healthcare organizations using password-protected access.

Another example of electronic verification can be seen with the database that verifies DEA certification. This database is operated by the National Technical Information Service (NTIS), and access to it is available through an annual subscription to the service. Access to updates depends on the level of subscription that is purchased. The data received by the NTIS are actually downloaded from the DEA's files.

Board certification can be verified through some, but not all, specialty boards. The American Board of Family Medicine, for example, makes verification data available through its Web site. Again, an agreement is required before a password is issued to access board Web sites. A word of caution is in order when considering electronic board certification: Not all specialty board Web sites are acceptable primary sources. Users should research the requirements for a particular accrediting or certifying agency before using an electronic database to be certain that the database is acceptable to the applicable agency.

Verbal Verification (Telephone)

Verbal verification—that is, confirmation by telephone call (most likely) or personal contact—is an acceptable form of verification under NCQA standards. Verbal verification can significantly reduce the time required for obtaining verification data. Documentation of the verification should include the information verified, the name and/or title of the person supplying the information, the date of verification, and the signature/initials of the person who verified the information.

Process Management

Because the entire credentialing process in an MCO is driven by the 180-day rule, process management becomes pivotal to a successful credentialing program. Efficient process management is directly tied to the ability of the department to complete processing of each file within NCQA's 180-day time limit, or to recognize when an application is outside the allotted 180 days and bring it into compliance. Numerous other processes must also be considered as part of credentialing management, such as synching recredentialing dates throughout the system (if the system is centralized), managing expiring information/documents, and complying with health plan reporting requirements.

Organization of the Credentialing Department

The organizational structure of a credentialing department will vary among MCOs. Most commonly, the credentials function is organized within the quality management department, reflecting the fact that it is viewed as a quality function. It is not unusual for a credentialing department to be organized as part of the provider relations department, however, so that the contracting and credentialing functions have the same reporting pathway. Because contracting and credentialing goals conflict with each other, having one executive take responsibility for both functions is not always practical, however.

Examples of descriptions of the credentialing manager and credentialing specialist positions are included on the CD that accompanies this book. The size of the organization, along with management decisions about how to best manage the process, will inevitably drive the actual organizational structure of the credentialing department.

Credentialing Manager

The credentialing manager is the individual who has overall management responsibility for the entire credentialing process. This position requires an individual with knowledge and experience in credentialing and process management, as well as the ability to assign and reassign duties so as to carry out the entire process in the most efficient way possible. The credentialing manager interacts with external customers, including physicians, allied health practitioners, potential delegated entities, and physician organization management. He or she also shoulders the responsibility of complying with mandates established by regulatory agencies such as NCQA, the Joint Commission, URAC, and state and federal entities.

Credentialing Coordinator

The credentialing coordinator may be assigned team leader responsibilities in larger organizations, or he or she may assume many responsibilities of the department manager if the reporting structure assigns these responsibilities to the coordinator rather than to the manager. Credentialing coordinators need extensive knowledge about credentialing functions and should be able to efficiently manage a group of credentialing specialists or verifiers. This position may provide oversight to credentialing specialists and verifiers and assist in that process as necessary.

Credentialing Specialist or Verifier

This position is filled by the true "foot soldiers" of the credentialing verification operation. Individual credentialing specialists may be assigned to handle an application from its receipt to completion of the credentialing process, or they may work in specialized teams for verification. Examples of roles on verification teams include members who verify only hospital privileges, members who verify only licenses, and so on. This kind of teamwork is common in very large organizations that receive thousands of applications for credentials, such as large CVOs and centralized credentials operations. In most MCOs where credentialing is done internally, one or two credentialing specialists or verifiers process an application from receipt to completion.

■ State and Federal Requirements

Once NCQA, the Joint Commission, or URAC requirements are met, the credentialing professional might assume that the credentialing program would withstand any inspection, review, or criticism by other regulating agencies. Unfortunately, this is not always the case. Most states have requirements governing credentialing activities, and federal programs have their own requirements. These requirements may not always be in sync with one another. The same rule that applies to conflicts between accrediting agencies also applies to local, state, and federal law: The higher rule always takes precedent. Just as state law takes precedent over municipal code, and federal law takes precedent over state law, so does state and federal law take precedent over NCQA, the Joint Commission, and URAC standards.

Remember, accreditation is voluntary—that is, the law does not require it even though it may be recognized as evidence that an organization is in compliance with state or federal law if all accreditation standards are met. This qualification is known as "deemed status." The federal government grants deemed status to hospitals with the Joint Commission accreditation; these institutions are deemed to be in full compliance with Medicare's Conditions of Participation.

Deemed status is not automatic and is not granted by all states to entities operating within their jurisdiction, or by the federal government to all entities covered by its standards and requirements. It is important to research state and federal regulations covering the activities and to review policies and procedures to ascertain that they are in compliance on all levels.

■ Notes

1. The Joint Commission., *2009 Hospital Accreditation Standards.* Oakbrook Terrace, IL: Author; 2009: Medical Staff Standards, MS .06.01.05, Element 9, p. 205.
2. National Committee for Quality Assurance (NCQA). *2009 HP Standards and Guidelines, Credentialing Standards,* July 2009.
3. National Committee for Quality Assurance, note 2.
4. Council for Affordable Quality Healthcare (CAQH). "Universal Provider Datasource." Available at: http://www.caqh.org/ucd.php. Accessed August 17, 2009.

Health System Credentialing and Credentials Verification Organizations

CHAPTER 10

Margaret Palmer, MSA, CPMSM, CPCS

■ Credentialing in a Healthcare System

Many healthcare systems have established centralized credentialing organizations. The first section in the chapter explores some basic principles of credentialing in a healthcare system.

What Is a Healthcare System?

For purposes of this chapter, a healthcare system is defined as an integrated delivery system consisting of hospitals, other facilities, and services (which may include ambulatory care facilities, long-term care facilities, home health, medical groups, and health plans, among others) that are related by a corporate structure or through management agreements. Healthcare systems can be either for-profit or not-for-profit ventures. Governance takes place through a corporate structure that may consist of one governing body or multiple boards that ultimately report to a single governing board.

What Is a Centralized Credentialing Organization?

A centralized credentialing organization provides credentialing services to all or defined components of a healthcare system. For the remainder of this chapter, the component of the organization that provides credentialing services is referred to as a centralized credentialing service (CCS) or department (CCD). For ease of reference, this department will be referred to as a credentialing department in this chapter.

Why Establish a Centralized Credentialing Department?

Healthcare systems that are interested in establishing a credentialing department usually do so because a number of hospitals or other entities within the system are

With thanks to Vicki Searcy and Madeline Schneikart, who wrote the versions of this chapter that appeared in previous editions of this book.

required to perform credentialing, and these hospitals (and other entities) may have practitioners in common. As a consequence, each entity is required to credential the same practitioners. When there is significant overlap of practitioners, it usually becomes apparent that it would be sensible to establish some type of centralization of credentialing to avoid constant duplication of effort. This structure is also appealing to the practitioners within the healthcare system, who must make applications to multiple facilities for credentials and privileges. For example, assume a healthcare system with six hospitals and one governing body in the same geographic area has a combined medical staff of 3000 practitioners. The more overlap that exists, the more compelling the rationale for establishing a credentialing department. It would not be unusual for 50% or more of the practitioners to overlap (i.e., one practitioner might have multiple relationships within the six-hospital system).

A second reason to establish a shared credentialing department is to pool the talent that it takes to perform credentialing functions. For example, each hospital in a 12-hospital system would have to employ individuals skilled in credentialing (the number needed would depend on the size of the medical staff organization of each hospital, among other factors). These individuals can be difficult to find and train. consequently, it may make sense to the system to set up a credentialing department to attract the best credentialing staff and provide training for new credentialing recruits. Each organization that makes credentialing decisions in a healthcare system, however, needs to have credentialing staff who are skilled in working with practitioners during the evaluation and decision-making process. Usually the staff who remain in the hospitals and other entities are skilled in the privileging aspect of credentialing, as well as other key functions required to be maintained at the local hospital level. In contrast, the staff who work in the credentialing department are skilled at data management and verification procedures.

A third reason that healthcare systems create credentialing departments is to establish consistent credentialing methods for all entities within the system. Consider once again the example of the six-hospital system in the same geographic area with a single governing body. If there is no credentialing department, that governing body would most likely receive multiple recommendations for the same practitioners (e.g., one practitioner might apply to three of the medical staffs). One hospital might have more extensive credentialing procedures than other hospitals in the system. Perhaps one of the hospitals requires four peer references for initial appointment, another hospital requires three, and the rest require one. Many other inconsistencies could crop up that would not make sense to the governing body. These inconsistencies could lead to disparate recommendations from the various entities for the same practitioner. When these circumstances occur, governing bodies frequently recommend that, at the very least, credentialing policies and procedures be consistent among all the entities within the system. In many cases, this leads to establishment of a credentialing department.

How Does an Organization Establish a Shared Credentialing Department?

It is critical that the organization's intent be clear from the beginning concerning which services will be provided by the credentialing department, how it will relate to the facilities/entities within the healthcare system, and what its major roles and responsibilities are to set the expectations for the scope of services to be provided by the credentialing department and how the credentialing department will function from the very beginning. Many credentialing departments have failed because the organization failed to clarify its intent in establishing a centralized credentialing operation. The following key issues must always be addressed:

- Customers of the credentialing department
- Regulatory requirements that must be met
- Scope of services to be provided by the credentialing department
- Relationship of the credentialing department to its customers
- Location of the credentialing department
- Credentialing software
- Operating policies and procedures
- Ability/potential to expand services

Customers of the Credentialing Department

The customers of the credentialing department may include hospitals, long-term care facilities, a physician–hospital organization (PHO) that contracts with managed care entities, and ambulatory care facilities. All customers must be identified so as to carefully craft the "work product" that will be provided to all the customers of the credentialing department.

The customers of the credentialing department often form a users group that meets periodically (at least annually) to review operating manuals, scope of data required, verification sources to be used, changes in accreditation standards and/or state or federal laws or requirements, policies, procedures, and other issues that the users group has in common.

Regulatory Requirements

Once the customers of the credentialing department are known, the regulatory requirements that relate to credentialing should be fairly easy to determine. In most organizations, these regulatory requirements will include the Joint Commission accreditation requirements for the specific type of organization (e.g., hospital, long-term care, ambulatory care), Medicare's Conditions of Participation (COP) for hospitals, and the National Commission on Quality Assurance's (NCQA's) requirements for the managed care components. Additional accreditation bodies could be factored in as well, such as the Accreditation Association for Ambulatory Health

Care (AAAHC), URAC, Healthcare Facilities **Accreditation** Program (HFAP), and a relatively new entrant on the accreditation scene, Det Norske Veritis (DNV). See Chapter 2 for additional information on accrediting bodies.

The regulatory requirements will be one of the drivers of the services that are provided by the credentialing department. If a healthcare system is required to meet, for example, Joint Commission, Medicare COP, hospital licensing, and NCQA requirements, all of these requirements will be factored in when the scope and methods of verifications to be performed by the credentialing department are determined.

Scope of Services of the Credentialing Department

One of the mistakes that healthcare systems frequently make when establishing credentialing departments is to place within the credentialing department at least some credentialing processes that cannot be standardized across all the customers of the organization. The more work that the credentialing department performs that is unique to one or more facilities, the more likely it is that the credentialing department will fail to achieve the organization's goals. Those portions of the credentialing process that can be performed by the credentialing department include items that are standardized across participating organizations (customers of the shared service). Therefore, the two elements that are most often successfully shared are application management and verifications. Other elements of the credentialing process that are unique to each customer (i.e., pre-application screening, privileging, practitioner quality profiling, proctoring, and the mechanism for evaluating practitioners' current competence as it relates to privileges requested) should remain with the customers of the shared service.

Once a shared service is established that meets all regulatory requirements (e.g., those established by NCQA and the Joint Commission), and the quality profiling processes and decision-making mechanisms are well defined and functional, the healthcare system can seek delegation from health plans. Delegation is a process through which a health plan reviews the organizational process for credentialing and agrees to delegate decision-making authority to the organization. If properly managed, it can result in more rapid contract activation and earlier initiation of revenue streams.

Because the focus of the credentialing department is collection of practitioner information, data entry, data verification, and dissemination of results, the organization has an opportunity to create a service that yields excellent data integrity. The credentialing database can be utilized to drive other business applications such as referral services, contracting, claims processing, and billing functions, thereby eliminating duplication of effort in other departments. Additionally, use of a single database can assist in the elimination of reconciliation problems.

FIGURE 10-1 shows an example of the scope of services for a shared credentialing department.

Scope of Services and Functional Organization Chart

Participating Programs
Medical/Professional Staff Services

Services Provided

- Requisition and receive credentials work product from centralized credentials department
- Coordinate receipt of quality profiles, medical record reviews, and site audits for each practitioner on required Joint Commission and/or NCQA standards, as applicable
- Coordinate and oversee documentation of credentialing evaluation and decision-making process
- Manage proctoring requirements (if applicable)
- Manage hospital privileges/peer review information and process (as applicable)
- Maintain assigned data elements in accordance with data dictionary policies and procedures
- Committee meeting management support
- Management of CME activities (if applicable)
- Financial management of application fees/dues
- Medical/professional staff administrative support

Centralized Credentials Department

Services Provided

- Application management using common application forms
- Provide credentials verification per Joint Commission and NCQA standards for initial appointment and reappointment using a blended standard
- Tracking of expirables
- Maintenance of a consolidated credentials verification file for each practitioner
- Distribution of credentials work product (i.e., audit summary report) to participating programs
- Process hospital verification requests from outside organization

Manager

- Assure that management reports and file audits reflect compliance with operating standards
- Assure that staff are well trained and knowledgeable
- Assure that systems support and sustain operating objectives
- Perform quality control on closed credentials files
- Assure customer service commitments are met

Clerical Support (1)

- Telephone
- Maintain supplies
- Open mail
- Filing

Credentials Specialists (2–3)*

- Outbound letters, requests, and queries for source verification
- Sends application (initial and reappointment) to practitioners who meet criteria for credentialing
- Assess closed practitioner files against standards

Data Entry Clerks (2)

- Data entry of application and incoming mail responses

Database Administration

- Database administrator

*May need three during start-up, depending on data cleanup, conversion aftermath, and backlogs.

FIGURE 10-1 Score of Services and Functional Organization Chart

Relationship of the Credentialing Department to Its Customers

Appropriate organizational positioning of the credentialing department can ensure its support by all current and future entities within the healthcare system enterprise. Typically, most healthcare systems seek some neutral organizational position for this unit, rather than having the credentialing department report to an administrator or medical director in one of the customer organizations (i.e., a credentialing department set up within a medical staff services department [MSSD] of one of the hospitals). In a large healthcare system, the credentialing department might report to a corporate chief medical officer or other executive. Alternatively, the credentialing department could be set up as a cost center at the corporate level, with some appropriate corporate reporting relationship on administrative matters and to a users group or joint management oversight group for purposes of monitoring quality of services provided.

Location of the Credentialing Department

Locating a credentialing department at one of the participating organizations is almost always a mistake, because roles and responsibilities often become blurred when this approach is taken. As an example, imagine a hospital MSSD that shares space with the credentialing department. Perhaps one of the key MSSD employees is sick and an important meeting needs to be covered. A staff member from the credentialing department fills in for the meeting. On the surface, this may seem to be an appropriate deployment of resources. However, when the credentialing department staff member is filling in for the MSSD employee, there is credentialing department work that isn't getting done—and it affects all the customers of the credentialing department.

For this and other reasons, the other customers of the credentialing department may feel that the participating organization where the credentialing department is located gets preferential treatment. To overcome this problem, it is recommended that the credentialing department be located in a neutral position. If the work product that is being delivered by the credentialing department to the participating organizations is electronic (the recommended medium), the credentialing department can be located most anywhere. It can truly be a "virtual" organization.

Credentialing Software

The mechanism for sharing the services provided by the credentialing department is credentialing software that operates on a wide area network or on a Web server. It is critical to obtain software that is capable of providing a central database that supports systemwide practitioner processing, with the ability to partition practitioner databases and have added functionality at each participating program.

The healthcare system should make a listing of which functions need to be supported by software and then evaluate potential products against that list.

Operating Policies and Procedures

An overview of a sample process for requisitioning and providing services follows:

1. A practitioner contacts a participating program (customer organization) with a request for membership or affiliation. The participating program performs pre-application screening via telephone interview to assess whether the practitioner meets organization-specific criteria to receive an application. If these criteria are not met, the practitioner is sent a refusal letter. If the criteria are met, the participating program forwards an e-mail to the credentialing department to initiate an application to the practitioner.
2. The credentialing department sends an application to the practitioner. When the practitioner's application is returned to the department, the staff in the credentialing department performs complete and accurate data entry/document scanning and initiates all verifications in accordance with methods that all customer organizations have agreed to, and that are in compliance with the Joint Commission, NCQA, and other regulatory requirements. This process leads to the creation of a master file on that practitioner that can be shared with other customers of the credentialing department that may also need to credential the practitioner. Additionally, the staff in the credentialing department maintains practitioner files with regard to address changes and reverification of expiring information (e.g., medical malpractice insurance, license, DEA prescribing privileges, and board certification).
3. The participating program is notified of the completion of the file and can print an audit report with scanned documents at its site. The participating program will then add additional organization-specific elements to the practitioner's file (e.g., delineation of privileges, quality profile) and route the file through its evaluation and decision-making process.
4. The use of stratified data security ensures that each participating program can view only those practitioners assigned to the program.

These policies and procedures need to be detailed in an operations manual and must be approved by all participating programs. The operations manual describes the services that will be provided by the credentialing department, the manner in which the deliverables will be provided, time frames for providing services, and the roles and responsibilities of the participating programs (i.e., how the credentialing department and the participating programs will interact).

It is beyond the scope of this chapter to provide a complete operations manual. A brief description of each item and sample language are included in the CD that accompanies this book.

Additional Tools

Scripps Health, a healthcare system located in California, has kindly agreed to share some documents that are used by its credentials verification service. The following policies are included on the CD that accompanies this book:

- Authorizing Centralized Credentialing Service
- Initial Application Processing
- Primary Source Verification
- Expirables, Ongoing Monitoring, and Global Database Management

MSSPs who have not performed credentialing within a healthcare system will note that these policies and procedures are necessarily more operational in nature than most credentialing policies and procedures written for a single medical staff organization. They are closely linked to the use of the database because it is a shared service, and all participants have to understand how the operation works and each party's role in the use of the database.

Summary of Healthcare System Credentialing

Many innovations in credentialing, such as "paperless"—or, perhaps more appropriately, "paper on demand"—credentialing, are used within healthcare systems. Indeed, a healthcare system that sets up a credentialing department that serves a large number of hospitals and other entities usually has more resources than a single medical staff services department for a hospital. Shared credentialing departments in healthcare systems often have greater access to information services within the system because the healthcare system has determined (back in the "organization's intent" phase) that the success of the shared credentialing department is a vital service to the overall success of the healthcare system.

Technology offered by credentialing software vendors has advanced over the past few years, and many features are now available to help shared credentialing departments be successful. These features include online applications, Web crawlers that automatically update specific information, and tracking mechanisms that allow large credentialing departments to track the productivity of credentialing staff. These features may very well be of interest to the single MSSD and should be investigated, particularly if the hospital has large numbers of practitioners to manage.

Sharing of peer review information also becomes a factor when a healthcare system establishes a shared credentialing service. Each state may have specific laws governing which types of information can or cannot be shared and the circumstances under which it can be shared. Healthcare systems would be well advised to check with forward-thinking, innovative legal counsel regarding these issues.

Credentials Verification Organizations

History of Credentials Verification Organizations

Many of the first credentials verification organizations (CVOs) were started by local medical societies to provide centralized credentialing services to hospitals within a limited geographic area. Physicians who were burdened by the duplication of credentialing that occurred at each hospital in which they held membership and privileges usually supported the establishment of these early CVOs. In addition, many hospitals welcomed the opportunity to participate in centralized credentialing to reduce their investment in these labor-intensive, costly, and redundant services.

The growth of centralized credentialing services was limited by several factors. One problem was the perception that the use of a centralized service would jeopardize the hospital's accreditation status. Until the late 1980s, the Joint Commission had been silent on whether information collected by a third party would be acceptable as primary source documentation. In addition, some medical staff services professionals perceived these services as a threat to their job security. Moreover, concerns about confidentiality of sensitive credentialing documents meant that many organizations were hesitant about working with CVOs.

When managed care organizations (MCOs) that sought NCQA accreditation began credentialing their practitioners in the early 1990s, the need for centralized credentialing services exploded. At that point, commercial CVOs entered the market to compete with existing medical society and healthcare association–sponsored verification services.

In addition, CVOs have been created by many healthcare systems and networks to provide credentialing services to components of their organization. For example, a healthcare system that includes multiple hospitals, a provider network, an ambulatory care center, a surgery center, and a home health agency may find it more cost-effective to create its own proprietary CVO that provides services only within the health system.

A large opportunity remains for improvement in true centralization. Thousands of hospitals and MCOs continue to duplicate requests for information on practitioners. At the same time, there are so many players that it becomes very difficult to obtain the broad level of cooperation needed to agree on processes, forms, and cycles to achieve an optimal level of centralization.

What Is a CVO?

The acronym "CVO" initially was loosely interpreted as "centralized verification organization." It eventually became defined as "credentials verification organization" when NCQA introduced a certification process for CVOs in 1996. In reality, neither term is truly accurate: CVOs can and do provide a much broader range of services than purely credentials verification.

Services Provided by CVOs

A CVO provides services to a wide variety of customers. Those customers may include hospitals, health plans, medical groups, ambulatory care facilities, insurance companies, and all derivations of MCOs.

With the use of Web-based technology, today's CVOs are not limited to providing services in a limited geographic area. Currently available technology includes many primary sources, including electronic databases that can be accessed through Internet-based queries. Other technology utilized by larger CVOs today includes electronic applications submitted online through Web-based software, electronic lookup that enables clients to view in brief or in detail the status of in-process work, and ongoing electronic monitoring for incoming sanctions against licensure and/or fraud and abuse against federally sponsored healthcare programs.

A wide variety of services are offered by CVOs, including primary source verifications for initial and recredentialing, application management services, maintenance of information subject to expiration, allied health professional credentialing, physician office site surveys, software sales and service, evaluation of files, and consulting services. Other types of services that can be provided include oversight and follow-up on the proper completion of the initial or reapplication packages, file maintenance of time-sensitive documentation, and ongoing monitoring of sanctions from licensure agencies, the Office of the Inspector General (OIG), and the General Services Administration (GSA) government-wide exclusion list.

The services that are described next are often provided by commercial CVOs as well as CVOs that are proprietary to a health system.

Monitoring of Licensure and Governmental Agency Sanctions

NCQA requires that organizations conduct ongoing monitoring of all practitioners to ensure they have not been sanctioned by either the state licensing agency or any federal agency. Data on federal sanction can be found in several federal databases, which identify providers who have been excluded from any of the federally assisted or sponsored medical insurance programs. No federal healthcare program payments may be made for any items or services furnished by an excluded provider. Providers may be excluded for a multitude of reasons, the most common of which are license revocation or suspension, program-related convictions, and patient abuse and neglect.[1] A sanction is a penalty that acts to ensure compliance with Medicare or Medicaid regulations.

Federal law requires that both the OIG (http://oig.hhs.gov/fraud/exclusions/exclusions_list.asp) and the GSA (http://epls.gov) databases be queried to confirm the good standing of practitioners participating in all federal programs, including Medicare, Medicaid, Federal Employee Health Benefits (FEHB; also known as Champus), the U.S. Department of Veterans Affairs (VA) or U.S. Department of Defense TriCare program, and the Government Employees Health Association

(GEHA). In addition, NCQA, URAC, and the Centers for Medicare and Medicaid Services (CMS) have incorporated this requirement in their respective sets of standards for both initial and recredentialing activities for practitioners and organizational credentialing. All of the previously mentioned organizations have also established standards that mandate ongoing monitoring for newly excluded provider status on a periodic basis. Given that the OIG database is updated monthly and the GSA database is updated every business day, a query of both databases every 30 days would ensure compliance with these requirements. In addition, licensure status must be checked monthly for new sanctions posted on whatever periodic basis and through whatever methodology is available in all states.

The National Practitioner Data Bank (NPDB), Healthcare Integrity and Protection Data Bank (HIPDB), Fraud and Abuse Control Information Service (FACIS), Sanction Check, and Federation of State Medical Boards (FSMB) databases identify excluded providers, as reported from the OIG, on a regular monthly basis. The GSA reports its data to the OIG. However, the OIG reports only OIG-initiated sanctions to the NPDB-HIPDB and FSMB, and the GSA data are not reported to either of these databases. Consequently, to thoroughly comply with the federal regulations, the GSA database should be queried separately at its primary Web site (http://epls.gov).

It is incumbent upon a commercial CVO to be aware of the variations in the standards that might affect the client's accreditation or certification status (whether through NCQA, the Joint Commission, URAC, Medicare's Conditions of Participation, or all of these) if the CVO is asked to assist the client with development of a primary source verification program.

Application Management Services

Application management services refer to initial application or reapplication distribution and the collection and tracking of these documents prior to performance of the verification process. The CVO will perform these services either online or via paper-based correspondence.

Management of Information Subject to Expiration

Many CVO customers find it beneficial to contract with a CVO to maintain information related to providers that expires in the intervals between credentialing decisions. For example, malpractice insurance, licensure, DEA registration, and other critical information are all subject to expiration. Healthcare organizations obviously have an interest in making sure that current information is continuously maintained. Although accreditation standards for managed care do not require maintenance of expiring documentation during the interim between recredentialing cycles, some state statutes do require this kind of ongoing monitoring.

It is interesting to note that CMS has a different standard for acute care facilities on this issue. CMS has published its intent to maintain its managed care standards in sync with NCQA and URAC. Although they have certain differences, CMS more or less follows the NCQA industry standard.

Categories of Providers to Be Credentialed

NCQA reviews the categories of providers that a CVO credentials as part of the CVO certification process. URAC expects to find a credentials verification process for all providers listed in member directories. The CMS requirements mirror the NCQA requirements. Medicaid, state statutes, worker's compensation systems, state regulations, and state departments of insurance may also have requirements for credentialing these professionals.

URAC has developed new standards for credentialing in preferred provider organizations and health maintenance organizations. This issue is discussed more fully in Chapter 9.

Physician Office Site Surveys

A CVO may be contracted to perform office site surveys for an MCO.

Evaluation of Files

Some CVOs contract to perform evaluation of files for clients. Many of these organizations are reluctant to assume the potential liability associated with file evaluation because the CVO customer may make decisions solely based on the CVO's evaluation and recommendation. Liability generally lies with recommendations for decisions and decision making, which is typically performed by the MCO.

Consulting Services

CVOs employ competent, experienced, and credentialed staff who can offer expert consulting services on designing systems and programs for credentialing activities.

■ To Outsource or Not to Outsource to a CVO

The decision whether to outsource a service traditionally performed in-house frequently involves both raw economics and more ephemeral philosophical considerations. There are numerous cost benefits to outsourcing. Even so, some believe that these advantages are outweighed by the potential for some loss of control over processes.

Cost Benefits

The cost benefit of outsourcing a labor-intensive administrative function is easy to justify. A larger CVO will have already expended the capital outlay necessary to obtain access to numerous electronic databases, which are, in some cases, expensive to install and keep current. In addition, these electronic connections require critical access to competent information systems technologists who are not always available in-house for smaller organizations. The obvious benefit is that the overhead for these installations can be shared among numerous clients rather than having individual organizations duplicate these expenses.

Costs are reduced for health plans and hospitals when the verified information can be resold numerous times. The practitioners benefit because they avoid having to complete numerous applications and provide duplicative documentation to multiple entities. Likewise, healthcare organizations benefit because their costs are lowered, and typically they receive verified information in an expedited manner.

The true potential savings to healthcare facility clients from outsourcing the credentialing function can be enormous. Time and effort must be taken to calculate the actual costs attached to the credentialing process in each healthcare organization and to perform a cost analysis that weighs the internal costs against the fees associated with a fully outsourced proposal from an external (certified) CVO.

When access to databases is shared, the fees can be spread out among numerous participating organizations rather than just one, resulting in savings for all participants. There is also the ability of a larger staff to be shifted to accommodate workflow volume fluctuations.

Turnaround Time

Turnaround time for credentialing applications is generally improved in a CVO, as individual employees are assigned certain tasks as full-time jobs. In a hospital MSSD, one individual often performs multiple tasks and, therefore, is subject to chronic distractions. In contrast, CVO credentialing staff tends to be organized functionally, thereby assuring that no other tasks are being performed and sole attention is given to the completion of the specific task assigned.

While NCQA and URAC require a 180-day turnaround time from signed attestation date by the applicant for completion of all primary source verification to the final decision by the credentialing committee, the industry standard in managed care is quite a bit less than a 180-day turnaround time. NCQA has stated that the time frame for reporting or submitting applications back to clients has changed from 120 days to 305 days. Therefore the attestation date can be older than 120 days, but not the other items of information or verification. In addition, some state statutes actually require no longer than a 60-day turnaround time, as measured from attestation date to notification of the provider of the final credentialing committee decision. Most MCOs strive for less than a 30-day turnaround time for the verification process.

■ NCQA CVO Certification Standards

In 1996, NCQA introduced a certification program for CVOs. The intent of this process is to identify CVOs that perform credentialing activities in a manner that meets NCQA credentialing standards. Managed care organizations can then contract for services with a certified CVO and be relieved of the obligation to conduct audits of the CVO's compliance with NCQA standards. The NCQA certification places a stamp of approval on the operations of the CVO, signaling that the CVO's standards for quality and choice of sources of information are consistent with NCQA's credentialing and recredentialing standards.

CVOs are surveyed by NCQA and may receive certification for a maximum of two years. They are resurveyed every two years thereafter. Limited certifications may also be issued for shorter cycles, based on the quality of the survey. In the event a CVO's certification expires while it is awaiting resurvey, NCQA extends the certification period until the new survey has taken place. The CVO is "certified" for various elements of the credentials process, with a maximum of 10 elements being approved (these elements are described later in this section). The individual elements cannot be certified if the overall survey of the CVO shows noncompliance with good business practices or an inadequate quality program. The oversight activity of the contracting entity is obviated only for those portions for which the CVO is certified. For example, if a CVO is not certified for the element of current, valid licensure to practice, then a contracting organization would have to provide oversight for the licensure verification portion of the process outsourced to the CVO.

There are 13 standards on which the CVO is reviewed.[2] The first standard relates to the CVO's written policies and procedures for verification, frequency of reporting, and data management of credentials. It is under this standard that the organization's operational activities, methods, sources, and processes are reviewed. NCQA has approved certain sources for the verification of various elements of the verification process. The certified CVO must adhere to those approved sources in its processes of verification. The CVO is required to complete all verifications within 120 days so that the client has an additional 60 days to complete the evaluation, decision making, and implementation of a practitioner into its network.

A second standard relates to the CVO's internal continuous quality improvement program. To assess compliance with this standard, the survey team reviews the CVO's written quality improvement plan or policies and procedures, looking for a defined scope of activities, defined goals and objectives, and a defined process for assessing performance. In addition, this standard requires the CVO to have a written client complaint process, an analysis of activities and the complaints process, and documentation of follow-up of identified opportunities.

A third standard requires protection of credentialing information. This standard addresses the policies and procedures related to confidentiality of both paper-based and computerized information; disposal of information; physical access security of the office and the files; appropriate orientation of staff to security and confidentiality and obtaining a signed confidentiality statement from each employee; mechanisms for electronic data management, such as password protection; systems for tracing historical changes to the database; and data backup and recovery.

Six standards relate to the verification and reporting of licensure, DEA or CDS certification, education and training, work history, malpractice history, medical board sanctions, and Medicare and Medicaid sanctions. Other standards cover the CVO-developed application and attestation processing. These standards specify elements of information to be collected from applicants and include areas of concern such as illegal drug usage, Americans with Disabilities Act (ADA) requirements concerning accommodation for disabilities, loss of licensure or felony convictions, loss or limitation of privileges, disciplinary activity, current malpractice and insurance coverage, and an attestation statement of correctness and completeness.

In addition, NCQA standards require the CVO to have policies and procedures in place for the ongoing monitoring of practitioner sanctions between recredentialing cycles related to Medicare and Medicaid sanctions and sanctions/limitations on licensure. Some healthcare organizations contract for such monitoring on an ongoing basis between recredentialing cycles; other organizations may perform this function on an in-house basis. In any event, there must be a mechanism for capturing new information on previously processed practitioners. The CVO must advise all clients under contract for this service of its receipt of new information on any of the client's previously processed practitioners. This is not a required component of a CVO service, but if it is offered as a service, the NCQA standards are applicable. Before contracting to provide this service, CVOs should determine that notification of these actions is not in conflict with state or local regulation or local peer review statutes.

Elements for Certification

A CVO may receive certification on the following elements:

- License to practice
- Drug Enforcement Agency registration
- Education and training
- Malpractice claims history
- Medical board sanctions
- Medicare/Medicaid sanctions
- Practitioner application processing
- CVO application and attestation
- Ongoing monitoring of sanctions
- Work history

A CVO may be surveyed by NCQA surveyors on any or all of these elements. Therefore, when a healthcare organization contemplates using a CVO, the organization must match the elements it wants to outsource with the elements for which the CVO is certified. If the organization contracts with a CVO for an element that is not NCQA certified, it must comply with the due diligence and oversight requirements for the noncertified element only.

The NCQA CVO Survey

The NCQA survey is typically scheduled after an application is received and a pre-survey assessment is completed, which includes a description of the business, standard contract forms, lists of practitioners credentialed during the previous six months, employee job descriptions, policies and procedures, marketing material, and other information. A CVO must have been in business with policies and procedures in place at least six months before it is eligible for NCQA survey.

The survey team consists of an administrative and credentialing surveyor. The credentialing surveyor must meet one or more of the following criteria:

- Maintain current National Association Medical Staff Services (NAMSS) certification as a Certified Professional Medical Services Management (CPMSM) or Certified Professional Credentialing Specialist (CPCS)
- Have knowledge of and experience with credentialing programs, especially in MCOs
- Have substantial experience in NCQA survey processes
- Have no financial conflict of interest with the CVO to be surveyed

NCQA has initiated an interactive, Internet-based survey process. As part of this process, the initial application and supporting documents and relevant policies and procedures are submitted online. All administrative review takes place off-site and via conference calls.

The on-site survey is scheduled for one day. It includes the review of credentials files and assesses compliance with the security standard. The survey also include the review of CVO records, policies and procedures and documentation, surveyor on-site observations, and information gained from interviews with the CVO staff, both on- and off-site. It concludes with an exit conference during which the surveyors summarize their findings. No indication of the outcome of the survey is discussed at the exit conference. Instead, the survey team's written findings are forwarded to NCQA, where they undergo executive review.

A survey draft report is forwarded to the CVO within a few weeks, at which point the CVO may comment on the reported findings. This exchange presents an opportunity to correct any factual omissions prior to the issuance of the final report. After the reply is received by NCQA, the full report is forwarded to NCQA's review oversight committee (ROC), which makes a final determination of whether certification is warranted. The final decision by the ROC is forwarded to the CVO approximately 90 days after the survey takes place.

Successful surveys result in certification for a maximum period of two years. If the CVO does not meet the standards that pertain to overall business operations such as policies and procedures or the quality improvement program, it cannot be certified in any of the elements. However, having met the baseline criteria, the CVO can be certified for the number of elements it qualifies for within the certification process, based on survey findings in the review of each element.

The NCQA survey process is voluntary on the part of the CVO. Given that the surveys are costly, however, it is undertaken with serious intent of success. The survey process has become extremely vital to the success of any commercial CVO that plans to contract with any type of MCO. Reflecting the significance of certification within the managed care industry, it is virtually impossible to obtain a managed care CVO contract without maintaining CVO certification. NCQA is clearly the leader in the industry in terms of general acceptability among managed care clients, although URAC also has a strong following in certain areas, and several states mandate compliance with NCQA standards for organizations as a prerequisite for doing business in those states.

■ URAC CVO Certification Standards

In 1998, URAC approved standards for the accreditation of CVOs. These standards closely resemble NCQA's certification standards and are designed to assess the same areas. They cover the scope of services, the credentialing process, CVO personnel, quality improvement, delegation of responsibilities, confidentiality, and grievances and complaints.[3]

URAC accreditation is much less prevalent than NCQA accreditation, although many larger CVOs expend the effort and expense needed to achieve certification by both agencies in an attempt to attract a wider circle of clients. There does not seem to be any substantial difference between NCQA and URAC in terms of performance expectations of the CVO.

■ The Joint Commission CVO Guidelines

The Joint Commission does not have an accreditation program for CVOs, but acknowledges that hospitals and other healthcare organizations may choose to use the services of a CVO. The Joint Commission standard states:

> *Verification from the primary source: any hospital that bases its decisions in part on information from a CVO should have confidence in the completeness, accuracy, and timeliness of that information. To achieve this level of confidence in the information, the hospital should evaluate the agency providing the information initially and then periodically as appropriate. The principles that guide such an evaluation include the following:*
>
> - The agency makes known to the user the data and information it can provide.
> - The agency provides documentation to the user describing how its data collection, information and development, and verification process(es) are performed.

- The user is given sufficient, clear information on database functions including any limitations on information available from the agency (such as practitioners not included in the database); the time frame for agency responses to requests for information; and a summary overview of quality control processes relating to data integrity, security, transmission accuracy, and technical specifications.
- The user and agency agree on the format for transmitting credentials information about an individual from the CVO.
- The user can easily discern what information transmitted by the CVO, is from a primary source and what is not.
- For information transmitted by the agency that can go out of date (licensure, board certification), the CVO provides the date the information was last updated from the primary source.
- The CVO certifies that the information transmitted to the user accurately represents the information obtained by it.
- The user can discern whether the information transmitted by the CVO from a primary source is all the primary source information in the CVO's possession pertinent to a given item and, if not, where additional information can be obtained.
- The user can engage the CVO's quality control processes to resolve concerns about transmission errors, inconsistencies, or other data issues that may be identified from time to time.
- The user has a formal arrangement with the CVO for communicating changes in credentialing information.[4]

■ CVO Operating Models

There are many operating models for CVOs, and the various models reflect issues of client base, technological sophistication, size, capitalization, profit status, commercial status, public status, and captive status. With numerous CVOs in the marketplace with varying levels of technical sophistication, it would be an exhaustive exercise to try to review the wide range of variations and permutations that characterize these varying businesses. Following are the major types of operating models:

- Initiated in and by the managed care (MCO) industry and built for big-business, high-volume, streamlined services with no ability to customize the deliverables based on individual client requests.
- Initiated by professional physician organizations and primarily intended to service hospitals. These CVOs are sponsored by medical societies as nonprofit, value-added adjuncts to professional organizations.
- Created in an integrated delivery system and proprietary to entities within the healthcare systems (multi-entity).

- Sponsored by hospital trade organizations and developed as value-added services in a nonprofit environment to member organizations (multi-system).
- Established by large insurance companies offering healthcare network insurance, which have built in-house service departments. Some have undergone CVO certification status, but service only their internal organizations. In some cases, they may offer the service to physician groups with whom they have contracts.
- Created by commercial organizations with private or public financial backing, which offer services as a for-profit business unit or organization to various categories of clients.
- Established by the small independent CVO operator, which contracts with a small number of clients in a low-overhead environment (cottage industry) to provide services to a much smaller client base with less sophisticated needs.

■ CVO Computer Operations

Use of information systems technology within the various models of CVOs is as variable as the technology and financing used to support those models. All CVOs need automation. The decision that all CVOs have to make, then, is whether to design and build a system in-house or whether to purchase a software program that is available on the open market.

A good working system, at a minimum, should include a solid database design with a well-planned number of fields for maintaining pertinent information. This will allow for the end result of report writing and processing that can be performed on a timely and convenient basis. The system also needs to be able to capture a full complement of information from application processing for reporting and tracking staff productivity and accuracy. Open memo fields are also desirable so that notes can be placed in the files to capture data from telephone contacts and other non-computerized functions of the process. If extremely high volume is anticipated, a scanning and indexing operation might also be in order for document management and retrieval. The latest technology allows for receipt of documents through computer faxing, with the software being able to convert these documents to PDF formats that can then be transferred to an electronic storage system, rather than having workers manually scan and index the documents.

A prospective client should assess all of its information needs and capabilities and compare the available technology with the receptive technology of the CVO to determine if the situation will enhance information maintenance and exchange or make it more difficult.

Electronic Transfer Capabilities

A wide variety of systems are available for transferring information, visual files, and application forms in an electronic format. Methods used to carry out this function include Internet transportation of documents as files via cable or DSL.

Many hospitals are anything but technically advanced in their ability to receive data electronically through programmed software interfaces. The more salient questions to address are feasibility, cost-effectiveness, and ability to access the level of technology already developed and available.

Client Access to the CVO Database

Many CVOs allow clients to enter the CVO's database via the Internet through a hosted Web site with appropriate security access; the client can then search the database to obtain the status of various elements of information that pertain to its practitioner base. The important information to query regarding these systems would be how often the database information is refreshed, how the database is updated, and what the sources of the updated information are. This type of information seeking allows the prospective client to fully understand the quality and timeliness of the information being provided.

■ Security of Practitioner Data

The security of practitioner data covers several areas of concern for a prospective client. Initially, the security of the practitioner data in the database applications is of prime concern.

In addition, the CVO must ensure the security of paper-based information that passes through potentially many hands from the primary source that verifies the information to the housing of the information at the CVO. This process should be governed by policies that cover storage protection of the paper, copies of the completed files, access to the physical storage as well as building security, disaster recovery plans, and appropriate disposal of paper and information.

Some CVOs developed by business-minded individuals seem to be totally unaware of the legal implications, case law, or legislative climates regarding traditional medical staff protections of peer review information. Procedures to take advantage of the protections to safeguard confidential and sensitive peer review information are usually well understood and followed in the hospital environment. Caution should be exercised in dealing with CVOs where it is apparent that there is inadequate knowledge and expertise in this area.

■ Conclusion

The decision to use a CVO or to form a centralized credentialing service must be well thought out, and the priorities of the organization considering the CVO or centralized credentialing department must be defined. When considering whether to contract with a CVO, access and maintenance of data in a secure and confidential manner, and compliance with the relevant accrediting agencies' standards should be the primary concerns. When considering the formation of a centralized credentialing department, it is very important to have consensus from all components of the system about its operation.

■ Notes

1. Jackson B. "Protecting a Practice from Excluded Providers." *Physician News Dig*. Available at: http://www.physiciansnews.com/law/103jackson.html. Accessed August 5, 2009.
2. National Committee for Quality Assurance (NCQA). *2009 HP Standards and Guidelines: Credentialing Standards*. July 2009.
3. URAC. "Credentials Verification Organization Standards: Accreditation Standards Summary." Available at: http://www.urac.org. Accessed August 17, 2009.
4. The Joint Commission. "Medical Staff Standards," in 2009 *Hospital Accreditation Standards*. Oakbrook Terrace, IL: Author; 2009.

CHAPTER 11

The Role of the Medical Staff in Quality Improvement

Curtis Pullman, MHA

■ Introduction

The traditional boundaries that once separated a healthcare organization's medical staff services department (MSSD) and quality department are today much less defined. Each department now plays an important role in providing practitioner-specific performance information to the leaders of both the healthcare organization and the medical staff charged with the responsibility of review, assessment, and, when necessary, intervention. As a result, the role of the medical staff services professional (MSSP) is becoming increasingly important as it relates to the organization's quality improvement program: These professionals are now charged with facilitating the processes associated with the evaluation of practitioner-specific performance.

This chapter introduces the MSSP to this role and the role that the medical staff performs with the organization's quality improvement efforts. Additionally, the basic accreditation standards that relate to this area are addressed, albeit briefly—this chapter is *not* intended to provide a compendium of all accreditation requirements regarding the medical staff and its role in quality improvement functions.

It is fundamentally important that MSSPs understand their organizations' quality improvement program, the committee structure used to support this program, and the processes used to capture both aggregate and practitioner-specific performance information. It is also important to acknowledge that each organization's internal quality improvement program operates in an increasingly transparent world, meaning that internal performance will be accessed by individuals external to the organization.

■ The Transparent Environment of Health Care

The expectation of government agencies, accrediting organizations, insurance providers, employers, and consumers of high-quality health care that strict attention

With thanks to Wendy R. Crimp, BSN, MBA, CPHQ, and Vicki L. Searcy, CPMSM, who wrote the version of this chapter that appeared in the previous edition of this book.

will be paid to costs and the appropriate utilization of resources has placed both healthcare organizations and practitioners in a challenging position. These expectations, combined with consumers' immediate access to information on the Internet, have meant that the healthcare industry now operate in an increasingly transparent environment.

One result of this transparent environment is that healthcare organizations no longer consider their quality improvement programs to be something that must be implemented just to comply with accreditation standards. The quality improvement program and data on the organization's performance with respect to key performance metrics are now vital to the organization as it is compared against other organizations by accrediting agencies, insurance payers, and healthcare consumers. Healthcare organizations that perform well with comparative metrics can use this information for marketing purposes and when negotiating reimbursement rates with payers. Healthcare consumers, in turn, can evaluate and compare both organization- and practitioner-specific performance information via Internet access. This instant and continuous access provides the opportunity for consumers to become educated and informed about their selection of healthcare providers.

Internet sites provided by HealthGrades, the Leapfrog Group, and the Joint Commission provide organization-specific and comparative performance information in areas such as patient safety, the Joint Commission's core measures (national quality improvement goals), and accreditation status. With increasing frequency, individual states in the nation are now providing the public with organization-specific data related to volume, mortality, and complication rates. Additionally, some states are providing practitioner-specific information on the Internet in areas such as volume, mortality, and complication rates.

Performance and Finance

Through their submission of claims data to payers, healthcare organizations disclose the details of a hospitalization or an outpatient visit. Utilizing the diagnosis, procedure, and billing codes on the claim, payers are able to identify the complications or unexpected events that may have occurred during the patient's encounter.

Building on this ability to identify unexpected events, the Centers for Medicare and Medicaid Services (CMS) has implemented a new program commonly referred to as the "Never Events" program under the Deficit Reduction Act of 2005.[1] The agency has identified a listing of complications or "never events" that are considered to be unacceptable as part of any patient's healthcare encounter—for example, complications such as a surgical site infection following specific procedures, a patient fall, and a foreign object unintentionally retained after surgery. Hospitals that receive Medicare reimbursement are now required to report the defined "never events" with the understanding that CMS will not reimburse the additional costs associated with intervention required to care for the complication. It is anticipated that state-funded programs and private insurance carriers will implement similar programs to limit their reimbursement for care associated with events that should not occur within a healthcare setting.

Another example of the increasing correlation between performance and finance is the work being done by the Leapfrog Group. Formed in 1998, The Leapfrog Group represents major companies and other agencies that purchase healthcare services for their employees and enrollees. It encourages hospitals to participate in its survey to assess the individual hospital's performance with initiatives to improve quality and safety.[2] The Leapfrog Group educates employees and enrollees on various quality and patient safety initiatives, and provides the hospitals' survey results on its Internet site to encourage employees and enrollees to compare performance. Hospitals that perform well on the survey may be seen as the preferred providers by healthcare consumers.

It is within this environment of transparency that healthcare organizations must implement and maintain a quality improvement program that provides performance information at both aggregate and practitioner-specific levels if they are to effectively compete in the market.

Historical Overview: Form Versus Function

A variety of approaches have been used to structure, organize, and direct the participation of medical staff in quality initiatives at healthcare organizations. Depending on the prevailing management philosophy, shifts in the strategies and operational approaches used to support quality initiatives have occurred over time.

At one time, nearly all quality measurement and improvement activities that required medical staff participation were processed within the structured medical staff organization using the medical staff department committees and the medical executive committee (MEC) as vehicles for participation. Medical staff organizations provided adequate support when processing issues located exclusively within their domain (credentialing, privileging, peer review) but were largely ineffective as vehicles for addressing interdisciplinary issues that crossed over or outside of medical staff organization boundaries.

As increasing emphasis was placed on interdisciplinary quality improvement, the typical medical staff organization structure did not provide an adequate platform for support. As a result, the industry saw the emergence of other participative structures such as quality improvement teams, quality councils, hospital quality management committees (as opposed to medical staff quality committees), and others. These committees and teams may report to the MEC but may also be positioned more neutrally under administration or a board quality committee. Because some of the new structures have been created around the medical staff organization (often in an effort to gain protection under state peer review statutes), some healthcare organizations are experiencing duplication of effort or generally awkward flow of quality information and decision making across the organization. Healthcare organizations continue to struggle as they seek to determine which organizational approach is most effective and beneficial.

Generally, MSSPs and quality improvement professionals have been organized in separate departments. In many organizations, these two groups work independently, with minimal collaboration. Functions and work flow across departmental lines only when absolutely necessary. This "silo approach" has proved detrimental to the medical staff organization, however, because *both* skill sets need to work in an integrated approach to support quality improvement initiatives so as to optimize the results realized from the organization's efforts. When medical staff services and quality improvement professionals work separately, they lose the opportunity to synergize their efforts. For example, the quality improvement department may measure and report compliance with core measures. If these personnel worked in tandem with MSSPs to formalize the commitment of the medical staff organization to both monitor and enforce practitioner compliance with national benchmarks, the core measures initiative would have more effective mechanisms to drive up compliance rates and achieve superior results.

The complexity and nature of current expectations no longer permit quality improvement professionals and MSSPs to focus on their assigned functions separately, with collaboration occurring only "as needed." It is essential that both types of professionals jointly support the medical staff organization's participation in quality improvement by integrating their roles and efforts. The efforts of both groups are synergistic, and results will be amplified when they work together.

Clinical privileging provides another good example of the overlap of the two groups. On the one hand, MSSPs possess the required skills and knowledge and are in a perfect position to support the credentialing and privileging process that is conducted within the medical staff organization. This process includes building credentials verification data sets, associated record keeping, support of evaluation by medical staff leaders, and dissemination of results. On the other hand, most MSSPs do not possess the skills and knowledge required to support the clinical performance profiling required at reappointment (e.g., identification of key clinical indicators, data planning, aggregation of data, risk adjustment, benchmarking). The quality improvement professional is better positioned to provide this type of support. By working together, both kinds of professionals can build a coherent, integrated data set for delivery to decision makers.

It is important that the two groups carefully define outcomes and the roles that each group will undertake to support medical staff participation in quality improvement activities. This effort will result in the development of agreed-upon policies and procedures that will be shared by both departments. The ensuing alignment of expectations will minimize conflict, promote good working relationships, ensure that roles and relationships are well understood, and decrease duplication of effort.

If an activity is deemed to be "mission critical," then it requires attention to structural elements that ensure the service is delivered in the most efficient, consistent, and effective manner possible.

Healthcare organizations need to take a step back from their current operating design and identify the specific outcomes that they are trying to achieve. Once this has occurred, the organization can design the best structure for supporting its targeted outcomes. This modus operandi is completely different from the historical approach of trying to make the organizational approach "fit" existing structures. Hence the old axiom reads, "Form follows function," not "Function follows form."

Once the organization has designed a processing approach that fits with its desired outcomes and culture, it is important to remember that the new structure is not necessarily permanent. To stay "on its toes," the organization needs to be facile and mobile in responding to new challenges in a rapidly changing environment.

■ Quality Functions That Involve the Medical Staff

A vast array of quality functions are performed in hospitals today—some required, some discretionary. An overview of all possible functions is not possible within the scope of this chapter. Nevertheless, it is important to understand that the Joint Commission requires the medical staff to be involved in certain functions:[3]

- Medical assessment and treatment of patients
- Use of information about adverse privileging decisions for any practitioner privileged through the medical staff process
- Use of medications
- Use of blood and blood components
- Operative and other procedures
- Appropriateness of clinical practice patterns
- Significant departures from established patterns of clinical practice
- Use of developed criteria for autopsies
- Sentinel event information
- Patient safety

Medical staff organizations may also be involved in other quality improvement functions not included in the preceding list. For example, many hospital organizations have an infection control committee (or a multipurpose committee that encompasses the infection control function) with medical staff organization representatives. Many quality improvement functions may be assigned to committees that MSSDs support and facilitate. The MSSP may provide support to some of these committees in areas of agenda planning, issue tracking, or taking minutes. The following sections provide examples of quality functions that may be assigned to committees supported by MSSPs.

Medical staff committees involved in quality improvement functions are usually involved in measurement and assessment. Measurement of quality involves the collection of data about the important processes that are related to the quality function. Assessment involves the analysis of measurement data to determine if performance expectations were met and where additional improvements might be necessary.

An excellent source of quality measures and indicators can be found at a Web site sponsored by the Agency for Healthcare Research and Quality (AHRQ): http://www.qualityindicators.ahrq.gov. This Web site contains current indicators that relate to many quality functions in which the medical staff organization takes a leadership role, such as medication management, blood use, and operative and invasive procedures.

■ The Role of the Medical Staff in Quality Improvement

Because members of the medical staff play leading roles in the delivery of patient care, it is the expectation of accrediting organizations such as the Joint Commission and CMS that the medical staff will also support, participate, and sometimes lead the activities associated with an organization's quality improvement program. This section discusses the traditional areas of practice in which accrediting agencies require the medical staff to actively evaluate performance. Additionally, this section provides an overview of the committee structure typically used to support the work of the organization's quality improvement program.

Medication Management

The most important reason for evaluating the use of medications in hospitals is that essentially 100% of inpatients (and outpatients undergoing procedures) receive one or more prescribed drugs as, or in conjunction with, their primary treatment. Another reason for the medical staff to engage in evaluation of the use of medications is that the ongoing introduction of a multitude of potent new drugs, the increasing need for hospitalization and treatment for untoward drug reactions (two or more drugs may lead to an untoward drug reaction or there may be a food–drug reaction), the related litigation, and the ever-increasing cost of drugs. In addition, the Joint Commission has long required that the medical staff organization oversee functions related to medication management.

Some hospital organizations have one or more committees charged with carrying out various components of the Joint Commission's requirements related to medication management. For example, a pharmacy and therapeutics committee, a patient safety committee, and/or a medication management committee may be engaged in various aspects of medication management. In addition, various departments of the medical staff organization may be involved in receiving and reviewing information related to medication management.

In the past, medication management primarily consisted of adding and deleting drugs from the formulary (the listing of medications available within the organization for practitioner use) and identification of a few drugs (often antibiotics) that were subject to more intensive scrutiny (usually through some type of periodic audit process). Medication management is now much more complex and involves not only the practitioners, nurses, and pharmacy staff, but also risk management professionals because of patient safety issues. Medical staff services professionals who support and facilitate committees charged with carrying out medication management activities should do so in close collaboration with a representative from the pharmacy—and potentially an individual from the quality management department will be assigned to this function as well. The pharmacy representative (often the pharmacy director in a smaller hospital and a clinical pharmacist in a larger organization) will take the lead on making sure the committee is meeting Joint Commission and other regulatory and accreditation requirements associated with medication management.

The medication management function can be broadly described as collecting and analyzing data so as to monitor and improve the performance and safety of processes and outcomes related to the use of medications. Medication processes include selection and procurement, storage, ordering and transcribing, preparing and dispensing, administration, and monitoring.

The Joint Commission expects that an effective medication management system will be supportive of patient safety and will improve the quality of care by doing the following:

- Reducing practice variation, errors, and misuse
- Monitoring medication management processes in regard to their efficiency, quality, and safety
- Standardizing equipment and processes across the hospital to improve the medication management system
- Using evidence-based good practices to develop medication management processes
- Managing critical processes associated with medication management to promote safe medication management throughout the hospital
- Handling all medications in the same manner, including sample medications
- Managing look-alike/sound-alike medications and the implementation of systemic interventions to reduce the risk of selecting and administering the incorrect medication

In addition, the Joint Commission requires that the medication management system include mechanisms for reporting potential and actual errors, and for using this information to improve medication management processes and patient safety.

Review of Use of Blood and Blood Components

Because blood is a precious, sometimes life-saving, and not always harmless commodity, the Joint Commission requires that the medical staff organization take a leadership role in the evaluation of blood and blood product use. Guidelines are readily available to determine whether a patient meets the criteria to receive blood or a blood product. The criteria selected for this purpose should be recognized nationally and not based on a "community" level unless the latter equals or exceeds the national criteria. The medical staff should evaluate its members' blood ordering practices against these criteria to determine how blood and blood products are being used in the facility and act on opportunities for improvement. Criteria supported by the American Association of Blood Banks are readily available through it publications.

The processes that are addressed through blood and blood product use include ordering; distributing, handling, and dispensing; administering; and monitoring effects on patients. The following are the basic components involved in implementation of blood and blood product use:

- Criteria for use of blood and blood products are approved via the medical staff organization.
- There is a method to apply criteria and report results. Review of individual cases may be required through the peer/case review process.
- When necessary, there is intensive review of all confirmed transfusion reactions.
- The medical staff organization provides for oversight of the function.

The oversight function may be performed by a medical staff committee (although it is becoming rare for contemporary medical staff organizations to have a single-purpose "blood use committee") or through some type of a quality or performance improvement committee that periodically receives data that measure the performance of a variety of functions—including blood use. If the medical staff organization makes a performance improvement committee responsible for oversight of blood and blood product use, a pathologist typically provides periodic written reports that allow the committee to make a determination of where improvements in processes related to blood and blood product use are possible.

The medical staff services professional who is involved in supporting a committee or group charged with oversight of this function will work closely with a representative from the quality management department as well as an assigned individual from the organization's blood bank.

Review of Operative and Other Procedures

The review of operative and other invasive procedures has long been a fundamental component of a medical staff organization's quality improvement activities. This emphasis precedes the requirements for "surgical case review" that have, for many years, been a Joint Commission–required function of the medical staff organization. Looking back in history, in 2000 BC, Hammurabi, a Babylonian emperor, wrote extensive laws that governed society. The Code of Hammurabi stated:

If the surgeon has made a deep incision in the body of a free man and has caused the man's death or has opened the caruncle in the eye and so destroys the man's eye, they shall cut off his forehand.

To our knowledge, this is the oldest example of surgical case review that exists (as well as spelling out the consequences of a surgical complication). More than a century and a half later, in 400 BC, the Hippocratic Oath included the Latin phrase "*primum non nocere,*" which means that the physician should "first do no harm."

Today, review of operative and other invasive procedures remains a cornerstone of hospital quality improvement functions. This function is required by both the CMS and the Joint Commission as part of their standards.

The CMS defines an invasive procedure as "any procedure that clearly involves an incision, excision, amputation, introduction, endoscopy, repair, destruction, suture, or manipulation. Invasive procedures also include any procedure that affects, or has the potential for affecting, the DRG."[4] The CMS standards focus on the criteria for performance of surgical and invasive procedures as well as the setting in which the procedures are performed (e.g., inpatient versus outpatient).

The Joint Commission requires that the organization collect data that measure the performance of processes related to operative and other invasive procedures. The current emphasis of the Joint Commission is on issues related to patient safety—and there are a myriad of issues in operative and other invasive procedures that involve patient safety (e.g., procedures done on the wrong patient, wrong procedures performed, and wrong-site surgery). The Joint Commission does not specify exactly which data are to be collected, with the exception that an analysis must be performed for all major discrepancies between preoperative and postoperative (including pathologic) diagnoses.

Settings where operative and other invasive procedures are often performed include traditional operating rooms, cardiac catheterization suites, endoscopy suites, radiology departments, emergency departments, renal dialysis units, and others. The purpose of the operative and other invasive procedures function is to collect and analyze data that are used to monitor the stability of existing processes related to the performance of operative and other invasive procedures in all of these settings. Data collection and analysis are performed to assist in identification of specific areas where further study could lead to improvements and increased patient safety.

In the past, operative and other invasive procedures evaluation was conducted via case review. For example, if a surgical case did not meet criteria for the performance of the procedure or if some type of complication occurred during a procedure, the case would be reviewed by a committee. More recently, many organizations have migrated toward using aggregated and trended data that are compared to established national benchmarks (for example, complication rates associated with specific procedures might be reviewed, rather than each individual case). This approach assures equity in evaluating the performance of identified procedures regardless of which medical staff member performed the procedure (and, therefore, also addresses level of care issues). The old focus on "complication rates" is rapidly being replaced by analysis of data that show improved functional status or other positive outcomes—in contemporary terms, did the procedure address the problem that it was intended to address (e.g., decreased pain or improved mobility)? Additionally, this committee may review other performance metrics associated with work processes in the surgical area, such as operating room turnaround times (the time necessary to prepare the operating room for the next case); delayed start time with the first case of the day, which can affect the scheduled start times for all subsequent cases; and the use of blocked time (time set aside for a specific surgeon that may or may not be utilized).

Medical staff services professionals who support groups or committees charged with oversight of operative and other invasive procedures (and there could be any number of groups that look at various aspects related to this function) will work closely with a quality management department partner to assure that accreditation and regulatory requirements are addressed and that the activities associated with this function are appropriately documented.

Oversight of Quality Functions

Although not required by CMS or the Joint Commission, many organizations provide for oversight of quality functions via a committee, such as a quality council, quality oversight committee, or similarly named group. This group provides oversight of quality functions in much the same way that a credentials committee coordinates and provides oversight of credentialing and privileging activities. Small organizations may elect to have the MEC provide direct oversight of quality functions. For the purposes of this chapter, this oversight group is called the quality committee.

The organization's quality committee provides the mechanism for a final review of the actions and recommendations of other quality-related committees and groups prior to review by the MEC and governing board. It typically has the ability to modify recommendations of other quality-related committees or to request further review and evaluation. The chair of the committee is usually a member of medical staff leadership or a physician who serves in a medical director role for performance improvement. The membership of the committee is typically multidisciplinary and includes organization leaders who have the ability to direct and implement change.

The quality committee may also oversee and direct the organization's initiatives related to patient safety, patient satisfaction, and accreditation. The committee reports its recommendations to the MEC and to the governing board (the governing board often establishes a quality committee of the board in large organizations).

The MSSP must be aware of the practitioner-specific information produced by quality committees. He or she must facilitate the availability of this information for use in the evaluation of practitioner performance at reappointment and through the medical staff's ongoing professional practice evaluation (OPPE) and focused professional practice evaluation (FPPE) processes.

Ongoing Professional Practice Evaluation/Focused Professional Practice Evaluation

As mentioned at the beginning of this chapter, the boundaries separating the roles and responsibilities of a healthcare organization's quality and medical staff services departments have become blurred in recent years. This overlap becomes especially evident when discussing the role of the MSSP in supporting the processes associated with the provision of effective evaluation of practitioner performance. The same blurring of boundaries was also emphasized with the Joint Commission's implementation of the OPPE and FPPE standards for medical staff. These standards created the immediate need for the two departments, whose staff members possess specific skill sets, to work together to successfully meet the standards' intent.

The OPPE standards, which were implemented in 2008, call for the practitioner-specific evaluation process to be ongoing and presented to medical staff leadership more frequently than once a year. As a result, most organizations present practitioner-specific OPPE reports at intervals of every three, six, or nine months. Because these OPPE reports must reflect practitioner-specific and comparative data, the medical staff services and quality management departments must work together to identify the performance metrics where practitioner-specific data are available.

The OPPE standards provide the following examples of metrics that may be included in the evaluation process:

- Review of operative and other clinical procedures performed and their outcomes
- Pattern of blood and pharmaceutical use
- Requests for tests and procedures
- Length of stay patterns
- Morbidity and mortality data
- Practitioner's use of consultants
- Other relevant criteria determined by the medical staff

While some healthcare organizations are data rich and have established practitioner performance profiling systems, others do not. Even in the latter cases, an effective OPPE report that provides a meaningful evaluation of a practitioner's performance can be developed using metrics that have been traditionally reported with practitioner-specific information. Examples include the following:

- Medical record suspensions
- Medical record deficiencies (late history and physical reports, incomplete orders, and late signatures)
- Core measure performance
- Peer review results
- Citizenship/professionalism/practice issues requiring an investigation by the MEC
- Failure to renew licenses, certifications, or professional insurance in a timely manner
- Lawsuit settlements and licensing board actions

EXHIBIT 11-1 shows examples of the types of information that can be collected for OPPE purposes.

FIGURE 11-1 provides an example of a template used for an OPPE report. Its format allows for easy identification of those practitioners who have a performance concern in more than one area. Analysis of the data and details regarding specific performance issues must also be included in the OPPE report. One important element of performance data is which privileges have actually been exercised by each practitioner, as compared to which privileges have been granted. The organization will need to justify continuation of privileges to a practitioner who does not use them in the healthcare organization

In addition to providing ongoing status report of the performance of practitioners, the OPPE report should identify those practitioners who demonstrate potential competency issues. Medical staff and hospital leadership are responsible for identifying performance issues from OPPE data and determining the appropriate intervention. An option for intervention may be to place the practitioner on an FPPE.

The FPPE standards were implemented in 2008 by the Joint Commission and require a focused evaluation to be implemented whenever a quality or performance concern is identified through the OPPE process. Additionally, all initially appointed practitioners and current practitioners granted new privileges must complete a period of focused evaluation (see Chapter 7 for information about FPPE used to validate competency for newly granted privileges). The remainder of this chapter's discussion of FPPE concerns the use of FPPE when questions of competency or performance need to be addressed. Note that although these requirements have a new title (FPPE), the requirement to evaluate performance or competency issues is not new and was previously referred to as "focused evaluation and peer review" by the Joint Commission.

The medical staff's policy on FPPE should identify the performance criteria that will trigger the implementation of a FPPE, the circumstances when an FPPE may be extended, and the circumstances when a failed FPPE may lead to corrective action as defined in the medical staff bylaws. Communication to a practitioner being placed on a FPPE should include the reason for the review, the time frame

Exhibit 11-1 General Competencies as a Framework for OPPE (Examples of What Type of Information to Collect)

Competency	Data and Information

Volume/Demographics (Provides comparative information to support analysis)	◊ Volume
	  ▪ Admissions—inpatient
	  ▪ Ambulatory cases
	  ▪ Consultations
	  ▪ Surgical cases/procedures
	  ▪ Length of stay
	◊ Demographics
	  ▪ Specialty
	  ▪ Department
	  ▪ Leadership positions and committee participation
	◊ Risk-adjusted mortality

Patient Care The provision of care, treatment, and services is
—Appropriate
—Timely
—Safe
	◊ Ongoing professional practice evaluation
	  ▪ Appropriateness of clinical practice patterns
	  ▪ Review of operative and other clinical procedures performed and their outcomes
	  ▪ Pattern of blood and pharmaceutical use
	  ▪ Requests for tests and procedures
	  ▪ Length of stay patterns
	  ▪ Results from department specific indicators (high-volume/high-risk/problem-prone activities)
	◊ Evaluation by peers/department chair
	◊ Evidence of substantive information for full range of privileges, particularly those considered "high risk"

Exhibit 11-1: General Competencies as a Framework for OPPE (Examples of What Type of Information to Collect) (continued)

Competency	Data and Information

Medical/Clinical Knowledge
—Knowledge
—Application of knowledge
—Effectiveness
	◊ Licensure status
	◊ Board certification
	◊ Experience
	◊ Individual results from core measure data
	  ▪ Acute myocardial infarction
	  ▪ Heart failure
	  ▪ Community-acquired pneumonia
	  ▪ Pregnancy and related conditions
	◊ Infection control data
	◊ Morbidity
	◊ Results of open and closed medical record review/audits
	◊ Use of new technology/testing/medication
	◊ Focused review outcomes
	  ▪ Identified concern/actions
	  ▪ Information from tracking and trending activities
	  ▪ Number of cases reviewed with findings (grading system)
	  ▪ Significant departures form established patterns of clinical practice

Practice-Based Learning and Improvement —Use of scientific methodology —Education —Efficiency	◊ Participation in hospital sponsored CME/education programs related to granted/requested privileges ◊ Completion of CME related to granted/requested privileges ◊ Development/presentation of educational programs ◊ Completion of continuing education to maintain licensure/certification ◊ Completion of education to obtain/maintain certification ◊ Use of consults ◊ Response to calls regarding change in patient status, results of diagnostic testing

Exhibit 11-1 General Competencies as a Framework for OPPE (Examples of What Type of Information to Collect) (continued)

Competency	Data and Information
Interpersonal and Communication Skills —Professional relationships —Compassion —Service	◊ Results of patient surveys ◊ Compliments ◊ Noncompliance with requirements: no-use abbreviation, universal time-out ◊ Complaints, comments from patients/dissatisfaction ◊ Confirmed documented behavioral issues ◊ Information from patient services/marketing ◊ Compliments from hospital staff

Professionalism
—Citizenship
—Ethical behavior
—Respect/caring
	◊ Compliance with bylaws
	◊ Compliance with policies, rules, and regulations
	  ▪ Compliance with timelines for completion of H&P and operative reports
	  ▪ No-use abbreviation compliance
	  ▪ Illegible medication orders
	  ▪ Legibility of medical record entries
	  ▪ Timely completion of records (delinquency rate)
	◊ Validated reports of disruptive behavior
	◊ Meeting attendance (if required)

Systems-Based Practice
—Resource use
—Timeliness
—Teamwork
—Continuity
	◊ Participation in hospital administrative functions
	◊ Medical record suspension/delinquent records
	◊ Persistent nonformulary use
	◊ Participation in PI activities/sponsorship or member of quality team or committee
	◊ Resource use—overuse, misuse
	◊ Trend late-start surgery
	◊ Utilization
	  ▪ Inpatient denials
	  ▪ Outpatient denials

Exhibit 11-1 General Competencies as a Framework for OPPE (Examples of What Type of Information to Collect) (continued)

Competency	Data and Information
Other	◊ Risk management • Trending of occurrence/incident reports • Verification of liability coverage • Litigation information: judgments and settlements • Data Bank report • Involvement in sentinel/reviewable events ◊ Cost of care

Source: Courtesy of Sheryl Deutsch, Quality Management Options, LLC, September 2009.

and methodology of the review process, the expected performance outcome, and the actions that may be taken if the desired level of performance is not achieved. The results of FPPE should be reviewed by the practitioner's department chair, as the chair will make the recommendation for additional review or indicate successful completion of the evaluation process. The FPPE findings should then be shared with the appropriate medical staff committees, as outlined in the FPPE-related policies and procedures.

■ Patient Safety

The immense focus on patient safety in the healthcare industry is evident by the number of journal articles dedicated to the topic, the implementation of new practice standards to improve safety, and the use of new technology that promotes the delivery of safe patient care. The Joint Commission's National Patient Safety Goals (NPSGs) have also increased the focus of patient safety goals, and the "Quality Check" section of the Joint Commission's Internet site displays hospitals' performance in terms of the NPSGs.

Medical staff members have been asked to lead and facilitate the implementation of many of the initiatives associated with NPSGs. For example, to promote the correct communication of a practitioner's order to a nurse or other professional

Physician Performance Report: Cardiology

Indicator	Type	Actual	Excellent	Acceptable	Notes
Patient Care					
Activity					
Number of admissions	#				
Number of consultations	#				
Number of inpatient procedures	#				
Number of outpatient procedures	#				
Number top five DRGs	#				
a.	#				
b.	#				
c.	#				
d.	#				
e.	#				
Outcomes					
Case reviews deemed care controversial or inappropriate	Review	#	#	#	
Mortality (discharge disposition)	#	#	#	#	
Severity-adjusted mortality index (if they have APR DRGs)	Rate	%	%	%	
Unanticipated deaths					
Medical DRGs	Review	#	#	#	
Surgical DRGs	Review	#	#	#	
Death within 24 hours of cath lab procedure	Review	#	#	#	
Unexpected transfers to CCU,ICU, or CVICU	Review	#	#	#	
Surgical site infections	Review	#	#	#	
Excessive blood loss	Review	#	#	#	
DVT/PE (deep vein thrombosis/pulmonary embolism) while in-house	Review	#	#	#	
Stroke during or following procedure	Review	#	#	#	
Unexpected return to surgery	Review	#	#	#	
Unexpected readmission within 24 hours	Review	#	#	#	
Patient requiring reversal agent for conscious sedation	Review	#	#	#	
Medical/Clinical Knowledge					
Use of Evidence-Based Guidelines					
AMI bundle	Rate	%	%	%	
Heart failure bundle	Rate	%	%	%	
Eschemic stroke/TIA bundle	Rate	%	%	%	
Pneumonia bundle	Rate	%	%	%	
SCIP (Surgical Care Improvement Project: CMS and Premier)	Rate	%	%	%	
Practice-Based Learning and Improvement					
Failure to Rescue					
Unanticipated cardiopulmonary arrest outside ICU, PACU, or OR	Review	#	#	#	
Avoidable transfers to a higher level of care	Review	#	#	#	
Complications					
CHF readmissions < 31 days	Rate	%	%	%	
Postop MI	Review	%	%	%	
Discrepancies					
Blood usage not meeting criteria	Review	%	%	%	
Cross-match to actual transfusion	Review	%	%	%	
Interpersonal and Communication Skills					

FIGURE 11-1 Physician Performance Report: Cardiology

Documentation					
History and physical not documented within 24 hours of admission	Review	%	%	%	%
Verbal orders authenticated within 48 hours	Rate	%	%	%	%
Postoperative/postprocedure not documented within 24 hours	Rate	%	%	%	%
Medical record completed within 30 days of discharge	Rate	%	%	%	%
Chart Entries					
Legible	Rate	%	%	%	%
Dated/timed	Rate	%	%	%	%
No unapproved abbreviations	Rate	%	%	%	%
All essential chart documents available within expected time frames	Rate	%	%	%	%
Satisfaction Ratings					
Patient	Rate	%	%	%	%
Staff	Rate	%	%	%	%
Validated incidents of inappropriate physician behavior	Review	#	#	#	#
Professionalism					
Responsiveness					
Validated incidents of physician nonresponse to nurse request	Review	#	#	#	#
Validated incidents of nonavailability for ED call for on-call MD	Review	#	#	#	#
Suspensions					
Medical records	Rate	%	%	%	%
Education					
CME compliance	Rate	%	%	%	%
System-Based Practice					
Length of Stay (LOS)					
LOS index by medical DRG: severity adjusted	Rate	%	%	%	%
LOS index by surgical DRG: severity adjusted	Rate	%	%	%	%
Avoidable patient days due to physician decisions or practice	Review	#	#	#	#
Medicare patients with certain medical DRGs with 1-day LOS	Number	#	#	#	#
National Patient Safety Initiatives					
Wrong procedure/patient/surgical site	Review	#	#	#	#
Validated noncompliance with presurgical/invasive procedural safety	Review	#	#	#	#
Number of pharmacy interventions	Review	#	#	#	#
Critical Hospital Policies and Procedures					
Start-time delays	Rule	#	#	#	#
Risk management referral for significant clinical concern	Review	#	#	#	#
Referral from external source for quality of care issues	Review	#	#	#	#
Nonresponse to medical staff committee request	Review	#	#	#	#
Sentinel events	Review	#	#	#	#

FIGURE 11-1 Continued

member of the care team, a read-back process must now be completed. That is, if a practitioner calls in an order for a medication to be given to a hospitalized patient, the nurse taking the order must document the order and then read it back to the practitioner for confirmation that it has been correctly communicated. Additionally, prior to the start of a procedure, a "time-out" is to be performed to confirm the patient's identification, the procedure, the procedure site, and the availability of necessary equipment. The practitioner must actively participate in or lead the time-out process.

Sentinel events and the technique used to review the occurrence of the event represent another activity where medical staff participation is expected. Sentinel events are defined by the Joint Commission as "an unexpected occurrence involving death or serious physical or psychological injury, or the risk thereof. Serious injury specifically includes loss of limb or function." The Joint Commission notes that the phrase "or the risk thereof" includes any process variation for which a recurrence would carry a significant chance of a serious adverse outcome." The term "sentinel" signifies an immediate need for investigation and response.[5]

The method used to review sentinel events is called root cause analysis. Such analysis breaks down the processes associated with the sentinel event to determine its cause. Processes associated with communication, equipment, the environment, and staff orientation and education are reviewed as part of this scrutiny. The findings are shared with the appropriate committees, and the appropriate actions are implemented to reduce the risk of the event occurring in the future.

In another measure intended to increase patient safety, practitioners and other members of the care delivery team are transitioning to the use of electronic medical records to write orders and clinical documentation, so as to reduce the risk associated with illegible handwriting and the use of confusing abbreviations. Moreover, bar coding technology is now used as part of the processes associated with dispensing and administering medications and blood products.

At the time of this chapter's writing, a new initiative associated with patient safety was being implemented: Patient safety organizations (PSOs) are being established and registered through the Agency for Healthcare Research and Quality, which is the lead federal agency charged with improving quality and safety in health care.[6] The PSOs will provide a structure for hospitals, doctors, and other healthcare providers to voluntarily report information on patient safety events in a confidential manner. Aggregated information will then be shared with healthcare organizations and providers in an effort to identify safety issues and promote safe practice.

■ Reporting Quality Functions

EXHIBIT 11-2 indicates the scope of routine indicators that might be reported to a medical executive committee in an average hospital. This sample MEC quality

Exhibit 11-2 Medical Executive Committee Dashboard Report

Medical Executive Committee
Dashboard Report
2010

Dashboard report	A dashboard report is a concise snapshot of key indicators related to clinical care, service, and safety. Dashboard reports are used to flag potential quality problems and to identify successes, both of which can then be further investigated and studied. Dashboards establish expectations (via the targets) and facilitate evaluation of performance.
Purpose	To identify key indicators of quality for issues that directly affect the success of the strategic objectives of the organization.
Performance measures (indicators)	In health care, as in other arenas, that which cannot be measured is difficult to improve. Performance measures have been selected that are key measures of healthcare quality that can serve as the starting point for further investigation.
Benchmark	Benchmarking may be internal or, more likely, external, as in comparing one organization's outcome or service standard with another organization's or with a national standard.
Target	Established internally by the organization. National standards or benchmarks are useful to help organizations establish their own targets.

Performance Measure	Benchmark	Target	2009	Q1 January–March 2010	Q2 April–June 2010	Q3 July–September 2010	Q4 October–December 2010	2010 YTD	Status
Access									
ED waits									
Autopsy									

282 CHAPTER 11 The Role of the Medical Staff in Quality Improvement

Percentage of autopsy reports that show a significant discrepancy between the patient's treatment and cause of death	Percentage of deaths that result in an autopsy	Blood Usage Evaluation	C/T ratio	Significant transfusion reaction rate	Case-Specific Review	Percentage of hospital discharges that resulted in case-specific review by the hospital medical staff organization

Exhibit 11-2 Medical Executive Committee Dashboard Report (continued)

Performance Measure	Benchmark	Target	2009	Q1 January–March 2010	Q2 April–June 2010	Q3 July–September 2010	Q4 October–December 2010	2010 YTD	Status
Percentage of cases reviewed by the hospital medical staff organization in which significant practitioner problems were identified									
Clinical Practice Guidelines									
Core Measures									
Infection Surveillance									

				Medication Management		Patient Complaints		Operative/Invasive Procedures		Outcomes of Resuscitation	Codes per 1000 discharges	Codes outside ICU	Utilization of rapid response teams	Post-cardiac arrests

Exhibit 11-2 Medical Executive Committee Dashboard Report (continued)

Performance Measure	Benchmark	Target	2009	Q1 January–March 2010	Q2 April–June 2010	Q3 July–September 2010	Q4 October–December 2010	2010 YTD	Status
ICU bed utilization									
Percentage of coded patients surviving at discharge									
Safety Issues									
Restraints/ Seclusion/Behavior Management									
Utilization Management									
Number of denials appealed via QMD									
Number of denials overturned (could include $)									

summary is commonly referred to as a "MEC dashboard report." It relies on measures of central tendency—for example, rate-based means, medians, and percentiles—to identify undesirable trends. This dashboard of indicators typically provides aggregated performance results rather than the practitioner-specific information found on the OPPE report. The reporting of aggregated data in this manner is an effective way to identify possible improvement opportunities that might require intervention by the medical staff.

This type of a dashboard has been in use for many years and should be regarded as the minimum standard for performance reporting that every organization should meet. Some organizations, however, are using more contemporary report formats to provide data to the MEC. These newer formats move beyond the traditional rate-based reporting illustrated in Exhibit 11-2 and may include application of more advanced statistical tools that lend relevance and validity to the analysis. The newer formats are more visual and dynamic, which assists in directing the attention of the user to critical issues that require attention and thoughtful consideration. Examples of these descriptive statistical methods including the following items:

- Analysis of dispersion—for example, standard deviation and the Z-score
- Use of statistical process control in determination of special versus common cause variation
- Application of risk adjustment methodologies or adjustment for adverse selection
- Regression and correlation analysis
- Other inferential and descriptive statistics applications
- Use of graphical illustrations with or without color as visual communications tools

■ Case Review

Peer review (also known as ongoing professional performance evaluation) provides a mechanism for members of the medical staff and other practitioners with clinical privileges to take an active role in activities that measure, assess, and, where necessary, improve performance of practitioner practice within the organization. Peer review programs provide practitioner-specific data for use in evaluating practitioner performance and competency at appropriate intervals (i.e., at the time of reappointment or at other appropriate times).

"Case review" is the term most commonly used to describe retrospective review of a health professional's performance of clinical professional activities by peers through formally adopted written procedures. Case review is used to describe review of a patient record, or single event, by an individual peer or group of peers, to evaluate issues that have been deemed important by the group overseeing the process. Typically, practitioners who are considered subject to case review include those with clinical privileges (MD or DO), dentists, podiatrists, psychologists, nurse practitioners, certified nurse-midwives, physician assistants, and certified nurse anesthetists. Depending on the role to be assumed, clinical nurse specialists may also be included on this list.

Definition of a Peer

In the past, it was believed that to qualify as a peer, one must be an individual who, to the fullest extent possible, has equivalent qualifications and privileges. For example, even though an orthopedic surgeon and a pediatrician are peers, two orthopedic surgeons would meet the definition of a peer more completely than would an orthopedic surgeon and a pediatrician. Attitudes in this area are changing, however, as participants have come to realize that the definition can be flexible depending on the issue or data under review.

When a specific case is the subject of review, individuals functioning as peer reviewers should not have performed any medical management on the patient whose case is under review. Competitors and partners, by virtue of being in the same specialty as the reviewee, may at times act as peer reviewers. If it is suspected that the outcome of the review may have been influenced by a competitor or partner relationship, a secondary review (internal or external) should be sought. External reviewers may be contracted or compensated for their peer review service (see the later discussion of external peer review).

Case Review Structure

Clinical departments provide a structure for organizing practitioners into peer groups for the purpose of conducting case review. Department chairs oversee and facilitate case review within their department and may collaborate with other departments as needed. Some organizations may elect to set up cross-departmental case review teams.

The medical staff organization (through its departments and committees and confirmed by the MEC) typically defines the indicators and types of situations and data that will be reviewed through the case review program. The organization is required to devise specific methods for participation in the review by the reviewee.

Staff Support of the Case Review Process

It is important that both the MSSP and the quality improvement professional work hand in hand to support case review. The quality improvement professional will be able to assist the medical staff in the identification of indicators, identify cases for review in accordance with indicators, act in a screening capacity, prepare reports, and interact with the practitioners and committees involved in the case review program. The MSSP can support the flow of information across programmatic structures and participants and assure that outcomes and actions are well documented and are in compliance with medical staff bylaws and procedures. In addition, the MSSP can assure that actions (e.g., limitations on privileges, suspension) are appropriately documented and disseminated, and that National Practitioner Data Bank reports are filed when the appropriate criteria are met. Professionals from both disciplines will need to assure that program information is well represented in professional profiling associated with evaluation of competency at reappointment and on an ongoing basis as specified in policies and procedures documenting OPPE requirements.

It is essential that a database be used to manage the case review process and track and report on results over time. Professionals from either discipline can maintain the database that the organization uses for case review.

TABLE 11-1 is an example of screening scores that might be used by the quality improvement professional and final scoring by the department chair to organize and classify the results of case review. In this scenario, the quality improvement professional who is screening a case referred for case review uses a screening score to organize the case for trending in the peer review database or for evaluation by the peer; the score represents the outcome of case screening. The next section of Table 11-1 illustrates scoring of the case by the evaluator. In this scenario, the evaluator would review only cases that received a screening score of 4. This approach helps the volunteer medical staff focus their time and effort on potential problem cases that might yield beneficial information as opposed to wading through stacks of cases where practice expectations were met.

The evaluation score suggests to what extent the case represents a significant departure from the standard of care, thereby indicating whether an action is needed. In both cases, low scores indicate positive peer review outcomes. It is important that positive outcomes are reported, for two reasons: (1) They provide affirmations of clinical competence, and (2) they serve to modify perceptions that reviewers are only looking for "bad apples."

It should also be noted that scores are not intended to be additive. Rather, patterns within scoring levels should be evaluated. For example, even though a score of 5 is not necessarily an adverse finding in and of itself, the practitioner with four times the number of 5 scores as his peers (rate based) might cause medical staff leadership to wonder why his clinical practice is so problem prone. This situation would likely be noted between the practitioner's appointments. It would be the responsibility of the quality professional and the MSSP to work together to identify these situations and facilitate further review.

External Peer Review

In some situations, the use of external peer review is necessary to assure the integrity of the peer review process. An external peer reviewer can be defined as a

Table 11-1 Classification Scores Used for Case Review

Screening Score	Description	Action Taken by Quality Professional
1	Screened by QI professional. No further review necessary.	Closed. Trend in database. No action necessary.
2	Finding expected and acceptable or minor problem with process or documentation.	Closed. Trend in database. No action necessary.
3	QI professional referral to other department/care provider issue. (Example: nursing unit manager.) No action necessary. Referred outside of peer review program.	Closed. Trend in database.
4	Referred by QI professional to department chair or designee for review.	Forwarded for further review. Trend in database.

Peer Evaluator Outcome Score	Description	Recommendation Made/ Action Taken
2	Finding expected and acceptable or minor problem with process or documentation.	Closed. Trend in database. No action necessary.
3	Refer to other department/care provider issue. (Example: nursing unit manager.)	Closed. Trend in database. No action necessary. Referred outside of peer review program.
5	Not necessarily routine, but not totally unexpected.	Closed. Trend in database. No action necessary.
6	Significant departure from established pattern of clinical practice. No adverse patient impact.	May implement focused review or investigation. Trend in database.
7	Significant departure from established pattern of clinical practice contributed to unexpected outcome. Adverse patient impact.	Implement focused review or investigation. Trend in database.

practitioner who is not a current member of the medical staff, is a peer of the reviewee, has no economic relationship to the reviewee, and has no personal knowledge of the reviewee or patient. External peer reviewers may be contracted for the peer review service. It is advisable to require that such reviewers sign a quality review participation agreement prior to performing peer review. In addition, risk management departments of hospitals sometimes use external review for assessing cases that have been classified as potentially compensable events (i.e., cases where a claim has been determined to be likely) or where a claim has already been filed.

As noted earlier, each medical staff organization should determine, as part of its policies, under which circumstances external peer review will be required or at least considered. Examples include the following:

- When there is no one on the medical staff with expertise in the subject under review
- When a peer review committee or the department chair determines that there is no comparable internal peer (related to the scope of service under review) or there is potential interference with the unbiased process needed for true peer review for improvement
- When there are conflicting recommendations from the medical staff committees or there is no strong consensus for a particular recommendation

Other considerations that relate to external peer review include the following:

- Which individual and/or group (i.e., a peer review committee or the MEC) must authorize external peer review?
- Where will the funds come from to pay for the external peer review?
- Can a practitioner under review obtain an external peer review at his or her own expense?
- How will the practitioner who is under review be notified that his or her case is undergoing an external review?
- What format and type of content are expected in the final report?

Evaluation of the OPPE Program

The organization should conduct periodic evaluations of the effectiveness of its OPPE program and report its findings to the MEC. In evaluating effectiveness, the following items (among others) should be considered:

- Timeliness of peer review
- Consistency of execution of the peer review process
- Defensibility of peer review conclusions and actions
- Availability of reports and documentation to support the ongoing competency process of medical staff members (i.e., reappraisal/reappointment)

Based upon the annual evaluation of effectiveness, revisions may be proposed to the OPPE program to make improvements in process and outcomes.

Notes

1. Centers for Medicare and Medicaid Services (CMS). "CMS Fact Sheet: Eliminating Serious, Preventable, and Costly Medical Errors—Never Events." May 18, 2006. Available at:http://www.cms.hhs.gov/apps/media/press/factsheet.asp?Counter=1863&intNumPerPage=10&checkDate=&checkKey=&srchType=1&numDays=3500&srchOpt=0&srchData=&keywordType=All&chkNewsType=6&intPage=&showAll=&pYear=&year=&desc=false&cboOrder=date???. Accessed August 4, 2008; "CMS Fact Sheet: CMS Improves Patient Safety for Medicare and Medicaid by Addressing Never Events." Available at: http://www.cms.hhs.gov/apps/media/press/release.asp?Counter=3219&intNumPerPage=10&checkDate=&checkKey=&srchType=1&numDays=3500&srchOpt=0&srchData=&keywordType=All&chkNewsType=1%2C+2%2C+3%2C+4%2C+5&intPage=&showAll=&pYear=&year=&desc=false&cboOrder=date???. Accessed August 4, 2008.
2. The Leapfrog Group. "The Leapfrog Group Fact Sheet." Available at: www.leapfroggroup.org. Accessed August 4, 2009.
3. The Joint Commission. *2009 Hospital Accreditation Standards*. Oakbrook Terrace, IL: Author; 2009: MS.05.01.01, MS-12.
4. Department of Health and Human Services, Centers for Medicare and Medicaid Services (CMS). "Basic Case Review Activities," in *Quality Improvement Organization Manual*. Washington, DC: Department of Health and Human Services; 2003: Section 4115.
5. The Joint Commission. "Sentinel Event Policy and Procedures." Available at: www.JointCommission.org/SentinelEvents/PolicyandProcedures. Accessed July 24, 2009.
6. Agency for Healthcare Research and Quality (AHRQ). "Patient Safety Organizations Overview." Available at: www.pso.ahrq.gov. Accessed August 8, 2009.

CHAPTER 12

Program-Specific Accreditation

Cindy A. Gassiot, CPMSM, CPCS

The major functions of a medical staff organization and healthcare organization accrediting groups have been discussed in earlier chapters. This chapter focuses on other medical staff functions—specifically, the functions performed by institutional review boards, cancer and trauma committees, continuing medical education programs, and graduate medical education, including how they are accredited.

■ Institutional Review Boards

Hospital institutional review boards (IRBs) are required to oversee protection of the rights and welfare of human subjects involved in clinical investigations of drugs and medical devices, which are ultimately regulated by the Food and Drug Administration (FDA). These boards were formed in many community hospitals for the first time in the 1970s, when intraocular lenses were invented but not yet approved by the FDA, and ophthalmologists began implanting them in conjunction with surgery to remove cataracts. In large teaching facilities, the IRB has a much older history.

Although there is no accreditation per se, the FDA has issued regulations that hospital IRBs must follow; these regulations govern the protection of human subjects involved in research on products regulated by the agency. Additionally, other federal agencies and departments, and some states, have established regulations that govern human subject protection. The medical staff services professional (MSSP) should be familiar with those regulations that apply to research being done at his or her institution.

Products under investigation include drugs that are being evaluated by the FDA and medical devices not yet fully approved by the agency. (The research must be based on adequately performed laboratory and animal experimentation and on thorough knowledge of the scientific literature.) When physicians use investigational products in the hospital setting (and sometimes on an outpatient basis), they must do so under carefully controlled, well-established scientific principles. The IRB's functions are to review and approve, require modification in, or disapprove research activities. Among its other duties, the IRB ensures that risks to subjects are minimized, that risks are reasonable in relation to the anticipated benefits and knowledge that is expected to result, that subject selection is equitable, that informed consent is obtained and documented, that appropriate data monitoring is in place, that privacy of subjects and confidentiality of data are maintained where appropriate, and that additional protections are provided for vulnerable subjects, such as individuals with acute or severe physical or mental illness or persons who are economically or educationally disadvantaged.[1]

Briefly, FDA regulations require the IRB to do the following:[2]

1. Be established at any institution engaging in any investigation, study, or research involving human subjects.
2. Be composed of no fewer than five members with voting authority. Members must be qualified by experience, expertise, and diversity of background to give advice for safeguarding human subjects. The IRB may not be composed of all men or all women or entirely of members of one profession, and it must have one member whose only affiliation with the institution is IRB membership. There must be one member whose primary concerns are in scientific areas and at least one member whose primary activities are nonscientific—for example, a lawyer, ethicist, or clergy. Also, no member of the IRB should have a conflicting interest with the issue under consideration.
3. Perform two primary functions:
   - Review and approve, require modifications in, or disapprove of any proposed investigational study.
   - Monitor any ongoing study. The IRB has a responsibility to ensure each study is carried out as stated in the protocol; any investigation must be followed until it is completed, discontinued, or suspended.
4. Follow written procedures and conduct business only if there is a quorum, which cannot consist of fewer than a majority of members of the committee.
5. Maintain records sufficient to clearly describe the results of any study.
6. Ensure that investigators obtain legal informed consent (the elements of which are specified by the FDA).
7. Receive, investigate, and act on complaints relating to any study under review regardless of their source (e.g., subjects, the sponsor of the study, members of the medical staff, and so on).
8. Make records available for inspection by authorized agents of the FDA.

To assist these committees in operating according to regulations, the FDA has developed a self-evaluation guide. The following guidelines, which are reproduced in part from that document, should be used by the institution to determine which written policies and procedures are needed.[3]

Policies and procedures are required describing the functions of the IRB with respect to the following:

1. Conducting the initial and continuing reviews
2. Reporting findings and actions to the investigator and institution
3. Determining which projects require review more often than annually
4. Determining which projects need verification from sources other than the investigators that no material changes have occurred since the previous IRB review
5. Ensuring prompt reporting to the IRB of changes in research activities
6. Ensuring that changes in approved research are not initiated without IRB review and approval
7. Ensuring prompt reporting to the IRB of unanticipated problems or serious or continuing noncompliance with the requirements or determinations of the IRB
8. Ensuring prompt reporting to the IRB of any suspension or termination of IRB approval

Additional policies and procedures should describe the operations of the IRB with respect to the following:

1. The review process:
   - All members should review the entire protocol.
   - One or more primary reviewers should review entire protocol, report to the IRB, and lead discussion on the protocol.
   - All members should have access to the entire protocol.
   - The role of subcommittees of the IRB should be delineated.
   - Emergency studies must be reviewed.
   - Procedures for expedited review should be followed.
2. Criteria for approval of investigation:
   - The risks to subjects must be minimized.
   - The risks to subjects must be reasonable in relation to the anticipated benefits.
   - The selection of subjects must be equitable.
   - Informed consent must be adequate.
   - Where appropriate, there should be adequate provisions to protect the privacy of subjects and maintain the confidentiality of data.
   - Appropriate safeguards must be included in the study to protect the rights and welfare of vulnerable subjects.
3. Voting requirements:
   - A quorum is required to transact business.
   - There must be quorum diversity requirements.
   - Approval or disapproval of a study should require a certain percentage of the vote.
   - All members must have full voting rights.

- Proxy votes should not be allowed.
- Investigators should not vote on their own studies.

4. IRB record requirements that the institution must maintain include the following:
   - Copies of all research proposals reviewed, consent documents, progress reports, and reports of injuries to subjects
   - Minutes of meetings:
     - Actions taken by the IRB
     - Record of voting, including the number of IRB members voting for, against, and abstaining
     - Basis for requiring changes in or disapproving research
     - Record of discussion of controversial issues
   - Record of continuing review activities
   - Copies of correspondence between the IRB and investigators
   - A list of IRB members and qualifications
   - Written procedures describing the function and operation of the IRB
   - Statements of significant new findings provided to subjects

5. Each investigator must provide information to the IRB. This information must include the following:
   - Professional qualifications to do the research (including a description of necessary support services and facilities)
   - The title of the study
   - The purpose of the study (including the benefit to be obtained by doing the study)
   - The sponsor of the study
   - Results of previous related research
   - Subject selection criteria
   - Subject exclusion criteria
   - The justification for use of special subject populations (e.g., mentally retarded persons, children)
   - The study design (including a discussion of the appropriateness of the research methods)
   - A description of procedures to be performed
   - Provisions for managing adverse reactions

FDA Institutional Review Board Inspections

In response to a Congressional mandate to expand its monitoring of biomedical research conducted under its regulations, the FDA developed the Bioresearch Monitoring Program and, as part of that effort, began an expanded review of IRBs in April 1977.[4] The aim of this program is to protect human subjects by ensuring the existence of well-organized and properly functioning local IRBs. The Bioresearch

Monitoring Program, which encompasses IRBs, clinical investigators, sponsors, monitors, and nonclinical laboratories, is also intended to ensure the quality and integrity of data submitted to the FDA for regulatory decision making, as well as to protect human subjects of research. For this reason, the IRB regulations note that the FDA may inspect IRBs and review and copy IRB records.

Institutional Review Board Program

Under the Bioresearch Monitoring Program, the FDA conducts on-site procedural reviews of IRBs. These reviews are intended to determine whether an IRB is operating in accordance with its own written procedures as well as current FDA regulations. They may consist of routine procedural reviews or be undertaken in response to a complaint or suspected investigator misconduct.

The FDA's *Compliance Program Guidance Manual for IRB Inspections* is available to the public by writing to the following address: Freedom of Information Staff, HFW-30, Food and Drug Administration, 5600 Fishers Lane, Rockville, MD 20857. This manual is also available on the Internet: http://www.fda.gov/oc/ohrt/irbs/operations.html#inspections. Information sheets and frequently asked questions about IRB operation can be found at the following Web site: http://www.fda.gov/oc/ohrt/irbs/default.htm. A self-evaluation checklist for IRBs is also available: http://www.fda.gov/oc/ohrt/irbs/irbchecklist.html.

The professional association for IRB coordinators—the Association of Clinical Research Professionals—sponsors seminars and training programs as well as a certification program for clinical research coordinators. The Web site for this association is http://www.acrpnet.org.

■ Approved Cancer Programs

The Commission on Cancer of the American College of Surgeons (ACS) sponsors a voluntary approval program for institutional cancer programs.[5] Although the tumor registry is the locus of a cancer program in the hospital, the MSSP may provide administrative support to the hospital cancer committee that is seeking approval for its cancer program. An understanding of the components of a hospital cancer program is helpful for performing these tasks.

Cancer programs are assigned an accreditation category that describes the services available at the facility. These services may include community hospital cancer programs, teaching hospital programs, network cancer programs, and pediatric cancer programs, among others. The goals of the ACS cancer program are to decrease morbidity and mortality of cancer patients and to improve the quality of patient care. Encouraging hospitals to improve cancer control efforts through prevention, early detection, pretreatment evaluation, staging, treatment, rehabilitation, and surveillance for recurrence of cancer, and to enhance the care of the terminally ill patient are key components of the pursuit of these goals. A cancer committee oversees these efforts.

To seek ACS approval of its cancer program, the facility must be accredited by a recognized authority, such as the Joint Commission, Hospital Facilities Accreditation Program, National Committee on Quality Assurance, Accreditation Association for Ambulatory Health Care, or American College of Radiology, depending on the services offered by the institution. The facility must also have specific resources available to ensure state-of-the-art diagnosis and treatment of cancer. In addition, the organization must have the following elements in place:

- Cancer program leadership, which may include a cancer committee
- Cancer conferences
- Quality control of cancer registry data
- Quality improvement
- Community outreach

The Cancer Committee

The cancer committee or another leadership body is a standing multidisciplinary committee, with defined authority. This committee, which has responsibility and accountability for the organization's cancer program, must have scheduled meetings. Membership on the committee must include physicians from both diagnostic and treatment services. Depending on the category of facility, the committee must have one coordinator designated for each of the four areas of cancer committee activity: cancer conferences, quality control of cancer registry data, quality improvement, and community outreach. The committee develops and evaluates the annual goals and objectives for the clinical, community outreach, quality improvement, and programmatic endeavors related to cancer care. It also must establish and implement a plan to evaluate the quality of cancer registry data and activity. This plan must include procedures to monitor case finding, accuracy of data collection, abstracting timeliness, follow-up, and data reporting on an annual basis.

Cancer Conferences

An approved cancer program includes conferences to educate the medical and ancillary staffs and provide consultative services to patients. The cancer committee must plan for the conferences on an annual basis and ensure that the required numbers of cases are discussed at the cancer conferences on an annual basis and that 75% of the cases discussed are presented prospectively. The cancer committee must establish multidisciplinary attendance requirements and attendance rates for conferences.

Cancer Data Management

A system to monitor all types of cancer diagnosed or treated in an institution is a critical element in the evaluation of cancer care. The quality of cancer registry data must be evaluated on an annual basis. Case abstracting must be performed or supervised by a Certified Tumor Registrar (CTR). For each year between surveys, 90% of cases must be abstracted within six months of the date of first contact. An 80% follow-up rate must be maintained for all analytic patients from the cancer registry reference date. A 90% follow-up rate must be maintained for all analytic patients diagnosed within the last five years or from the cancer registry reference date, whichever period is shorter. The facility must also participate in special studies as requested by the ACS's Commission on Cancer.

Knowledgeable personnel must staff the cancer registry. A national association for these individuals—the National Cancer Registrars Association (NCRA)—sponsors a certification program for cancer registrars.

Clinical Management

An approved cancer program must have appropriate facilities, equipment, and specialized staff. Radiation treatment services must be available on-site or by referral. Based on the facility, an inpatient medical oncology unit or a functional equivalent must exist to provide specialized care to patients. Staging must be assigned on a staging form in the medical records of at least 90% of eligible annual analytic cases. Nurses with specialized knowledge and skills in oncology should provide care for patients treated in the program, and their competency must be evaluated annually. The guidelines for patient management and treatment currently required by the Commission on Cancer must be followed. Rehabilitation services must be provided on-site or by referral. This is evaluated on an annual basis.

Research

The ACS standards may require the institution to conduct research, depending on the nature of the organization. Information about the availability of cancer-related clinical trials must be provided to patients through a formal mechanism. As appropriate to the organization, a specific, required percentage of cases must be enrolled in cancer-related clinical trials on an annual basis.

Community Outreach

The approved cancer program must reach out to the community through education and supportive services that are provided on-site or coordinated with local agencies and facilities. Two prevention or early detection programs must be provided on-site or coordinated with other facilities or local agencies on an annual basis.

Professional Education and Staff Support

Other than cancer conferences, the cancer committee must offer one cancer-related educational activity each year. All members of the cancer registry staff must participate in a local, state, regional, or national cancer-related educational activity each year.

Quality Improvement

The standards require that the quality of cancer patient care be measured, evaluated, and improved. Each year, the cancer committee must complete and document the required studies that measure quality and outcomes. Two improvements that directly affect cancer patient care must be implemented annually and documented.

Cancer Program Approval

Eligible programs that meet the requirements set out in the standards may initiate the approval process by requesting consultative services by a trained Commission on Cancer consultant or other cancer registry professional. A consultant must evaluate all institutions seeking initial approval of their cancer programs. Regionally based field staff members provide consultative services and conduct cancer program surveys. After the consultant visits the institution, a status report is prepared. If the organization is found to be compliant with all standards, the program will be ready for a survey, which will then be scheduled.

Cancer program surveys entail a comprehensive evaluation of the entire scope, organization, and performance of a cancer program. A physician surveyor who is specially trained to evaluate compliance with the 36 standards that are required for approval performs this survey, which takes place every three years. Each program being surveyed must complete a Web-based survey application, which provides background on the structure of the program and activity since the last survey. The application also lists the evaluation standards and allows the program and surveyor to rate compliance with each standard. Cancer program staff members perform an independent review of a program's application and supporting documentation. The multidisciplinary program review subcommittee may also review program-related activity and standard ratings before an accreditation award is assigned.

Approval Awards

Approval awards are based on compliance with the 36 standards. Programs with deficiencies in mandatory standards are allowed 12 months to document changes for administrative review in an attempt to receive full approval. Four types of accreditation awards are possible: three-year accreditation with commendation, three-year accreditation, three-year approval with contingency, and nonapproval. Deferred status is given for one year when a new program is rated deficient in one standard. Programs that do not resolve this status at the end of a 12-month period must reapply for a new survey.

National Cancer Registrars Association

As mentioned earlier, the NCRA is the professional association for tumor registrars. It supports a certification program that allows an individual to become a CTR. Information on this association and its certification program is available on its Web site (www.ncra-usa.org).

■ Approved Trauma Centers

The ACS's Committee on Trauma has long been committed to reducing trauma morbidity and mortality; it first published guidelines for care of injured patients in 1976. A natural result of the establishment of trauma guidelines was the development of a verification process whereby a hospital can be surveyed by ACS trauma surgeons to determine whether the facility meets ACS criteria.[6] The approval (verification) program was initiated in 1987, and by mid-1993 ACS completed more than 200 surveys and consultation site visits. According to the ACS, the goal of a trauma system "is to match a health care facility's resources with a patient's medical needs so that optimal and cost-effective care is achieved."[7] Its approval program continues to grow, with more and more hospitals seeking ACS verification of their trauma services.

The MSSP may assist in supporting this effort. He or she should be familiar with the designations made by ACS for trauma centers and have some knowledge of the respective requirements for his or her own facility's trauma level.

Trauma Center Levels

Because hospitals have varying resources and capabilities, depending on their size and location, the ACS has designated four levels for trauma services.

Level I Centers

The Level I facility is a regional resource trauma center that serves as a tertiary care facility. Because of the large number of personnel and facility resources required for patient care, most Level I facilities are university-based teaching hospitals.

Level II Centers

The Level II center is a hospital that is expected to provide initial definitive trauma care regardless of the severity of the injury. It may be an academic institution or a public or private community facility located in either an urban, suburban, or rural area.

Level III Centers

The Level III center serves communities that do not have immediate access to a Level I or II institution. Level III trauma centers can provide prompt assessment, resuscitation, emergency operations, and patient stabilization, and can also arrange for possible transfer to a facility that can provide definitive trauma care.

Level IV Centers

The Level IV facility provides advanced trauma life support in remote areas where no higher level of care is available prior to patient transfer.

Hospital Criteria

To be an ACS-approved trauma facility, each hospital must meet certain level-specific criteria. Criteria are designated as "essential" or "desired" for the respective levels. In other words, all criteria are essential for a Level I trauma center, most criteria are essential for a Level II center, and some criteria are desirable for Level III and IV facilities.

Hospital Organization

The medical staff must establish the trauma service, which is responsible for coordinating the care of injured patients, the training of personnel, and trauma quality improvement. Privileges for physicians participating in trauma care are determined through the medical staff credentialing process. A board-certified surgeon must be designated to serve as the trauma service director. A multidisciplinary trauma committee is required for centers rated at Levels I and II. In addition, Level I and II trauma centers must have hospital departments or sections of general, neurologic, and orthopedic surgery; emergency services; and anesthesiology. Neurosurgery and orthopedic surgery departments are not required for Levels III and IV, and an emergency service is not required for Level IV. Criteria also spell out the various clinical capabilities of the hospital according to level.

Criteria for ACS approval also address the facilities, resources, and capabilities that each level must meet. These criteria address the need for specially trained personnel, resuscitation equipment, operating room capabilities, postanesthesia recovery room capabilities, intensive care units, radiology and laboratory capabilities, and rehabilitation service staff and equipment, with specific requirements applying to each level.

All ACS-approved trauma centers must establish a quality improvement program. The quality improvement activities undertaken as part of this program must include a trauma registry, special audits for all trauma deaths, morbidity and mortality conferences, and other reviews. A criterion that applies to Level I, II, and III trauma centers is that an on-call schedule must be published for surgical and other major medical specialties. Other criteria pertain to outreach programs, prevention and publication education, a trauma research program, continuing medical education, trauma support personnel, organ procurement activity, and transfer agreements.

The Approvals Process

The designation of trauma facilities is a political process performed by the local governmental emergency medical service (EMS) authorities. The ACS approvals and consultation program is designed to assist hospitals in evaluation and improvement of trauma care, but it does not officially designate a facility as a trauma center. At the request of an appropriate local or state authority and of the hospital, the ACS will perform a verification review.

To obtain a trauma level designation, the facility applies to the ACS, completes a presurvey questionnaire and hospital resources checklist, and has a survey scheduled. A team of two surgeons from the ACS performs the site visit and reports their findings to the ACS trauma department. This final report, which is confidential, is then sent to the requesting governmental agency or to the hospital by the ACS's Committee on Trauma. Maximum approval for successful facilities is for three years, and reverification is accomplished through the same review process.

The ACS's Committee on Trauma also provides consultation to hospitals, communities, and state authorities for the purpose of identifying areas for improving trauma care or preparing for a verification visit.

American Trauma Society

The American Trauma Society is a leading organization for trauma care and trauma prevention in the United States. The American Trauma Society's Registrar Certification Board (ATSRCB) endorses the concept of voluntary, periodic certification by examination for all trauma registrars. Its certification program allows an individual to become a Certified Specialist Trauma Registrar (CSTR). Information on this association and its certification program is available on its Web site (www.amtrauma.org).

Continuing Medical Education Programs

A large number of states have mandatory continuing medical education (CME) requirements for physician relicensure or for membership in the state medical association. Some malpractice insurance plans and physician specialty organizations also require participation in CME. As there is a significant cost to practitioners who participate in CME—not only in tuition but also in time away from practice—many healthcare facilities provide accredited CME programs for their medical staffs. Medical staff services departments frequently support such programs.

CME should play a role in a practitioner's delineation of clinical privileges. In addition, the choice of CME programs offered should be based in part on results of the medical staff's performance improvement findings, as required by the Joint Commission.

Depending on the sophistication of the CME program, medical staff services personnel may spend a significant amount of time assisting the CME committee with curriculum development, contacting speakers for conferences, notifying medical staff members, compiling and analyzing program evaluations, and recording CME credits for reporting to medical staff members. If the CME program is accredited, a full-time employee may be required to support the program and its documentation requirements.

The Physician's Recognition Award

To provide additional motivation to pursue CME, the American Medical Association (AMA) offers the voluntary Physician's Recognition Award (PRA). Applications are based on one, two, or three years of CME, and certificates issued are valid for one, two, or three years from the date of application. Criteria for the awards are described in the following sections.[8]

Educational Options for the PRA

Activities designated by accredited sponsors as category 1 or category 2 include the following:

1. Publishing articles
2. Preparing a presentation for a category 1 designated conference
3. Obtaining a medically related advanced degree
4. American Board of Medical Specialties Board certification
5. Formal activities such as lectures, seminars, and workshops offered by accredited organizations
6. Approved international conferences
7. Approved AMA pilot projects

Physician-designated activities for category 2 include the following:

1. Consultation with peers and experts concerning patients
2. Medical research and study online
3. Using nondesignated enduring materials
4. Teaching residents or other health professionals
5. Reading authoritative medical literature, and other activities

The AMA offers two PRA certificates: the standard award and an award with commendation. The requirements for the certificates are listed in the next subsection. Reading authoritative literature an average of two hours per week is required for all certificates.

AMA PRA Standard Certificates

The following requirements must be fulfilled to obtain PRA certificates:

Three-year certificate: 150 hours—60 hours category 1; 90 hours category 1 or 2 credits

Two-year certificate: 100 hours—40 hours category 1; 60 hours category 1 or 2 credits

One-year certificate: 50 hours—20 hours category 1; 30 hours category 1 or 2 credits

Category 1 credit refers to programs accredited by the Accreditation Council for Continuing Medical Education (ACCME). The ACCME, through its recognition process, allows state or territory medical societies to accredit CME providers. This organization is composed of representatives from AMA, American Board of Medical Specialties, American Hospital Association, Association for Hospital Medical Education, Association of American Medical Colleges, Council of Medical Specialty Societies, and Federation of State Medical Boards. All accredited providers have demonstrated an ability to meet the accreditation requirements. Accreditation, either directly by the ACCME or through a recognized state medical association, affords the CME provider with the ability to designate activities for AMA-PRA category 1 credit. State medical associations survey, evaluate, and accredit CME programs at community facilities whose programs meet the essentials and guidelines of approved programs. Only institutions accredited as CME sponsors by the ACCME or their state medical society may designate a CME activity for AMA-PRA credit.

Accredited CME

To be accredited, a healthcare facility must meet the ACCME's standards for accredited CME, called the "Essential Areas and their Elements." These standards are briefly described in the following subsections.[9]

Essential 1: Purpose and Mission

The provider must have a written statement of its CME mission, approved by the provider's governing body, which includes the CME purpose, content areas, target audience, type of activities provided, and expected results of the program.

Essential 2: Educational Planning and Evaluation

The CME provider must use a planning process that links identified educational needs with a desired result in its provision of all CME activities. The provider must use needs assessment data to plan CME activities. The provider must also communicate the objectives of the activity so that the learner is informed before he or she participates in the activity. The CME activities must be in compliance with policies for disclosure and commercial support.

Essential 3: Evaluation and Improvement

The provider must evaluate the effectiveness of its CME activities in meeting identified educational needs. It must also evaluate the effectiveness of its overall CME program and make improvements to the program.

The provider must have an organizational framework for the CME unit, which provides the necessary resources to support its mission. The provider must operate the business and management policies and procedures of its CME program so that its obligations and commitments are met.

CME Accreditation Through State Medical Associations

A healthcare facility seeking accreditation of its CME program can obtain information and application forms from the state medical association or society. The first step in the accreditation process is completion of a preassessment questionnaire. If the responses on this questionnaire demonstrate significant compliance with the essentials, the state medical association then invites the facility to complete the application forms. Completion of these forms is time-consuming, but provides an exhaustive look at the CME program of the facility. If the application meets with approval by the state medical association's CME committee, a site survey is then scheduled. Representatives of the state's CME committee conduct the site survey, meeting with the CME committee chair and members and CME support staff, visiting educational facilities, and reviewing documentation.

Provisional accreditation is awarded for two years to an initial applicant that successfully completes the accreditation process. Full accreditation is awarded for a maximum of six years to an accredited institution following completion of the provisional period and a second review and site survey. Non-accreditation is designated for an initial applicant following a review that reveals the institution is not in substantial compliance with the essentials. Non-accredited organizations may reapply later when they can fully comply with the essentials.

■ Graduate Medical Education

Most academic medical centers and many community hospitals participate in graduate medical education (GME) programs. Formal graduate medical education programs seek accreditation by the Accreditation Council on Graduate Medical

Education (ACGME). The ACGME is a private professional organization that is responsible for the accreditation of nearly 8,734 residency education programs. Residency education is the period of clinical education in a medical specialty that follows graduation from medical school; it prepares physicians for the independent practice of medicine.

The ACGME's volume of accredited programs makes it one of the largest private accrediting agencies in the United States, if not the world. The ACGME accredits residency programs in 130 specialty and subspecialty areas of medicine, including all programs leading to primary board certification by the 24 member boards of the American Board of Medical Specialties. Completion of an ACGME-accredited residency program is a prerequisite for certification in a primary board. Completion of an ACGME-accredited subspecialty program is also required before an individual can sit for board certification in the majority of subspecialties. Twenty-eight specialty-specific committees, known as residency review committees (RRCs), periodically initiate revision of the standards and review accredited programs in each specialty and its subspecialties.

To gain and maintain accreditation, residency programs are expected to comply with the accreditation standards for their discipline. In addition, institutions sponsoring residency programs are expected to adhere to a set of institutional requirements.

Compliance with the ACGME's standards is measured through periodic review of all programs. Each year, the RRCs review nearly half of all accredited programs. Approximately 2200 of these reviews involve a formal on-site visit to the program; the remaining reviews are based on documents that each program provides to the ACGME. On average, each accredited residency program receives a visit to the site every 3.7 years. Sponsoring institutions are also visited periodically. The interval between site visits ranges from one to five years, with a longer period indicating that the ACGME and RRCs are more confident about the ability of a given program or institution to provide quality education.[10]

Besides each individual residency program accreditation process, the healthcare facility must comply with institutional requirements and undergo a survey for compliance with issues such as the institution's commitment to GME, as evidenced by the following achievements:

- Maintaining the appropriate agreements and documentation for oversight of each program
- Maintaining the Joint Commission or a comparable accreditation
- Maintaining policies and procedures that outline what has to be in place for all residents, such as financial support, benefits and conditions, work hours, conditions of appointment, expected competencies, and the work environment
- Establishment of a GME committee along with its composition, responsibilities, and meetings

- Required communication among the residency programs and the organization and the leadership of any other organization that supports the program by allowing training on its site
- Establishment of processes and protocols for internal reviews and reporting on all programs[11]

Typically an academic center with multiple GME programs will have a coordinator dedicated to the administrative aspects of the institutional accreditation; it may also have individual coordinators in charge of each residency program. In community hospitals, GME consists of rotating periods through specific units or areas of service. If the base program is located at another facility, however, the MSSP may be in charge of maintaining the administrative function that supports the rotating residents and students. A database of information concerning these individuals needs to be maintained, as well as documentation such as copies of the agreements with the original program stating who will be on-site, what they are expected to do, who will provide supervision, and whether the originating program will provide the professional liability insurance for those individuals while on-site.

National Board of Certification for Training Administrators of Graduate Medical Education

The National Board of Certification for Training Administrators of Graduate Medical Education Programs has been created to establish standards for the profession, to acknowledge the expertise needed to successfully manage GME programs, and to recognize those training program administrators who have achieved competence in all fields related to their profession. Information about this certification program can be found on its Web site (www.tagme.org).[12]

■ Notes

1. Food and Drug Administration. *Guidelines for Institutional Review Boards and Clinical Investigators, 1998 Update* (21 CFR Part 6, 1998). Washington, DC: U.S. Department of Health and Human Services; 1998. Available at: http://www.fda.gov/oc/ohrt/irbs/default.htm. Accessed July 9, 2009.
2. Food and Drug Administration, note 1.
3. Office for Human Research Protections. *Institutional Review Board Guidebook*. Washington, DC: U.S. Department of Health and Human Services. Available at: http://www.hhs.gov/ohrp/irb/irb_guidebook.htm. Accessed January 31, 2006.
4. Food and Drug Administration. *Guidelines for Institutional Review Boards and Clinical Investigators, 1998 Update: A Self-Evaluation Checklist*. Available at: http://www.fda.gov/ScienceResearch/SpecialTopics/RunningClinicalTrials/GuidancesInformationSheetsandNotices/ucm118063.htm. Accessed July 9, 2009.
5. American College of Surgeons, Commission on Cancer. "Cancer Program Standards, 2009 Revised Edition." Available at: http://www.facs.org/cancer/coc/cocprogramstandards.pdf. Accessed July 9, 2009.

6. American College of Surgeons, Committee on Trauma. *Resources for Optimal Care of the Injured Patient: 2006.* Chicago, IL: Author; 2006.
7. American College of Surgeons, note 6.
8. American Medical Association. *Physician Recognition Award Booklet.* Chicago, IL: Author; 2006. Available at: http://www.ama-assn.org. Accessed July 9, 2009.
9. Accreditation Council for Continuing Medical Education. *Essential Areas and Their Elements.* 2006. Chicago, IL: Author. Accessed at: http://www.accme.org. Accessed July 9, 2009.
10. Accreditation Council on Graduate Medical Education. *The ACGME at a Glance.* Chicago, IL: Author. Accessed at: http://www.acgme.org. Accessed January 22, 2010.
11. Accreditation Council on Graduate Medical Education. *Institutional Review Committees.* Chicago, IL: Author. Accessed at: http://www.acgme.org. July 9, 2009.
12. Training Administrators of Graduate Medical Education Programs. Available at: http://www.tagme.org. Accessed July 9, 2009.

Practitioner Health and Behavior Issues

Cindy A. Gassiot, CPMSM, CPCS

CHAPTER 13

■ The Impaired Practitioner

The American Medical Association (AMA) defines an impaired physician as a physician who is "unable to practice medicine with reasonable skill and safety to patients because of physical or mental illness, including deterioration through the aging process or loss of motor skill, or excessive use or abuse of drugs including alcohol."[1]

The exact number of practitioners who are impaired by drug or alcohol abuse in the United States is unknown, but the rate of substance abuse among healthcare providers has been estimated to be the same as that for the general population, approximately one in ten.[2] Adding to the problem, aging physicians may be impaired by senile dementia or some other illness that is progressively debilitating. Medical staff and credentialing services professionals will more than likely encounter this difficult problem sooner or later in their careers. Healthcare organizations are now required to have in place guidelines and procedures to follow in motivating impaired practitioners to seek treatment and a monitoring program that allows rehabilitated practitioners to return to practice. "Ignoring the value of documented recovery or correction of prior problems only causes attempts to hide disabilities, thus delaying treatment and recovery. The risk of harm to patients treated by a disabled practitioner increases unless the credentialing process recognizes rehabilitation."[3]

The Joint Commission has a standard requiring medical staff to establish a process to identify and manage matters of individual practitioner health that is separate from the medical staff disciplinary function. The rationale for the standard acknowledges that assistance and rehabilitation, rather than discipline, aids a practitioner in seeking treatment and rehabilitation, and provides protection for patients. Medical staff services departments (MSSDs) should have a policy addressing this matter. A sample policy on practitioner health can be found in the CD that accompanies this book.

This chapter examines the causes of practitioner impairment and the programs available to assist practitioners and healthcare facilities with treatment, rehabilitation, and monitoring of impaired individuals. The tough problems of the aging practitioner and disruptive practitioner are also addressed.

Causes of Practitioner Impairment

Physicians work in a state of sustained stress. Despite their medical training, or perhaps because of it, they are prone to hazards such as physical and emotional stress, long hours, irregular sleeping schedules, and constant fatigue. As a result of these stresses, they often find themselves using substances such as alcohol or drugs or develop resultant conditions that may result in illnesses or impairments in their ability to practice.

The causes of practitioner impairment vary widely. Studies of practitioners who have become impaired suggest that one potential source of impairment may be the individual's inherent personality structure. Although obsessive–compulsive traits can be a professional asset, many individuals with these attributes also demonstrate basic insecurity, dependency, depressive features, and vulnerability to stress. A practitioner's self-imposed demands, combined with the expectations of his or her professional role, may prove very stressful. If the practitioner is unable to meet his or her needs for nurturing and intimacy, a framework for impairment may be established.

Many aspects of medical training and practice contribute to stress, including long hours with accompanying fatigue and the frustration of caring for chronically ill patients. Many practitioners are never taught how to keep an appropriate emotional distance between themselves and their patients. Practitioners give and give of themselves emotionally and, over a period of time, can experience burnout. At-risk practitioners may turn to alcohol, other drugs, or other compulsive behaviors for relief of this psychic pain. The interplay of stress, personality, and genetic factors may trigger a chemical dependency.[4]

The clues to impairment may be subtle. TABLE 13-1 lists symptoms that may be displayed by a physician who suffers from impairment.

Hospital-Based Programs*

A hospital has certain legal responsibilities to take action against an incompetent physician. With respect to an impaired physician, however, responsibility and liability are not as clearly defined. Administrators and colleagues often ignore or overlook signs of developing impairment in the hope that it will disappear. Only in cases of blatant impairment do they tend to intervene, and then usually in a punitive manner.

Preferable is a nonpunitive approach in which the hospital works as an advocate for the physician, rather than against him, while still safeguarding patients from

---

*The section "Hospital-Based Programs" is reprinted with permission of the American Medical Association from *Proceedings of the 4th AMA Conference on the Impaired Physician*. Chicago, IL: AMA; 1980:7–31.

Table 13-1 A Symptom Checklist for Detecting Physician Impairment

A Disturbing Metamorphosis	Deteriorating Job Performance
Embarrassing behavior at work and social functions	Absenteeism
Emotional volatility	Complaints about the physician's behavior from patients or staff
Evasiveness	Consistent lateness
Hostility	Inability to explain treatment plans
Inappropriate euphoria	Increased incidence of treatment errors
Uncharacteristic impatience or rudeness	Rounds late at night or at other odd times
Uncooperativeness	Unreachable when on call
Unpredictability	
Unreliability	
Unusually poor personal hygiene	
Withdrawal from routine activities	
Chaos at Home	**Numerous Trials and Tribulations**
Abuse	Arrests for driving while intoxicated
Continual discord	Frequent accidents
Inappropriate spending	Frequent hospitalizations
Obsessive involvement in an outside activity—for example, gambling	Frequent involvement in lawsuits
	Habitual self-prescribing of controlled substances
Sexual problems	
Unexplained absences	Multiple physical complaints

Source: Adapted from "What to Do When a Colleague Is Impaired," by Patrick H. Hughes, Martha Illige-Saucier, and Eric A. Voth, *Patient Care*, vol. 29, no. 12, p. 119, © by Advanstar Communications, Inc., 1995. Reprinted with permission.

harm. This type of program can detect emerging impairment, offer support to the physician and his family, and encourage early treatment. Helping the impaired physician is in the best interest of the hospital as well as the impaired physician himself and the hospital's patients.

Is a Hospital Program Necessary?

Whether a program at the hospital level is necessary or even feasible depends on several variables, including the following:

- State mandatory reporting laws
- Geographic location
- Size of state

- Activities and strengths of county medical society programs
- Activities and strengths of state medical society programs
- Size of the hospital
- Hospital constitution and bylaws
- Interest and level of awareness of the medical staff and administration

Generally speaking, impairment is more likely to be detected at the hospital level much earlier than it is at the county or state medical society level. This is particularly true in a large state or in a densely populated area.

Small hospitals, however, may be especially resistant to initiating programs because of their size, the intimacy among staff, or time constraints. This may necessitate the involvement of the county or state medical society program.

Ideally, hospital, county, and state medical society programs will complement one another. For example, if a hospital working in concert with a state program is unsuccessful in encouraging an impaired physician to seek treatment, the state society may become involved and thereby assure that the physician does not evade the issue even if he changes his hospital affiliation or practice mode.

Organization

No single model is applicable to all hospitals because of the many variables in medical staff bylaws, size, and state laws. These differences, however, give each hospital/medical staff the capability of establishing a program that is tailored to its individual needs. The local hospital association, county medical society, or state medical society may be able to identify programs operating in other hospitals in the area that can be used as a model.

A formal policy on practitioner impairment should be incorporated into the bylaws and should include a provision for immediate suspension of privileges if a physician is a threat to himself or his patients. Legal input will assure that due process elements, informed consent, confidentiality aspects, and the legal rights of both the hospital and an impaired practitioner are adequately addressed. Additionally, the bylaws should include a provision of immunity for those acting on behalf of the hospital program.

A program to aid impaired practitioners should be organizationally separate from credential review and peer review, although it is desirable that input from committees charged with carrying out these functions be utilized where feasible in case-finding activities.

The hospital should continually promote its advocacy program to assure visibility and use. In this regard, an ongoing education component encourages reporting from staff and other hospital personnel, and is beneficial in increasing levels of awareness, changing negative attitudes and stereotypical perceptions, and providing cognitive information on the nature and treatability of impairment. Where possible, educational programs for spouses should be initiated. The spouse is often aware, far earlier than hospital personnel, of a practitioner's impairment.

In addition to education and promotion, other components of a hospital-based program include case findings, intervention, rehabilitation, and reentry. It is generally recommended that treatment be arranged on an outpatient basis or in another hospital.

Case Finding

A hospital is responsible for implementing policies to assure that its staff members are capable of providing quality medical care, as well as procedures to assess their mental and physical health. These existing mechanisms can be the foundation for early case finding and prevention.

The medical staff monitoring process (note—impairment could be identified via evaluation of OPPE data) offers an avenue to review a practitioner's performance and discussing potential or existing problems.

Although credentialing, peer review, and medical staff (performance improvement) functions should be outside the purview of activities relating to helping impaired practitioners, members of these committees can help identify practitioners who are impaired or potentially impaired.

Reports about a practitioner who is having problems should be encouraged and accepted from nurses, colleagues, other hospital personnel, and family members. For this reason, a visible contact person or contact mechanism (e.g., special "hotline") is imperative. Whether reports are also accepted from patients, and whether reports may be made on an anonymous basis, is up to the discretion of the hospital. Anonymous reports can be valuable as well as detrimental. In any event, the identity of the person who reports a practitioner who may possibly be impaired should be kept confidential, and provision for such confidentiality should be emphasized to encourage reporting.

The Joint Commission standards require that a medical staff implement a process to identify and manage matters of individual health of licensed independent practitioners. Most medical staffs have opted to deal with this process by establishing a committee.

Several options are available with respect to the structure and composition of the specific committee to receive and act on reports of impairment and requests of help. Potential members might include the following:

- Well-liked, respected senior staff members
- Staff members or administrators recovering from impairment
- Resident and student representatives
- Hospital administrators
- Department heads
- Chiefs of staff

- President, past-president, and president-elect of the medical staff (to allow for ongoing knowledge and interest)

Four basic types of committees have been identified: (1) structured, with administrative and physician members; (2) nonstructured, with physician members only; (3) structured, with physician members only; and (4) nonstructured, with basic members plus others added depending on the individual case. Those programs that are defined as structured have standing committee status and an ongoing function, whereas nonstructured committees are constituted on an ad hoc, or as needed, basis.

Some people feel strongly that staff officers with disciplinary authority should not be included because their presence might deter reporting from those who fear punitive action. Others feel equally strongly that these people with "power" should be included because their responsibility for quality care cannot be abdicated or delegated.

The question of whether the committee should be a standing committee or be convened on an ad hoc basis is equally debatable. Both approaches have merit.

Regardless of how the committee is composed, it should focus exclusively on problems relating to impairment and practitioner well-being as opposed to incompetence or illegal activities. The name of the committee should also be positive, such as "Practitioner Health and Well-Being" versus "Practitioner Impairment Committee."

A mechanism for verifying allegations of impairment should be incorporated into any program. Options include verification by a solo member or by a subgroup of the committee.

Intervention

Intervention at the hospital level can emphasize the human factors that have been shown to be positive elements for encouraging a physician to seek treatment. If the committee finds its efforts are hampered by loyalty, embarrassment, or overprotectiveness, it may then be necessary to involve the county or state medical society in the intervention process.

If intervention is carried out within the confines of a hospital program, a special group or subcommittee should receive training in intervention techniques. The county or state medical society may be willing to provide training courses. The intervention team may also include a colleague of the impaired practitioner whom the "informer" has identified as the person most likely to induce the practitioner to get treatment.

Basically, the intervention process should be an organized attempt to persuade the practitioner to get help, while conveying the hope that treatment can be effective. Sources of help should be identified, a definite treatment plan presented, and a program for rehabilitation outlined. If the bylaws or a formal policy and procedure have been accepted/authorized, this fact can be used as leverage to encourage the practitioner to seek help promptly. During the period of rehabilitation, the medical staff must take action to assure that patients of the practitioner are not put at risk. In most situations, the practitioner does not see or take care of patients during a rehabilitation program because he has taken a leave of absence or privileges have been suspended during the rehabilitation period.

If the practitioner refuses help, it may be necessary to process the issue through the usual medical staff disciplinary channels. The medical staff/hospital has the "stick" of being able to restrict or suspend privileges. Even then, discipline should be applied in conjunction with a plan of rehabilitation wherever possible.

Reentry

The hospital/medical staff committee should monitor the practitioner's treatment and recovery and should continue its advocacy role through the reentry phase. Once the formerly impaired practitioner has returned to the hospital, the committee should recommend reinstatement of his privileges based on his current ability to practice. If monitoring of his activities is thought to be necessary for hospital, patient, or physician protection, the hospital/medical staff committee can delineate structured reentry points that allow for such monitoring (e.g., proctoring of surgical privileges, review of charts, supervised patient care, urine screening).

■ A Contract with an Impaired Practitioner

Once intervention has occurred and the practitioner has agreed to seek treatment, the hospital/medical staff or medical society committee should enter into a contract with the affected practitioner. The contract should specify the terms under which the hospital or medical society committee will act in an advocacy role to the state licensing board, hospital boards, medical societies, and the Drug Enforcement Agency, and should spell out terms of monitoring after the physician returns to practice. The purpose of this contract is to prevent any misunderstanding as to the terms and times specified. The contract should be specifically designed to meet the need of each individual and be uniquely suited to the particular circumstances. EXHIBIT 13-1 shows a sample contract.

When a practitioner agrees to seek treatment and enter into a voluntary rehabilitation agreement, the practitioner should agree to take a leave of absence from the medical staff to undergo rehabilitation. Because the leave of absence is neither corrective action nor a restriction of privileges, it is not reportable to the National Practitioner Data Bank.

Exhibit 13-1 Sample Contract with an Impaired Practitioner

Agreement

Name of Practitioner: _____ Date: _____

I, _____, agree to the terms of this contract for a period of two (2) years from the date of this contract.

I understand that all expenses connected with my treatment are to be rendered at my own expense and are my own responsibility.

I agree to cease the practice of medicine until clearance is received from the Well-being Committee.

I agree to enter a treatment center approved by the Committee for evaluation and detoxification on _____ (date).

I agree to Phase I of treatment, which will consist of a minimum of 28 days of treatment in an inpatient rehabilitation center.

I agree to Phase II of treatment, which will consist of an outpatient program, including attendance at regular AA meetings, and attendance at the weekly Physician's Recovery Group.

I agree to Phase III of treatment, which may consist of staff training if necessary, and gradually phasing into medical practice under the Committee's supervision.

I agree to completely abstain from any mood-altering chemicals (alcohol, sedatives, stimulants, narcotics, soporifics, over-the-counter drugs, and so on) except on a prescription from my primary care physician, after consultation with the Committee. I will not prescribe any medication for myself.

I agree to provide random urine or blood samples in the presence of another physician or designee, at the discretion of the Committee.

I agree to identification of a primary care physician before completion of Phase I. All aspects of my case history will be made known to this physician. He or she will receive a copy of this contract, and agrees to meet and consult with the Well-being Committee.

I agree to the following special terms as they apply to my illness (if any are stipulated).

I agree that should I leave treatment, the Committee will remove itself from an advocacy position with the Medical Licensing Board of the state of _____.

_____
Signature of Impaired Practitioner

Witness _____

Approved _____

Chairman, Committee Monitoring the Practitioner

Monitoring Recovery

When a practitioner completes a rehabilitation program and returns to the healthcare organization to resume practice, a process for monitoring must be put in place to assure that the practitioner can practice safely. Elements of a monitoring program should be included in the contract or agreement executed by the impaired practitioner, and should address at least the following points:

- Both inpatient and outpatient follow-up treatment
- Abstention from use of any mood-altering chemicals or drugs
- Provision of random urine and/or blood samples
- Identification of a primary care physician who will be authorized to consult with the well-being committee
- Any special terms that may apply to a specific case

Failure to abide by any of these provisions would result in the committee ceasing to act in an advocacy role for the impaired practitioner.

The well-being committee should gather and regularly review information about the practitioner's recovery. Ideally, one practitioner would be appointed to be a regular contact to support and advise the impaired practitioner during the period of monitoring and to report to the well-being committee. Confidential records (with the practitioner's identity protected) of the recovery and monitoring period should be maintained by the well-being committee. The medical staff may also want to proctor the recovering impaired practitioner during the period of monitoring.

The recovering practitioner may sometimes relapse or "slip" with the use of drugs or alcohol. Slips are not uncommon among recovering impaired practitioners, and one occurrence should not be a reason to terminate the monitoring plan. Treatment and monitoring should be intensified in such a case, and the practitioner may need to take a temporary leave from patient care responsibilities. Slips should be evaluated on an individual basis to determine the best course of action.

If the practitioner has privileges at more than one hospital, there could be an agreement between the well-being committees of the two hospitals that one will act as the primary monitoring facility and make regular confidential reports to the well-being committee of the secondary facility about the practitioner.

The Americans with Disabilities Act

The Americans with Disabilities Act (ADA) is a federal law designed to eliminate discrimination against individuals with disabilities. Hospitals and managed care organizations have modified credentialing procedures to conform to the requirements of the ADA. Healthcare organizations attempting to deal with issues of practitioner impairment due to drug or alcohol abuse as well as physical and emotional impairments must also keep in mind the provisions of the ADA.

The ADA's definition of an individual with a disability is very specific—namely, a person who has a physical or mental impairment that substantially limits one or more of his or her major life activities, has a record of such impairment, or is regarded as having such impairment. Alcoholism qualifies as an impairment under the ADA, whereas alcohol use that affects job performance is not impairment under this legislation. Indeed, unsatisfactory performance because of impairment due to alcohol or drug abuse is not protected by the ADA and must not be tolerated. When there is risk of an impaired practitioner causing harm to a patient, the hospital has a duty to take action to protect the patient. The ADA also specifically permits an employer to ensure that the workplace is free from the illegal use of drugs and alcohol. Nevertheless, it does provide protection from discrimination for practitioners who are recovering from drug and alcohol addiction.

The simple fact that a practitioner is recovering from alcohol or substance abuse is not a sufficient reason to deny appointment to the medical staff. The ADA allows medical inquiries and medical exams to be made prior to a practitioner's medical staff appointment if such inquiries are made after the completion of all other credentialing steps and the offer of appointment, but prior to actual appointment. If a healthcare facility decides to make the inquiries or order the medical exams, and based on the information received does not appoint the practitioner to the staff, the facility must be prepared to show in court that the practitioner could not exercise the requested privileges even with reasonable accommodations from the hospital.[5]

When dealing with issues of impairment, advice should always be sought from the organization's legal counsel.

■ The Aging Physician

To allow or encourage a physician to work beyond his or her physical or professional capacity is a great disservice to patients. Unfortunately, respect for age and long-standing service to the hospital and medical community often prevent organized medical staffs from addressing the aging physician who no longer has the skills to practice. In some cases, physicians continue to practice long after they have become prone to hearing and vision losses, memory lapses, cardiorespiratory disabilities, and loss of motor skills owing to their advancing age.[6] Although age alone is not a reason for curtailment of clinical privileges, it may suggest that the organization take a closer look to confirm that physical ability still matches privileges granted. Medical staffs should recognize the special needs of older physicians and develop policies to direct their actions.

A policy for the older physician could contain the following provisions:[7]

- All physicians older than the age of (65 or 70) must be reappointed annually.
- Physicians older than the agreed minimum age are required to submit with the reappointment application a letter from a private physician certifying that the physician is healthy enough to exercise the privileges requested.

- The credentials and medical executive committees have the authority to require the applying physician to undergo a physical examination following absence or disabling illness. The examining physician should be authorized by the applicant to report findings of the examination to the credentials or medical executive committee. The medical staff should also have the authority to require an examination as part of the evaluation of a physician who has demonstrated a performance problem.
- The physician health and rehabilitation committee of the medical staff will consider supportive options for a physician who needs help because of advancing age. These measures might include assistance in recruiting a younger associate to provide coverage for hospitalized patients or counsel in delineating clinical privileges commensurate with remaining ability.
- The medical staff will develop honors and awards that recognize long and valuable service as part of a structured program of withdrawal from hospital practice.

The Disruptive Practitioner

For too many years, healthcare facilities and their workers have suffered the antics, abuse, and disruptive behavior of a small number of temperamental practitioners. Examples of such behavior include throwing instruments in the operating room; verbal abuse of nurses and other healthcare professionals to the point that they cannot function in their jobs; disruptive behavior in meetings; and in a few cases, actual physical assault of other physicians, patients, or hospital staff members. These are not unusual occurrences. Unfortunately, the behavior of these practitioners gives new meaning to the term "hostile work environment." Such behavior can be costly to healthcare organizations. Low morale can lead to high employee turnover and additional costs for recruiting, orientation, and training. Additionally, dysfunctional teams can result in substandard healthcare delivery.[8]

The Joint Commission has finally acknowledged that disruptive behavior is a problem and has incorporated into its leadership standards requirements for a code of conduct that defines what disruptive or unacceptable behavior is. The standards also include language about managing conflict.[9] Additionally, a sentinel event alert has been issued warning that disruptive behavior can lead to preventable adverse outcomes and to decreased patient satisfaction.[10]

In the past, managers in healthcare facilities attempted to deal with these bad actors by counseling and cajoling them. Organizations are powerless to take definitive action until senior hospital managers, medical staff organizations, and governing bodies decide not to continue to tolerate this kind of behavior. A recent study found that, despite the fact that most hospitals now have a policy in place for dealing with disruptive behavior, definitive action is rarely taken. For example, a survey of

1627 physician executives conducted by the American College of Physician Executives in 2004[11] revealed that practitioners with disruptive behaviors were seldom punished. The survey noted that due to physician stature and revenue-generating ability, facilities are usually lenient when it comes to disciplining disruptive practitioners. The problem usually involves only a few practitioners and their interactions with nursing staff and other hospital staff members, or practitioners who do not want to participate in teamwork.

Experts say that practitioner behavior can be changed, if the organization has the will to act. Tactics for changing bad behavior include coaching practitioners on appropriate behavior, mediating disputes between practitioners and staff, referring troublesome practitioners for counseling, and taking strong disciplinary action. Some steps in this direction are discussed next.

Policy on Disruptive Behavior

The first step in managing disruptive behavior problems is the adoption of a zero-tolerance policy by the medical staff organization and governing body and inclusion of language in the medical staff bylaws to back up the policy. Most medical staffs have adopted these policies in the past ten years or so, but most of them advocate a step-by-step process that begins with collegial intervention and counseling and continues with progressive disciplinary action. The trouble with this type of policy is that there is no provision for instigating definitive action right away if a practitioner's behavior is egregious enough to warrant immediate disciplinary action by the medical staff organization. A practitioner who assaults a hospital staff member, patient, or another practitioner, for example, should not slide by with a collegial counseling session with a medical staff leader. Rather, the response to an occurrence of disruptive behavior should be commensurate with the degree of seriousness of the behavior.

There should always be a written report of all occurrences of disruptive behavior. In addition, an effort should be made to investigate and confirm the event.

When the behavior is not serious enough to warrant immediate definitive action, the most common approach is a collegial counseling session with one or more medical staff leaders and a warning that more serious consequences will follow if the behavior continues. These sessions should always be documented and follow-up letters should be mailed to the disruptive practitioner warning that more serious discipline will be applied if the behavior does not change.

If collegial attempts are not successful, the medical staff organization must take formal disciplinary action in accordance with the medical staff bylaws. If medical staff leaders are reluctant to meet with disruptive practitioners, the chairman or a member of the governing body could be requested to meet with the practitioner. This approach relieves medical staff leaders of an onerous chore that they may not be qualified or willing to address and puts the disruptive practitioner on notice that he or she is accountable to the governing body.[12]

If the procedure followed either through the medical executive committee or through the board is inherently fair and complies with the bylaws, and if there is a well-documented record of the practitioner's conduct and the hospital's and medical staff leaders' attempts to deal with it, the disciplinary action will be upheld. The courts have made it abundantly clear that the provision of patient care in an atmosphere of calm, order, and respect for the dignity of all need not be sacrificed to the disruptive proclivities of any appointee to the medical staff or any practitioner granted clinical privileges, regardless of his or her clinical abilities.

Policies on Disruptive Behavior and Sexual Harassment

Every MSSD should ensure that the medical staff has policies in place that address disruptive behavior and sexual harassment. All healthcare organizations have a duty to assure an appropriate work environment.

Most medical staff organizations do, in fact, have some type of policy and procedure on disruptive behavior and sexual harassment. Frequently, these topics are often covered in the medical staff bylaws. The problem is the failure of some medical staffs to deal with these issues as they arise. If a medical staff fails to take appropriate action to protect patients, employees, other practitioners, and other persons from a hostile work environment, the hospital cannot wait (and hope) for the medical staff organization to "do the right thing" but is legally obligated to intervene.

A sample policy on disruptive behavior and a sample policy addressing sexual harassment are included on the CD that accompanies this book.

■ Assistance in Dealing with Practitioner Behavior and Health Problems

If the local or state medical association or society does not offer assistance with chemical dependency, behavior issues, and mental health programs, physicians may be referred to private programs. Scribd's Web site (www.scrbd.com) has a nationwide listing of programs for anger management and disruptive behavior programs. Additionally, the Federation of State Physician Health Programs (www.fsphp.org) assists state well-being programs by providing education and resources to assist impaired practitioners. Its Web site includes guidelines for operation of state physician health programs. There is also a listing of each state medical society's program that includes information on staff, program structure, program services, funding, and monitoring requirements for chemical dependency and mental health.

■ Assistance for Other Professionals

The majority of this chapter has focused on physicians, their issues, and available resources. In fact, the Joint Commission's standards require that medical staffs have a process to address the health and well-being of *all* licensed independent practitioners who are granted privileges. Each hospital and medical staff will define which professional types of practitioners are considered independent and which ones are granted privileges. For example, sometimes privileges may be granted to dentists, oral surgeons, podiatrists, chiropractors, psychologists, and others. In the majority of situations, the local and/or state medical societies will only accept MDs or DOs into their health and well-being programs. Some of the other professional groups, such as the American Dental Association, have established similar programs at the state and local level to assist dentists with health issues; however, not all of the professions have developed such sophisticated programs. It will be the responsibility of the medical staff to identify other resources for these professionals, because all independent practitioners must be afforded the same type of assistance.

■ Notes

1. American Medical Association. "Definition of Impaired Physician." Chicago, IL: Author; June 28, 2004. Available at: http://www.ama-assn.org. Accessed September 1, 2005.
2. American Medical Association. *Substance Abuse Among Physicians*. Report 1 of the Council on Scientific Affairs; 1995.
3. Orsund CA, Wilcox DP. "Credentialing the New Applicant: Practical Advice." *Texas Medicine*. 1988;84:79.
4. Texas Medical Association Committee on Physician Health and Rehabilitation. *Do You Know a Doctor Who Needs Our Help?* Austin, TX: Texas Medical Association; 1996.
5. Janos EL. *Credentialing Under the ADA: Legal Overview*, 1999.
6. Lang DA, Jara GB, Kessenick LW. *The Disabled Physician*. Chicago, IL: American Hospital Publishing; 1989:17.
7. National Health Foundation. "Fair Treatment for Senior Physicians." *Medical Executive Committee Reporter*. 1990;5:5.
8. Kissoon N, Lapenta S, Armstrong G. "Diagnosis and Therapy for the Disruptive Physician: Behavior." *Physician Executive*. January–February 2002.
9. The Joint Commission. *2009 Accreditation Manual for Hospitals*. Leadership Standards LD.03.03.01.
10. The Joint Commission. "Sentinel Event Alert." July 2008. Available at: http://www.jointcommission.org/SentinelEvents/SentinelEventAlert/sea_40.htm. Accessed July 20, 2009.
11. American College of Physician Executives. "Poll Results: Doctors' Disruptive Behavior Disturbs Physician Leaders." *Physician Executive*. September–October 2004.
12. Greeley Company, The Credentialing Institute. *Disruptive Physicians: Enough Is Enough*.

CHAPTER 14

Effective Meeting Management

Jodi Schirling, CPMSM

As discussed in an earlier chapter, the role of the medical staff services professional (MSSP) includes providing assistance to the medical staff organization in meeting accrediting body requirements. A major part of this assistance involves management of medical staff meetings.

This chapter examines the purpose and various types of committees found in healthcare organizations. Preparation for effective meetings, documentation styles, listening skills, and the importance of meeting minutes are considered as well. Tools for effectively managing meetings are discussed at the end of the chapter.

■ When to Establish Committees

Aside from committees and clinical departments that are formed to comply with accreditation requirements, other medical staff groups are frequently formed for ad hoc (particular) purposes. When is it appropriate to have a team or committee work on a project? Groups are appropriate when there is a need to harness the creativity of a diverse population of members. Teams are also useful when time and resources allow for the group to proceed. In a situation when an urgent decision must be made, using a group may not be the best method to reach a decision. The group should also break into subgroups when there is an issue worthy of their attention. Other examples of when a group or committee is useful include the following situations:

- No one person has sufficient information to make a quality decision.
- Acceptance of an idea, program, or decision by the group is critical to its implementation.
- The topic is complex, and it is critical that everyone has the same understanding of the information and data.
- Conflicting views need to be reconciled.
- People receiving and having to act on the information are interdependent.
- The issue being faced is unstructured—what information is required, where is the information found—and the outcome is unknown.

- Information needs to be communicated and immediately processed among a number of people.
- A synergistic effect is likely to be produced from bringing a group together to process the issue.[1]

Groups or committees are not appropriate when there is a hostile culture—one that is autocratic or hierarchical—or when the leader or members are not willing to listen to dissent.

■ Understanding the Role of the Committee

Understanding the role and objectives of a group will assist the person responsible for coordinating the meetings and preparing minutes. Many different types of committees and groups hold meetings and document their proceedings. These groups can vary from a formal board of directors meeting to a time-limited quality improvement team.

Purpose of the Committee

What is the overall purpose of the committee? The committee's objective or primary goal should be clearly defined. Objectives of committees can be diverse and, in the healthcare setting, may include patient care management, operational or procedural development, administrative management, or research and education.

Once the committee's objective is known, it is helpful to understand the authority vested in the committee. Determine the scope or degree of authority. The degree of authority can be limited to a specific task, to a specific department or discipline, or to a multidisciplinary or multidepartment level, or it can extend hospital-wide. The committee's position or stature within the organization is also important. The level of authority of the committee can be either supervisory (i.e., one of oversight), subordinate (i.e., a group accountable for performing certain functions), or advisory or consulting.

The meeting coordinator should also be aware of the specific actions the committee is allowed to take. Some committees may simply report their findings. In other words, these groups collect and analyze data and report the results to others. Other committees are empowered to make recommendations or suggest specific actions. Still other committees—usually a small number—may actually implement the recommendations of other groups. The medical executive committee (MEC) fits into this latter category. The MEC implements policy and procedures, makes recommendations to the governing body (the final authority) on credentialing issues, and takes actions recommended as the result of peer review and quality monitoring activities.

Additional information that is helpful to those coordinating a meeting focuses on the characteristics of the committee: Is it a new committee or one of long

Table 14-1	Role of the Committee Chair
<ul><li>Calls the meeting to order</li><li>Keeps meeting to its order of business</li><li>Gives every member who wishes it a chance to speak</li><li>Tactfully keeps all speakers to rules of order and to the question</li><li>Gives pro and con speakers alternating opportunities to speak</li><li>Does not enter into discussion</li><li>States each motion before it is discussed and before it is voted upon</li><li>Puts motions to a vote and announces the outcome of the voting</li><li>May vote when his or her vote would affect the outcome or in any case when voting is by ballot</li><li>Should be familiar enough with parliamentary procedure to inform the committee on proper procedures</li><li>May appoint subcommittees when authorized to do so or if bylaws so provide</li><li>May assist in wording of motions if the motion maker requests assistance</li></ul>	

standing? Likewise, knowing the meeting frequency is useful. Committees that meet weekly will typically have shorter, more focused agendas than those that meet only monthly or quarterly. The efficiency with which the committee performs its assigned tasks can be determined by reviewing past meeting minutes. The effectiveness of the committee's activities can be determined by tracking recommendations or actions taken: Were the committee's recommendations approved and implemented, or were they sent back to the committee for further deliberations?

Knowledge of the leadership style of the chair is also useful. If the person serving as the committee chair has a long tenure with the committee, it can be assumed that he or she is aware of the committee's role and functions. Newly appointed chairs will need to be oriented to the committee's purpose and tasks as well as to the means used to manage a committee meeting. The committee chair should participate in the pre-meeting agenda planning as well as post-meeting follow-up. Effective chairs (see TABLE 14-1) focus on the responsibilities of the group and refrain from using the committee meeting as a forum for their own personal agendas.

■ Effective Meetings

Every effective meeting begins with careful planning. The three basic steps to follow when holding a meeting are listed here and described fully in the following sections.

1. **The preparation phase.** If the group that will meet is not a standing, regular committee, during this phase the purpose of the meeting will be defined. The context or environment in which the meeting takes place will also be clarified. The desired outcomes—results or products of the meeting—will be defined. Specific tasks to be performed during the meeting will be outlined. Resources for the meeting, flip charts, audiovisual equipment, data, information, and so on will be determined. Finally, the agenda will be planned.
2. **The conducting phase.** During this phase, the roles of the leader, facilitator, recorder, and timekeeper will be defined by the group. The committee will work through the agenda items and conduct an evaluation of the process prior to adjournment.
3. **The follow-up phase.** During this phase, the documentation from the proceedings is prepared and disseminated to members. Work to be conducted between meetings may have been assigned, and the leader should track the progress.

■ Preparation Phase

Scheduling

For efficient and effective scheduling, an annual calendar of medical staff meetings should be prepared and kept in the medical staff services department (MSSD). The MSSP must work closely with the chief of staff and all committee and department chairs and section chiefs so that the meetings are scheduled at a time convenient for the chair and the majority of the members; he or she will also facilitate the appropriate and timely flow of information between groups.

One method suggested for accomplishing this task is to think of the meetings as occurring on the face of a clock and then to plug that information into a calendar. Suppose the governing body meeting is at 12 P.M., the MEC at 1 P.M., the department of surgery at 2 P.M., the credentials committee at 3 P.M., the department of medicine at 4 P.M., the infection control committee at 5 P.M., and so on. Also suppose that there is not a smooth flow of information, because committees report to other committees, sections, and departments; sections report to departments; departments and most committees report to MEC; and the MEC reports to the governing body. Indeed, in this scheme of things there is considerable and unnecessary delay (FIGURE 14-1).

FIGURE 14-2 illustrates a far more reasonable schedule that allows for an expeditious flow of information. This schedule is transferred to a monthly calendar.

Of course, implementing such a meeting schedule might not always be possible. This clock system is simply suggested as one method to achieve timely information flow.

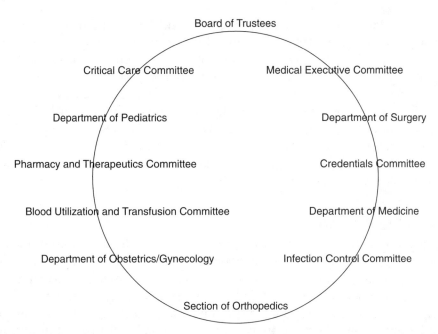

FIGURE 14-1 Clock System to Schedule Meetings: Poor Organization for Information Flow

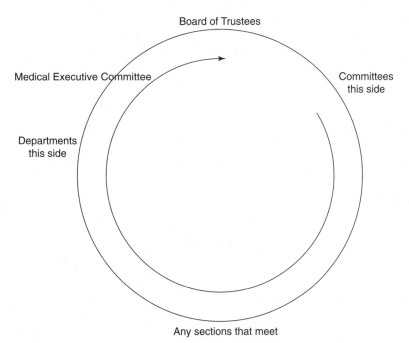

FIGURE 14-2 Clock System to Schedule Meetings: Ideal Organization for Information Flow

Once the master calendar is complete, it should be maintained in the MSSD. This calendar should be provided to all members of the medical staff as well as key hospital administrative staff. Distribution can be achieved in various ways. It is recommended that schedules be posted on the medical staff's Web site and that this be the primary communication mechanism related to scheduled meetings. Alternatively, paper copies may be mailed and e-mail or faxing can be used. It is helpful to ensure that the physician's office manager or whoever has control of the physician's schedule is made aware of the calendar—if you can get it on his or her calendar, it is more likely the physician will attend the meetings because the office staff will not schedule any patient activities during that time.

Meeting Room Arrangement

Two important components of meeting preparation are identification of an appropriate meeting place and setup of the room for the meeting. In many healthcare facilities, meeting space is limited, and meeting planners often have to try to overcome space and other logistics problems that make having an effective meeting difficult. For most meetings (except for extremely large meetings, where auditorium-type seating may be the only option available), there are three basic options, using two table shapes (rectangular and round).

Round tables should be used for informal meetings where discussion by all participants is the goal. The chair may sit in any position at a round table.

Rectangular tables are used for more formal meetings. The chair sits at the head of the table to indicate hierarchy. In this type of seating arrangement, the chair assumes an "arm's-length" distance from the participants (FIGURE 14-3).

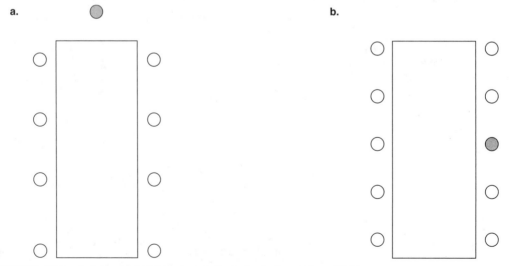

FIGURE 14-3 Chair Seated at Head and Chair Seated at Side of Table

If there is potential for negotiation or deliberation of important issues, the chair should sit on one side of a rectangular table. Many chairs find this location to be a more "powerful" position than the position at the head of the table. It allows the chair to play a more active role during the meeting (see Figure 14-3).

Meeting Notices

The MSSD (or the department that supports the committee) should send meeting announcements to the committee members. These notices should be sent at least one week in advance of standing committee meetings. Special meetings require additional notice as physicians have busy schedules, and short notice of an important committee meeting will have an impact on patient care. Three weeks notice is probably the minimum amount of notice for special meetings.

Use of e-mail is an effective way to distribute meeting announcements. Additionally, meeting notices and agendas can be posted on the medical staff's Web site. Members of a specific committee can be provided with a password to gain access to information related to the committee (e.g., agendas, minutes, documents to be reviewed prior to meetings).

Notices of standing and special meetings should include basic information such as the date, time, and location of the meeting. An agenda should also be provided with the meeting notice. If the members of the meeting are required to review supporting documentation, such documentation can be sent out to the members ahead of time, provided that steps are taken to assure the confidentiality of the materials.

Agenda Preparation

When used correctly, agendas are powerful tools. By organizing an agenda for the meeting, the chair can maintain control during the meeting. The mere placement of items on the agenda can influence the outcome either positively or negatively. For example, an item placed at the end of the agenda may be hurriedly discussed and voted on so the meeting can end. A well-known negotiating principle is that 80% of the decisions are made in the last 20% of the time. Also, placement of an item requiring lengthy discussion at the beginning of the agenda may mean that all items after it will not be discussed.

An agenda lets other committee members prepare for items to be discussed. For a committee to be most effective, the decisions it makes should reflect careful consideration. For example, the physician who will be asked to approve a policy closing the psychiatry section to new members will need to read the policy and think about questions and concerns before coming to the meeting. Providing an agenda promotes efficiency without losing valuable input.

Another benefit of having a well-planned agenda is improvement in meeting minutes. Minutes that are written around the agenda allow for easier retrieval of information.

An agenda should be clear and should state whether a given item is being presented for information, discussion, or action. In addition, the time allowed for discussion or action may be stated. When the formulation of the agenda occurs during the preliminary planning process, the chair can tailor the length of the agenda to match the length of the meeting.

To ensure that items from previous meetings requiring additional time for committee consideration are not omitted, previous minutes must be reviewed or a reminder placed in an agenda item file. Committee members should be contacted or instructed to submit agenda items far enough in advance to allow staff members to compile the agenda appropriately.

The specific agenda format will vary, but each agenda should include some basic elements such as approval of previous meeting minutes, committee and officer reports, old or unfinished business, new business, announcements, and the adjournment. When listing items under these headings, it is important that adequate information is included for easy understanding. Use of action verbs to emphasize the expected outcome of each item is helpful. A good tool for evaluating the contents of agenda is a form for that purpose.

An effective way of keeping track of what needs to be put on the agendas of the many committees supported by the office is to establish agenda files. The agenda file can be either a paper file or an electronic folder posted on a confidential shared drive on the organization's computer network. One file should be created for every medical staff group that meets regularly. Everyone in the facility and the leaders of the medical staff should be made aware of the existence of these files. Any item that anyone wants considered by a specific group can then be sent to the MSSD for placement in the appropriate agenda file. The MSSP also looks over minutes of previous meetings for referral items and places those in the files. The person compiling the agenda then consults the files prior to the agenda-planning meeting.

Consent Agendas

A consent agenda is a tool that can be used to save meeting time and to help ensure that committee time is spent on those items that require discussion. Consent agendas are used to expedite approval of routine, noncontroversial business brought before the committee. For example, medical executive committees often use them. The use of a consent agenda places responsibility on committee members to prepare prior to a meeting.

To use a consent agenda, the following steps should occur:

1. The committee members must understand how the consent agenda will work and agree to its use.
2. Consent agenda items must be distributed to committee members in advance of the meeting—far enough in advance for committee members to review all

the consent agenda items (and any backup documentation) and to determine if discussion at the meeting is necessary.
3. Any committee member may ask for any item listed on the consent agenda to be removed and addressed separately. This request can occur either prior to the meeting or at the meeting.

Consent agenda items are usually addressed toward the beginning of the meeting. This positioning allows any item removed from the consent agenda to be placed into the appropriate place on the agenda for discussion and/or action later in the meeting.

Some caveats do apply when consent agendas are used:

1. Do not use consent agendas to "hide" actions that are controversial or to push something through without discussion. If this kind of event occurs, the committee will usually never trust the items that are listed on a consent agenda again and may ban the practice.
2. Committee members must review items in advance of the meeting.
3. Committee members need to be committed to appropriate use of committee time. Items that are placed on a consent agenda are there because there is no need to spend valuable committee time on discussion. Sometimes committee members (or those attending a meeting) have submitted written reports for information—there is no action required. Nevertheless, they may feel compelled to speak about the report (or worse yet—read it to the committee). The committee members need to respect the time of all present and to refrain from discussion that serves no purpose.
4. It is beneficial for a committee that uses a consent agenda to have some rules about what can and cannot be placed on a consent agenda.

The use of a consent agenda can be an effective way to improve and streamline meetings—if and when it is understood and properly implemented.

Agenda-Planning Meetings

Prior to each scheduled committee meeting, an agenda-planning meeting should be held. The usual participants in the planning meeting include the MSSP responsible for the meeting, the chair and co-chair (if applicable), and a facilitator. This group finalizes the agenda for the meeting. To save time, this meeting can be held via telephone conference. Technology such as Web conferencing can be used to view the agenda, attachments, and other items necessary for planning.

When developing the agenda, the following questions should be answered for each item:

- What is the purpose of presenting this issue to the committee:
  - Information?

- Action required?
- Approval or endorsement required?
- Is there enough supporting documentation to accompanying the meeting agenda so that the committee members are well informed about the issue? If not, should the sponsor of the issue be invited to the committee meeting?
- How much time should be allotted for discussion? (Note: Many committees place time limits on discussion of the agenda items as a meeting management tool.)

The most efficient way to plan the agenda is to use a standard agenda format. Members of the committees will then become accustomed to this format, which makes the meeting flow more smoothly. Standardized agendas drive the meeting, in that business is conducted in a specific order. The standard agenda also encourages reporting by those groups required to do so. The agenda provides structure for the meeting as well as an outline for the meeting minutes.

A sample agenda format for the MEC meeting is shown in EXHIBIT 14-1. It allows for all required functions of the MEC, including acting on recommendations from medical staff committees and departments. An accompanying reporting schedule allows the committee to assure that periodic reports from committees and departments are received in the event that no MEC action is required. This type of agenda format can be modified to suit other committees as well. The format can be saved as an electronic template or extended to include page numbers, notebook sections, and so on, when paper documents are prepared. This allows for an easy flow of the meeting.

The CD that accompanies this book includes a sample agenda for a clinical department meeting. The topics reflect the required functions that must be performed by a clinical department of the medical staff.

■ Conducting Phase

The Four Processes During a Meeting

Four basic processes should occur during a meeting: participation, decision making, facilitating, and recording. All members of the group must participate. Each member is expected to contribute information and ideas and to discuss and improve upon ideas of others. Contributions to problem-solving and decision-making activities are the responsibility of each member. During the actual decision-making process, each member of the group must select from among the alternatives offered. Each member also plays a role in facilitating the meeting by keeping the group focused on the agenda and tasks at hand. Members should monitor the group process and use interventions to anticipate and moderate disruptive behavior. Finally, a record of the proceedings must be prepared.

EXHIBIT 14-1 Sample Agenda: Medical Executive Committee

Medical Executive Committee
Date/Location

Number	Item	Reason for Item Coming Before the Committee/ Action Requested	Responsible Person
I. 5 min.	Approval of Minutes		
II. 5 min.	Old Business		
III. 5 min.	Committee/Department Recommendations		
IV.	New Business		
V. 5 min.	Updates a. Administrative Report	Standing committee item— opportunity to provide information to medical staff	
5 min.	b. Medical Director Report	Standing committee item— as above	
5 min.	c. Nursing Director Report	Standing committee item— as above	
VI. 5 min.	Department Reports— Per reporting calendar	Medical executive committee must receive reports from all departments	
VII. 5 min.	Committee Reports— Per reporting calendar	Medical executive committee must receive reports from all medical staff committees	
VIII. 5 min.	Meeting Evaluation/ Future Agenda Items		
IX.	Adjournment		

To see that these functions are carried out, members of the group may take on specific roles. For example, one member will be identified as the leader; the role of the leader is to preside over the meeting and prepare the agenda. Another person may be assigned as the scribe or recorder; he or she writes down what is said and documents the decisions made by the group. In most cases, the recorder does not contribute to content discussion. In a medical staff committee, it would be appropriate for the MSSP to assume this role so that all medical staff members of the committee may participate in the discussions and deliberations. The facilitator is a consultant to the group who provides guidance on group process and dynamics—not on content.

Parliamentary Procedure

The support person attending medical staff meetings should be familiar with parliamentary procedure or at least have a reference ready at hand during the meetings to help facilitate the conduct of business. Some groups will appoint their own parliamentarian, but having a reference readily available will be very helpful if disputes arise.

Probably the most common reference work continues to be Robert's *Rules of Order*,[2] although some groups may prefer *Sturgis Standard Code of Parliamentary Procedure*.[3] A brief guide to the basics of parliamentary procedure can be found on the CD that accompanies this book.

The purpose of parliamentary procedure is to ensure that the majority rules while the minority is guaranteed a voice. In addition, following parliamentary procedure can assist in the orderly consideration of items and issues. Most medical staff meetings and performance improvement teams or groups are not so formal as to require a strict adherence of proper procedure. In fact, strict adherence might be a hindrance if the procedure becomes the overriding concern—a situation that must be avoided.

Forms

A meeting checklist is a useful tool in managing committee meetings. The staff members who are responsible for supporting the committee can use this checklist to ensure all preparations are made. There is a sample meeting checklist on the CD that accompanies this book.

An accurate record of attendance at each committee meeting must be maintained. An efficient way to keep attendance is to develop an attendance sheet for each committee. At the beginning of the meeting, members can be asked to sign in. Invited guests to the committee meeting should also sign in. The staff person supporting the committee should note who is present or absent so that the presence of anyone not signing the attendance form can be documented. For some medical staff organizations, attendance at medical staff committee meetings is considered a "citizenship requirement" for maintaining medical staff membership. The medical staff services office compiles the attendance records onto physician profiles that are used during the reappointment process. Although some medical staffs have removed the attendance requirement for their members, it is oftentimes useful to have a sense of the physician's interest and activity level; thus attendance information should be maintained and available if needed.

If a particular committee is operating at the supervisory or oversight level, other groups may be required to submit periodic reports to the parent committee. An annual reporting schedule is an effective management tool to assure that reports are submitted from each group on a periodic basis. Once the reporting schedule is prepared, it should be sent to the chairs of all committees and groups required to submit reports to the parent committee. The parent committee should review the schedule on an ongoing basis so that lapses in reporting can be addressed promptly. Two committees where this type of schedule is most helpful are the medical executive committee and the hospital quality committee. The CD that accompanies this book includes an example of a reporting schedule.

A standard format for submitting reports to the MEC may be especially useful. The standard format outlines basic information that would be required from each department, such as volume of activity. In addition, information can be requested on new procedures or services, personnel changes, equipment update, inspection or survey results, and performance improvement activities. Use of a standard report format ensures that all medical staff departments include relevant information in their periodic reports to the MEC.

Ground Rules

Medical staffs have a diverse membership, which is in turn reflected in the composition of committees and work groups in hospitals. The views and concerns of the many members of a committee add value to its deliberations. At the same time, this diversity can pose a challenge in managing a meeting. One easy way to deal with this concern is to have the committee members establish a set of ground rules by which they agree to operate. It is important that the committee members set the rules! Examples of some common ground rules for in person meetings include the following:

- Start on time
- End on time
- Follow the agenda
- No side conversations
- Pagers and cell phones on silent mode
- Refrain from "texting" during the meeting
- Only one person speaks at a time
- Take phone calls outside of the meeting room

Facilitated Meetings

In today's environment of continuous quality improvement in health care, the use of teams and task forces has increased dramatically. To avoid the risk of establishing a lot of new but ineffective committees, the use of trained facilitators is recommended. Trained facilitators can be extremely helpful in maximizing the performance of a committee's work. The facilitator participates in the agenda development meeting and attends the meeting, not as a member with voice and vote, but to assist the chair in meeting the objectives of the committee meeting, enforcing the ground rules, and moving the group through the agenda. Committees that use facilitators can be more productive, have more efficient meetings, and tend to have good participation from members.

■ Purpose of Meeting Minutes

Minutes of meetings of committees, department, services, or work groups are maintained for several reasons. It is important that the minutes be accurate and objectively reflect the proceedings of the meeting.

Historical Record

Minutes serve as documentation of the work of a group or committee. They provide background information on long-standing items. Minutes are used to educate new members of the committee or work group. By reviewing the minutes of the previous year, for example, the new members will know what was done and which hot topics or issues were addressed by the committee, and will have a better understanding of the structure of the meeting and the way in which the committee conducts its business. Minutes also serve as documentation of the accomplishments of the committee. Medical staff leaders can evaluate the effectiveness of medical staff and hospital committees' work through a review of the minutes.

Legal Document

Meeting minutes can also serve as a legal document. An example would be their use in providing evidence that due process was followed in the case of a peer review action. Additionally, minutes are used to demonstrate compliance with various regulatory and accreditation requirements.

Communication Tool

One of the most important functions of meeting minutes is to serve as a communication tool. The minutes are the formal record of recommendations, actions, and policy decisions made by a particular group. In addition, the meeting minutes can be used as a reporting tool—communicating issues or actions to another group.

Management Tool

Effective meeting minutes are a valuable management tool. They document actions to be taken and by whom, thereby affixing accountability and responsibility for particular tasks. They serve as a mechanism for tracking progress and follow-up on specific issues. Finally, minutes are used to help plan future meeting agendas. They facilitate the placement of unfinished business, deferred items, and so forth, on the agenda for future meetings.

■ Recording and Documenting Meeting Minutes

There is an art to taking minutes. The recording of the proceedings of any group deliberation is not simply a verbatim account of who said what. Instead, the writer must take care to provide an accurate and objective description of the meeting, and he or she must be able to listen and synthesize the discussion. The personal opinion of the writer must never be reflected in the minutes. Rather, minutes should reflect the consensus of the group (and not just the opinion of the loudest member). The writer should be able to transform personalized or opinionated statements into objective ones. For example:

> Member stated: "I think this is a stupid idea! There is no way the medical staff should stand for this!"
> Minutes reflect: "One member of the committee expressed concern with the proposed suggestion. The committee considered the concerns. The committee recommends that..."
> Member stated: "How in the *&%^$ are we supposed to comply with this new regulation. I may look into early retirement if this keeps up!"
> Minutes reflect: "Frustration was expressed regarding newly imposed regulations. No action was necessary."

The writer must be able to condense the discussion into one or two objective paragraphs. Conclusions drawn by the group, recommendations made, actions taken, and assignment of responsibility for such actions should be given special attention in the minutes.

Listening Skills

Imagine being in a room of 10 to 12 people. Papers are rustling, pagers are beeping, and doors are opening and closing. Dr. Jones comes in late and has a side conversation to determine what the group is talking about. Dr. Smith spills his coffee on his copies of the reports being reviewed. Administrator Brown is talking on the telephone. Sounds chaotic? This is probably an accurate description of any medical staff committee meeting. Healthcare professionals are busy people, and patient care issues always come first. As a consequence, committee and group meetings are subject to constant distraction and interruptions. So how does the individual recording the minutes stay focused?

It is easy to maintain focus if a trained facilitator is keeping the meeting on track. The facilitator would gently intervene to minimize distractions and side conversations. Unfortunately, not many medical staff meetings have the luxury of a facilitator in attendance, so the recorder must learn to focus on what is important and identify the intent of discussions.

The recorder of minutes must pay attention to all conversations. His or her notes should reflect the gist of the discussion. Keep in mind that while the minutes are not a verbatim recitation of the discussions, the recorder's notes from the meeting can be. Detailed notes are useful in constructing the final set of minutes. Over time, the recorder will be able to identify the key points of a discussion. The recorder should be familiar with the subjects being discussed.

In every group there will be participants who demonstrate particular types of behavior:

- *The dominator*: a person who likes to control the discussion and will not let anyone else get a word in. The chair of the committee or the facilitator needs to maintain control of the discussion and not allow one member to dominate the discussion.
- *The rambler*: a person who likes to hear himself or herself talk and will speak for a long period of time but say nothing. The chair of the committee or the facilitator can summarize the points made by the "rambler" and then redirect the discussion.
- *The arguer*: a person who will find fault or object to every idea presented. The chair of the committee should express empathy for the person's point of view and then remind the member that the goal of the meeting is to reach consensus.
- *The late arriver*: an individual who comes late, enters noisily, and expects the meeting to stop while he or she is brought up to speed. The chair of the committee should set the tone by welcoming the member and indicating that the chair will bring the late arriver up-to-date after the meeting is concluded.
- *The "shock jock"*: the person who makes off-the-wall comments and then sits back to watch the reaction of the group. The chair of the committee or the facilitator should redirect the discussion to the topic at hand. If the behavior persists, the chair should have a discussion about the behavior with the committee member outside of the meeting.

- *The introvert:* the more shy and introspective person who doesn't have a lot to say, but when he or she speaks, it is usually profound. The chair of the committee or the facilitate should make sure that every member of the group has had the opportunity to weigh in on an issue.

The recorder of minutes will begin to identify those committee participants who fall into certain of these categories. This insight into the person's group behavior will help the recorder in documenting the conversations.

The recorder must listen and then synthesize the conversation that places over the course of the meeting. This discussion then needs to be condensed, summarized, and organized in the minutes so that a reader will be able to follow a logical sequence in achieving understanding of the topic. For example, the minutes might follow this pattern:

1. What was the topic, and why was it presented?
2. What were the key points of the discussion? Were there specific pros and cons to the debates? Were supporting data presented and discussed?
3. What conclusion did the group reach?
4. Did the group make any recommendations?
5. Did it take action? If so, what action was taken, by whom, and when?

The "Evaluation of Content of Minutes" form shown in TABLE 14-2 can be a useful tool in assuring that the documentation contains all required elements.

The recorder must be careful not to twist or edit what is said. As mentioned previously, his or her personal opinions must be left out of the documentation. And remember, in most cases, the recorder is at the meeting to record the proceedings, not to participate in the discussions.

Identification of Speakers

In some meetings, controversial topics will be presented for discussion. There may also be close votes on recommendations. In such cases, the recorder may be asked to specifically identify a speaker. In most cases, however, it is best to keep names of speakers out of the minutes. The documentation can simply state, "It was moved, seconded, and carried that…" when an action is being taken. The exception would be when there are dissenting opinions or votes, and those members want the minutes to reflect their dissension or abstention from voting. When this situation arises, it is important to record the title or position of the person speaking in addition to the name because that information helps in later years when one is reviewing the minutes and is trying to re-create the situation and identify who was involved or who supported a particular idea or action.

When an informational report such as a department update is being given, it is appropriate to indicate who gave the report. For example, when the department of medicine's quarterly report is presented to the medical executive committee, the

Table 14-2	Evaluation of Content of Minutes		
		Yes	No
Are the functions of the committee accomplished? Review the committee's charge—did it conduct blood usage review, pharmacy review, and so on?			
Are issues addressed at the meeting? Issues can be raised through quality indicators, special studies, and peer review.			
Do the minutes include appropriate background information, such as how the evaluation is conducted, source of information, and threshold level for quality indicators?			
Are problems identified? Does the description of the problem/issue include enough information to determine its frequency and severity? The reason the problem is discussed is evident. Source of the issue is clear—department, committee, subgroup.			
Were conclusions drawn? After review and discussion of agenda item, did the group draw a conclusion?			
Are actions taken? No evidence of "rubber-stamping" an issue/report.			
Are actions appropriate to the problem/issue?			
Do minutes include who is responsible for the action?			
What will be done?			
When will action be taken?			
Are referrals to other department/committees documented?			
Are time frames for follow-up appropriate to the problem?			
Are minutes written so that an outside reviewer or department/committee member not in attendance can understand what happened?			
Is confidentiality maintained throughout content?			
Are patient and physician identities concealed?			
Are there issues that need follow-up or intervention by the president of the medical staff that weren't explicitly mentioned?			

minutes would state, "The department of medicine report was presented by Dr. Smith, chair. No action was required. Report was accepted."

What Must Be Documented

Most healthcare professionals will agree that the proliferation of medical staff committees was a direct response to the Joint Commission standards. Early Joint Commission standards identified functions that were to be performed, and most hospitals established a complex committee structure for accomplishing them. As a result, many hospital medical staffs have maintained the committee structure, sometimes even long after the requirement for such functions were removed from the Joint Commission standards. Keep in mind that the accreditation standards for hospitals require only the existence of a medical executive committee. The Joint Commission does, however, require that the hospital and medical staff measure, assess, and improve the following issues:

- Medical assessment and treatment of patients
- Use of medications
- Use of blood and blood components
- Operative and other procedures
- Appropriateness of clinical practice patterns (utilization review)
- Significant departures from established clinical patterns
- Patient and family education
- Coordination of care, treatment, and services
- Accurate, timely, and legible patient records

The Joint Commission also requires that the organization's medical staff use information gleaned from these activities as well as others in the ongoing evaluation of a practitioner's competence. Key additional information includes sentinel event data and patient safety data. Effective documentation of these activities will provide the medical staff with evidence of compliance with the Joint Commission standards.

Although the standards do not require committees to accomplish these functions, many hospital organizations use a committee structure to carry out the requirements. The documentation provided through committee meeting minutes remains an effective way of demonstrating the performance of the review. The Joint Commission continues to look for evidence of the conclusions, recommendations, actions, and evaluation in documentation, whether in a report or a set of meeting minutes.

Conclusions

When the group reviewing data or information reaches a conclusion based on those data, it indicates that the function is being performed correctly. It would be difficult to argue that blood use evaluation is being accomplished if minutes reflect only that the statistics were reviewed. Even if no action is required, that fact should be documented in the minutes. It shows that the committee looked at information and concluded that nothing further needed to be accomplished. Other examples of conclusions might include that further investigation is required, that further data analysis is necessary, or that specific actions be taken. Minutes should clearly reflect the conclusions reached by the group.

Recommendations

Once the committee has reviewed all the information regarding a specific issue and reached a conclusion, any resultant recommendations need to be reiterated. Again, recommendations can range from taking no action to approving policies or initiating disciplinary action. Recommendations are most often reflected in the minutes in the form of motions.

Actions

Once a recommendation is made in the form of a motion (or more informally, if the group has decided not to follow *Robert's Rules of Order*), the committee needs to act upon the recommendation. Minutes of the meeting should reflect the results of that action. Was the recommendation approved, not approved, or deferred? If the recommendation was approved, who is responsible for implementing it, communicating it, or following up on the item? What is the time frame for accomplishing the action?

Keep in mind the old newspaper adage of "who, what, when, where, and how." Minutes should include that basic information regarding actions taken.

Evaluation

The committee's work does not stop after an action is taken. Part of the Joint Commission's performance improvement philosophy is that the effectiveness of actions taken must be evaluated. In turn, part of the committee's role is to request follow-up to see that the action was indeed carried out and to determine how it was received. In addition, the committee should participate in an annual evaluation of its work. During that evaluation, the committee will be asked to determine whether its functions were carried out, which improvements were made, and which opportunities for improvement still exist. Accurate documentation of the effectiveness of each of its actions will allow the committee to conduct its annual evaluation with a minimum of work.

■ Minutes Formats

There are many accepted formats for documenting meeting minutes, each of which has both positives and negatives. Regardless of the format used, keep in mind that the end result should be professional in appearance and free of typographical errors. An "Evaluation of Formats of Minutes" form is a useful tool in ensuring that the minutes contain all required elements. (There is a sample on the CD that accompanies the book.) Minutes, regardless of their format, can be maintained in the traditional, paper-copy files or in an electronic file.

Examples of formats of minutes typically used follow in the next sections.

Two Columns

In this format, the page is divided into two columns. The first column contains the narrative discussion of each agenda item; the second column outlines the actions taken by the committee. This style is useful in meetings where detailed documentation of the discussions is necessary, as in the medical executive committee. The negative aspect of using this type of format is that the reader must scan through the entire narrative to identify conclusions and recommendations.

Three Columns

While otherwise similar to the two-column format, the three-column format adds a column to identify the issue. This format allows for ease in searching for a particular agenda item. Again, this format lends itself to more detailed descriptions of the discussion. The reader again must review all of the discussion to determine conclusions and recommendations.

Four Columns

Some committees find it useful to expand the column format to four columns. The fourth column pulls out from the body of the text the conclusions and recommendations made by the group. Groups use the four-column format most widely where detailed description of the discussion is not always needed.

■ Legal Aspects of Minutes Documentation

As stated earlier, meeting minutes can be used as a legal document. The minutes provide evidence that the peer review process has been followed or that regulatory and accreditation standards have been met. As peer review documents, medical staff committee minutes are accorded various levels of protection from discoverability under state statutes. The MSSP responsible for medical staff committee management should be keenly aware of the respective state laws governing protection of peer review documents. In addition, medical staff and performance improvement meeting minutes should be well protected from unauthorized access.

In writing minutes, a balance must be reached between providing the precision and detail required by the Joint Commission and other accrediting agencies to demonstrate compliance, and the instructions by healthcare attorneys to be concise and brief in documenting peer review activities. In addition, the organization needs to maintain meaningful records. This balance can be accomplished if the recorder is judicious in constructing the minutes.

The confidentiality of the meeting minutes should be protected within the organization. By demonstrating that minutes are treated as protected documents within the organization, the MSSP will help strengthen the healthcare attorney's argument that these documents are protected under the state statutes regarding peer review. The MSSD (or other hospital department responsible for meeting minutes) should have policies and procedures in place regarding control, distribution, and access to meeting minutes.

Here are some tips for helping to protect medical staff and quality improvement meeting minutes:

- Control distribution of meeting minutes by numbering each copy and collecting the copies after the meeting.
- Maintain only one file for minutes of meetings. Members of the committee should never establish their own files of minutes.
- Maintain a policy on access to minutes. Refer to your state statutes when creating this policy.
- Maintain the minutes in an electronic format on a confidential Web site or in a shared drive on the organization's computer network. Limit access to the electronic content to the members of the committee.
- Establish and maintain security for the documents. Maintain a separate, locked file cabinet for hard-copy documents; maintain secure, confidential, and access-restricted computer files for electronic documents.
- Develop a header or footer for your minutes that states "Confidential medical peer review/quality review document. Protected under (enter state statute number here)."
- Orient the members of the committee to the confidential nature of the discussions.
- Have members of the committee sign a confidentiality agreement. This agreement outlines the confidential nature of the meeting discussions and the expectations of the members to maintain confidentiality.
- Be aware that e-mail is discoverable, so use care when distributing medical staff peer review/quality committee minutes electronically. It is better to store the medical staff minutes electronically and provide updates to the committee members by sending an e-mail communication with a link to the secure site.

■ Follow-up Phase

Once the meeting ends, the work is just beginning for the support staff member and the committee chair. Committee meetings inevitably create a lot of follow-up activity. It is useful if the MSSD establishes standards for completion of the minutes and the time by which all follow-up correspondence is to be drafted, signed, and mailed out. Follow-up from the meeting should be in written form—either formal correspondence or printouts of e-mail messages. Documentation of follow-up actions should be attached to the minutes of the meeting as evidence that they were carried out.

■ Virtual and Paperless Meetings

A virtual meeting is a meeting that happens without the committee or group members coming together at one time. Typically the information is disseminated to the group, and then opportunities for subsequent comment are provided through a "chat room" environment or by documenting questions on a document in a shared computer drive or confidential Web page. Following an appropriate period of time for review and response, the group makes a decision or comes to consensus. Virtual meetings are effective when a small group needs to address a single issue—for example, when a group needs to develop or revise a policy. The group can review and comment on the document electronically. Once the document is finalized, the group can then use an electronic voting system to take action. Web conferencing can also be used for meetings where individuals will not come together, but still have the opportunity for discussion, review of documents, and other meeting functions.

Paperless meetings are exactly what the name implies—meetings that are conducted and recorded using electronic file transmission and documentation. There are varying levels of sophistication in running paperless meetings. The most simplistic approach is to create the agenda, minutes, and supporting meeting material and transmit them electronically to all members via e-mail; paper copies are not distributed to the members. Another method is to develop the agenda and documents and project them onto a screen in the meeting room using an LCD projector.

Organizations with a larger information technology budget and department may invest in the use of secure Web sites for meeting management. An example of such a Web site is Confluence (Atlassian Confluence, www.atlassian.com). This type of technology allows the meeting agenda, notes, planning documents, schedules, meeting attendees, and other information related to the committee or group to be posted on a secure Web site by a representative of the committee or group. Members are notified via e-mail of updates to the site and access the information using a link to the site. Use of this type of system keeps all meeting notes, agendas, and other documents together in one location to facilitate access to them.

A word of caution is in order regarding e-mail and other technological advances such as intranets as means of conducting meetings. A thorough consideration of the risks and benefits involved in use of new technology should be undertaken prior to embracing the use of electronic transmittal and interchange of information. Attorneys advise that organizations be proactive and attempt to build some safeguards into the process of using cyberspace to facilitate confidential communications. A specific policy or protocol should be developed that outlines the conditions under which electronic (e-mail) communications are permitted. For example, the following conditions might be established:

- Developing a convention to be used for the subject lines of e-mail transmissions (such as "Confidential and Privileged")
- Developing an appropriate confidentiality statement to be added to the text of such messages
- Never using a person's name (physician or patient) in the transmission, but rather some other confidential identifier
- Confirming by appropriate means that the proper recipient received the message
- Having the medical staff leaders who make use of this technology sign a confidentiality agreement that reflects these matters as well as others:
  - Agreeing to prevent unauthorized individuals from having access to the e-mails/information, whether at the office or at home
  - Agreeing to delete the e-mail information from their computers immediately after transacting the business at hand
  - Agreeing to inform the appropriate individuals at the hospital if there is a fear that the information was mistakenly sent to unauthorized individuals
  - Agreeing to update the hospital immediately if there is any change in the individual's e-mail address

Developing such a policy would help to foster a culture where confidentiality is respected. It would also be helpful in defending against allegations that peer review protections have been lost by the inappropriate or cavalier use of this technology when dealing with confidential matters.[4]

A "pending log" can be maintained listing the accomplishments of the group. This type of log is very useful for demonstrating the effectiveness of the committee to medical staff leadership. In addition, the accomplishment logs of all medical staff committees can be used to compile the reports that the medical staff periodically submits to the governing body. A sample format for a pending log is included on the CD that accompanies the book.

■ Tools for Effective Meetings

Forms

In preparing for a meeting, the recorder may find it useful to have a few handy tools available. One is a form for recording minutes. Many word processing programs have the capability to generate meeting minutes and agenda templates in a standard format. A form to be used for documenting the actions can accompany the agenda. If this type of software is not available in your facility, a minutes recording form can be easily created from the agenda. On this form, space is provided next to each item to summarize key points of the discussion, conclusions made, actions taken, the persons who are accountable for the actions, and the date when follow-up is due back to the committee.

Motion Cards

When conducting an in-person meeting, another useful tool is motion cards. The purpose of the motion card is to allow the person making a motion to write it out. By having the motion written out, there is no question that it will be reflected accurately in the minutes. Use of the motion cards also allows the committee member initiating the motion to track the amendments to the motion. A simple way to accomplish this is to use 3×5 cards. These cards can be distributed to the members at the start of the meeting. The recorder will have to prompt members to use the cards and to turn them in once the motion has been acted upon.

Flip Charts

Many committees and quality teams use flip charts or electronic whiteboards to record the discussions and actions taken by groups. Flip charts or the notes produced from an electronic whiteboard can be used to create more formal sets of minutes, or they can serve as the actual documentation of the activities of the group. Nevertheless, it is not recommended that flip chart paper be retained as the formal record of the group's activities. It is very cumbersome, takes up a lot of space, and usually is difficult to follow. In most cases, the group will prepare a storyboard or other report on their activities for the sponsoring department head or committee.

Other Tools

Many other tools can be developed to facilitate management of meetings. Medical staff services departments and quality departments usually have standard forms for tracking pending items, for communicating information from one committee to another, and for tracking results of peer review. These tools can be developed easily and, when put into use, make managing committees much easier.

The recorder or other support person should always make sure that basic supplies are available in the meeting room. Specifically, the table should be equipped with notepads, pens or pencils, and extra copies of the agenda. In addition, if audio-visual equipment is being used, additional supplies should be available, such as replacement bulbs for overhead projectors, masking tape for hanging pages from flip charts, marking pens, and extra flip chart paper.

Finally, the support person for each committee should bring appropriate reference materials to the meetings. These materials may include medical staff bylaws, credentials policies and procedures, and reference materials supporting key agenda items. Minutes of the previous meetings should also be on hand at the meeting. The meeting notebook with attached documentation of all follow-up activities is useful if a dispute arises regarding when an action was taken or other resolution of an issue.

Use of Technology

The availability of electronic technology can make the recording of meeting minutes easy to accomplish.

Use of Tape Recording Devices

Tape recording a meeting is an effective time management tool when there is no support person assigned to act as a recorder. It is appropriate to tape record the meeting and have someone else listen to the tape and prepare a set of minutes. A word of caution is in order, however: There must be safeguards in place whenever a meeting is recorded. First, members of the committee must consent to the use of recording devices. Second, the staff person who will have access to the tape recording must be clearly identified. Third, after the minutes are prepared, the recording must be erased. Recordings of meeting minutes should not be maintained on a permanent basis. Always consult with hospital legal counsel prior to implementing this practice.

Laptop Computers

Laptop computers can expedite the processing of preparing meeting minutes. Through the use of this technology, it becomes possible to have a draft set of minutes written within hours of the conclusion of the meeting.

To make most effective use of a laptop computer for developing minutes, some preparation is necessary prior to the meeting. At the very least, the agenda document or minute recording form should be created in the computer. The recorder then enters the key points of the discussion into the computer at the time of the meeting. After the meeting is over, the recorder reviews the rough information and turns it into readable text that will serve as the minutes.

Another way to use laptop computers is for the recorder to actually prepare the minutes ahead of time. Details regarding the place and time are entered. The attendance record can be a table; the recorder simply checks off those persons in attendance on the date of the meeting. The text can be prepared in advance as well. The issue, reason for its presentation, and action required of the committee could all be spelled out. The recorder will then enter brief, fragmented notes on the key points of discussion, conclusions drawn, and actions taken during the meeting. Within an established time frame, the text is cleaned up and the minutes are complete.

If meeting minutes are maintained in an electronic format (e.g., on a computer or on discs), the organization should establish policies to protect the confidentiality of the information. Policies should be in place that address use of computer passwords, access to minutes, distribution of meeting minutes, and retention of minutes. As previously discussed, care should be taken when transmitting information electronically.

A computer (either desktop or laptop) can also be linked with an LCD projector to limit the amount of paper that needs to be produced for a meeting. MSSPs will do themselves a service if they learn how to set up and use the LCD projector. When attached to a laptop computer or PC, the LCD projector can be used to display the current computer screen so that it is visible to all attendees at the meeting. This kind of technology is an effective way to display the agenda. If the group or committee is charged with creating a report or other document, the draft document can be displayed on screen and one member of the committee can be making the changes to the document in "real time" as the committee is in discussion. This method is highly efficient and allows the committee or group members to see the revisions or content as it is being developed.

Regardless of the type and sophistication of meeting audiovisual equipment that a healthcare organization uses, the MSSP needs to be proficient in the features and use of the system.

Fax Machines

It is easy to transmit data across the country and the world via facsimile machines. Meeting notices can be sent out with a few quick keystrokes and agendas distributed at the push of a button. But beware—caution must be used when documents are being sent via fax. In particular, the sender must ensure that the fax number is correct. A call ahead should be made to alert the physician's office staff that sensitive material is coming across the fax so that it can be picked up at their end and given directly to the physician.

Teleconferences and Videoconferences

Teleconferences and videoconferences are effective ways of working with people from across the city, across the state, or even across the country. Such conferences allow a group of people to discuss common subjects without incurring the effort and expense associated with traveling to an on-site meeting. Larger facilities may have the capability to schedule and manage conference calls in-house. Other groups may prefer to use an outside company to facilitate the call. In addition to telephone (voice only) conferences, reliable technology is available that supports face-to-face videoconferencing from several different locations.

To have effective long-distance conferencing (whether voice alone or voice and picture), careful advanced planning is required. Agenda items need to be solicited from all parties. The leader of the meeting must assign realistic time frames for discussing each item. It is useful to allow time at the end of the meeting for items that didn't make it to the agenda. It is also helpful to have everyone introduce himself or herself at the start of the meeting. When participating in voice-only conferencing, it is helpful for the recorder if participants identify themselves when they begin speaking. Depending on the technology, some voice and picture conferencing systems may experience a 3- to 5-second delay while the information is being transmitted. This delay can be a distraction, and parties at various ends of the conference must wait to speak until all parties have responded to issues.

Many types of electronic meeting systems are available. The most effective systems allow connection of multiple sites via phone or video and permit sharing of documents. Others include functionality that allows for capturing meeting notes or brainstorming results on a "virtual whiteboard." It behooves the MSSP to learn which videoconferencing and teleconferencing systems are available in his or her facility and to become facile in their use.

As with all technologies, some cautions apply to teleconferencing and videoconferencing. The conference should be held in a meeting room or office to limit the possibility of patients or visitors overhearing the discussion. Participants should identify themselves whenever they join or leave the conference.

Technology can be very useful in streamlining the work of the medical staff services department or other healthcare department charged with supporting committees. With the appropriate safeguards in place, there is no reason why these departments should not take advantage of technological advances.

■ Conclusion

Managing meetings takes thoughtful preparation and planning. A carefully considered agenda, an oriented and focused leader, and a setting conducive to conducting business will allow committees to be more productive and efficient. The use of technology such as videoconferencing or teleconferencing capabilities allows for meetings to occur without necessitating the expense of travel for those individuals at remote locations.

Support staff assigned to committees should understand the role of the committee. In particular, the recorder (often the MSSP) should understand his or her role in the proceedings. The opinions of the recorder should never be reflected in the minutes. The end product of clear, concise, and objective minutes, whether maintained in a paper system or electronic system, will serve as documentation that the medical staff is accomplishing its required functions.

■ Notes

1. Kayser TA. *Mining Group Gold: How to Cash in on the Collaborative Brain Power of a Group.* El Segundo, CA: Serif; 1990.

2. Robert HM. *Robert's Rules of Order*. New York: Berkley Books; 1993.
3. Sturgis A. *Sturgis Standard Code of Parliamentary Procedure*. 3rd ed. New York: McGraw Hill; 1988.
4. Horty, Springer, and Mattern. "Question of the Week." *Health Law Express* Web page. May 24, 2002. Available at: http://www.hortyspringer.com. Accessed June 2, 2002.

■ Bibliography

Orsund-Gassiot C, Lindsey S. *Handbook of Medical Staff Management*. Gaithersburg, MD: Aspen; 1990.

Winters B, Joseph E, Fox LA. *Documenting Healthcare Meetings: Tips, Tools and Techniques*. Chicago, IL: Care Communications; 1990.

CHAPTER 15

Introduction to the Law

Carla DiMenna Thompson, JD

■ The Legal System

The legal system affects all aspects of Americans' personal and professional lives. When a check is written, a car driven, or a street crossed, laws and regulations apply. There are laws, rules, and regulations concerning the manufacture, distribution, and labeling of almost everything bought, used, or consumed. Labor laws cover most workers, most buildings must conform to building codes, and fair credit laws govern every credit card purchase made. Laws govern and regulate almost every phase of life. The legal system also provides a forum for people to use to resolve their disputes.

Criminal Law and Civil Law

Law is often defined as social control. But whereas laws prohibiting murder, arson, and theft are obviously examples of social control through government legislation, there is more to the law than the administration of criminal justice. The law of torts, the law of contracts, and the rest of the body of law known as civil law is a complex system of rules that attach legal rights, responsibilities, and duties to various actions.

The criminal law segment of our legal system prohibits conduct that is contrary to the public order. Each state has its own laws defining what is a crime in that state. In the United States, there are laws dealing with the crimes of abduction, abortion, adultery, arson, bigamy, bribery, burglary, counterfeiting, disorderly conduct, dueling, embezzlement, escape, extortion, false impersonation, forgery, homicide, incest, kidnapping, larceny, malicious mischief, mayhem, murder, obscenity, obstructing justice, perjury, prostitution, rape, riot, robbery, suicide, treason, and vagrancy. This, of course, is not a complete list of all crimes prohibited by law in this country.

Crimes are divided into two major categories: misdemeanors and felonies. A misdemeanor is a crime that carries a maximum penalty of less than one year in jail and/or a fine. A felony is a more serious offense that carries a term of imprisonment of more than one year. The civil actions that healthcare professionals may be most concerned about are tort actions and contract actions.

In a criminal case, the plaintiff is always the state (sometimes called the People.)[1]

A general understanding of the law that applies to healthcare administration is important so that healthcare personnel can protect themselves, their employers, and even their patients. Healthcare professionals need to be aware of the laws and regulations that define what they may or may not do.

■ The Courts

The courts are probably the most familiar part of the U.S. legal system. Although few people have taken part in an actual trial, most people have seen a trial on television.

The court system is a complex structure of federal and state courts. In every state there is at least one federal court and an entire state court system.

Federal Courts

At the federal level, the trial courts are called U.S. District Courts. Each state has at least one federal District Court.

The intermediate level in the federal system is called the U.S. Court of Appeals. There are 13 federal Courts of Appeal, and each, except for the District of Columbia Circuit, encompasses several states.

Other federal courts include the Court of Claims and U.S. Customs Courts.

The United States Supreme Court

The final appellate court in the federal system is the U.S. Supreme Court. It hears appeals from the U.S. Court of Appeals and from the highest appellate court of each state. The U.S. Supreme Court also has jurisdiction to hear appeals involving the interpretation of a federal constitutional provision or a federal law or regulation. In very rare instances, the high court can hear appeals directly from the U.S. District Courts.

In some cases, the U.S. Supreme Court also has "original jurisdiction"—for example, when one state is bringing action against another state. In these rare cases the U.S. Supreme Court acts as a trial court.

FIGURE 15-1 outlines the hierarchy of the U.S. federal court system, with the Supreme Court sitting at the highest level.

State Courts

Within each state court system, there are several levels. Like the federal courts, most state court systems have three levels: the trial level, the intermediate appellate level, and the final appellate level. FIGURE 15-2 illustrates the organization of the state court system.

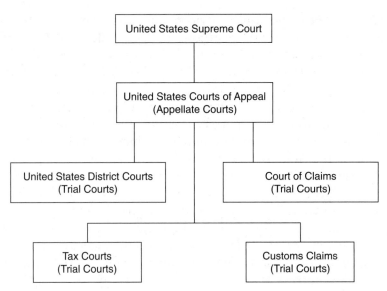

FIGURE 15-1 Federal Court System

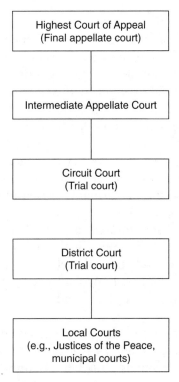

FIGURE 15-2 State Court System

In the state systems, the courts perform the same functions as their federal counterparts. Trial courts decide questions of fact, judge a defendant's guilt or innocence in criminal cases, and determine liability in civil cases. They also decide if a penalty should be imposed and whether it should be a fine or a jail term. In civil cases, they determine the amount of damages to be awarded.

Appellate courts in the state system, as in the federal system, review trial court decisions to determine if the court correctly applied the law to the facts. Only rarely do appellate courts review factual determinations made at the trial level. When the facts are reviewed, the situation is called a *de novo* review.

In a state system, local courts are usually specialized and are located all around the state. Municipal courts, traffic courts, police courts, and small claims courts are all examples of local courts. Their jurisdiction is very limited.

The courts of general jurisdiction are the basic trial courts for the community. In some states, these courts are called circuit courts or district courts. In California, they are called superior courts. In New York State, the basic trial courts are—oddly enough—called the supreme courts.[2]

■ What Happens in a Civil Lawsuit?

How Does a Lawsuit Begin?

As previously mentioned, court actions are classified into two categories: civil actions and criminal actions. Civil cases are those in which an individual, an organization, or a government agency sues for damages or injunctive relief from another party. Criminal actions are cases brought by the state or federal government against an individual who has been charged with committing a crime.

Civil actions are usually actions concerning the breach of a contract (ex contractual) or for a wrong, also known as a tort (*ex delicto*). Sometimes a suit is brought for equitable relief rather than money damages. Equity can prohibit certain wrongful conduct with an injunction or can compel the performance of certain action with an order for specific performance. Usually money damages cannot be obtained in an equitable proceeding.

When one person has been injured by another person, the injured party may consult an attorney to determine if the injury will give rise to a legal cause of action. The attorney will take the client's statement and may interview possible witnesses. The attorney will probably do some legal research to find the applicable laws and court decisions and will then determine if the client has a viable case.

If there is a cause of action and the client wishes to proceed with the suit, the attorney will then prepare a complaint or a petition and will file it in the appropriate court. The attorney's client is called the plaintiff, and the person or organization against whom the case is filed is called the defendant. The complaint states the facts of the plaintiff's action against the defendant and sets forth the judgment or money damages sought. The filing of the complaint does not prove that the plaintiff actually has a cause of action—that determination will be made by the court.

The plaintiff's attorney also files a document called a summons with the court. The summons directs the county sheriff to serve a copy of the legal papers on the defendant. In some states, the summons is served as a matter of course; in others, it must be served in advance of filing the complaint; in still others, only qualified process servers may serve the summons.[3]

After the summons is served, the original document is returned to the court, and it is noted whether the defendant was actually served. The serving of the summons is the defendant's official notification that a suit has been filed and that he or she has been named as a defendant. Filing the complaint and serving the summons officially commences a lawsuit. The defendant is then given a certain time period in which to file an answer to the plaintiff's complaint.

Venue and Jurisdiction

The attorney must file the case in the proper court. A court has no authority to hear a case unless it has jurisdiction over the persons or property involved.

Some actions, called local actions, can be brought only in the county where the subject matter of the jurisdiction is located. For example, a mortgage foreclosure can only be brought in the county where the property is located. Other actions, called transitory actions, can be brought in any county in any state where the defendant may be found and served with the summons. An action for personal injury is a transitory action.

The venue is the location, the county, or the district where the action will be tried. It may be changed (1) if there has been widespread pretrial publicity, (2) in an effort to find jurors who have not been exposed to that publicity, or (3) simply to provide a more neutral setting when there is a great deal of local sentiment about a certain case. A change of venue is requested by motion and is granted or denied by the judge.

Trial Preparation

Before the trial begins, both parties can file documents with the court. Sometimes a defendant may file a pleading called a *motion to quash service of summons,* which asserts that the defendant should not have been served or was improperly served. Defendants may also file a *motion to make more definite and certain,* which asks the court to order the plaintiff to describe the injury more fully or to set out the facts more specifically so the defendant can answer more accurately. Sometimes defendants ask the court to issue a summary ruling against the plaintiff with a *motion to dismiss* the case.

Before the actual trial, depositions are often taken. Depositions are out-of-court statements taken under oath. They are used for trial preparation and may be used in court. A deposition is not a public record.

Discovery is another legal term that refers to a party's attempt to find out more information about the case. Sometimes parties are required to produce books or financial or medical records or submit to a physical examination.

After the pleadings have been filed, a pretrial conference is often held. Sometimes a case is settled at this conference. If not, a trial date is set.

The Trial

Sometimes the lawyers involved in the lawsuit decide that a judge trial rather than a jury trial would be better for the case. In this circumstance, the right to a jury trial is waived.

When a jury is requested, the lawyers and the judge engage a process called voir dire to select the jury. In this process, the jurors are questioned to determine if they possess any prejudice or bias regarding the case. Each side has a certain number of challenges that can be made for any reason at all; these are called peremptory challenges. Each side also has an unlimited number of challenges that can be made for cause—that is, on the grounds that the juror cannot be termed impartial and is obviously prejudiced in some way.

Once the jury has been selected, each party makes an opening statement. Then witnesses are called to present evidence. The party calling the witness questions the witness first; this line of questioning is called direct examination. The opposing party then questions the witness in what is called cross-examination.

When all the witnesses have been called and examined, the parties are allowed to make summations or closing arguments. The judge then instructs the jury, and the members of the jury begin their deliberations. Sometimes the jurors are sequestered, or isolated, from the public when they are deciding a very controversial case.

After a decision is reached, the jury returns to the courtroom and the verdict is read in open court.

■ Statutes, Laws, and Regulations

The hierarchy of laws is as follows:

1. United States Constitution
2. Federal statutes and regulations
3. State constitution
4. State statutes and regulations
5. County and city ordinances
6. The common law

Statutory Law

Statutory law is the body of law created by legislative acts (in contrast to the law generated by judicial opinion and administrative bodies). Of course, the "supreme law of the land" is the United States Constitution.[4]

The structure of American government is probably familiar to all. It includes the U.S. Constitution, the national government, and the individual state governments. The three branches of government are known as the executive branch, the legislative branch, and the judicial branch. Administrative agencies that create administrative law are also important parts of the structure of government.

Common Law

Common law is the body of law derived from the ancient unwritten law of England. It consists of the principles, uses, and rules that do not rest upon any express declaration of the legislature.[5]

Courts attempt to decide cases based on principles established in prior cases. Prior cases that are similar to the case being considered are called precedents.

Decisions found to be unreasonable may be overturned.

Stare decisis is a legal principle that mandates adherence to decided cases. It is the policy of courts to stand by precedent and not to disturb a settled point.[6]

Lawsuits are resolved by applying decisions of previous cases. Sometimes the court will use a very slight factual difference to distinguish the present case from the previous cases.

Regulations

Federal Agencies

At the federal level, an administrative agency is created by an act of Congress. The president, with the advice and consent of Congress, appoints the agency's director or highest official.

Each agency makes rules (called regulations) that have the force of law; these regulations can be found in the Code of Federal Regulations (CFR). The agency can interpret and enforce the regulations through administrative hearings and decisions. Federal courts can review the decisions made at an administrative hearing and can also be asked to review the regulations.

State Agencies

At the state level, some agencies are created by statute and some are created by provisions in the state constitution. The governor may appoint the directors of these state agencies, although the statute or the state constitution might direct that the director or top agency official be elected. For example, in many states the attorney general is elected rather than appointed.

In state agencies, as in federal agencies, government policies are implemented through rules and decisions. Agency rules and decisions are subject to review by the courts.

Separation of Powers

No one branch of the government is dominant over another branch. Each affects and limits the functions and powers of the others. Thus the U.S. government is sometimes characterized as a "system of checks and balances." When Congress passes a bill, the president must sign it before it becomes law. If the president vetoes the bill, a vote by two-thirds of the Congress can override that veto. A law that has been passed by Congress and signed by the president can be declared invalid (overturned) by the U.S. Supreme Court.

The three branches of government (the executive, legislative, and judicial branches) work together to make, execute, review, and enforce the laws.

Statute of Limitations

Every civil and criminal case is subject to a specific statute of limitation, which is a time limit as to when a lawsuit may be filed. There is one exception: There is no statute of limitation for the crime of murder.

If a lawsuit is not filed within the required period of time, the right to sue is lost. The time to file a lawsuit will vary from state to state, and different times are prescribed for various types of cases.

■ Tort Law

A tort is a civil wrong; it is not considered a crime. The wrongdoer is called a tortfeasor. The purpose of tort law is to provide a method for peacefully determining liability and assessing damages to be paid to victims of wrongdoing.

Many different torts exist, and not all torts are recognized in all jurisdictions. In the United States, the most common torts are assault and battery, conspiracy, false imprisonment, forcible entry and detainer (this means keeping possession of real property), fraud, libel and slander, malicious prosecution, negligence, product liability, trespass, and a few others.

When a person is injured or his or her property is damaged, the rights and responsibilities of the parties involved are determined by the law of torts. Many torts involve negligence. When a judge, jury, or arbitrator determines that one party was negligent and that the negligent conduct caused injury or property damage, the negligent party is usually required to pay for the harm done.

Simply determining that someone caused injury to someone else is not sufficient. It must be proven that a defendant was at fault. Sometimes no one was at fault, as some accidents are unavoidable.

Usually a tort victim is compensated, with money, for the injury suffered. The sum awarded most often includes medical expenses incurred or reimbursement for lost wages. If the damage was to property, the victim is usually awarded the amount of money needed to repair or replace the damaged property. Sometimes people are compensated for their pain and suffering. Although it is very difficult to assign a dollar value to the loss of a leg or an eye, in our society it has been decided that monetary compensation is the best alternative.

Categories of Torts

Three categories of torts are distinguished: intentional torts, negligence, and strict liability torts. Most torts involve some sort of negligence, but in some cases there may be intentional wrongdoing. Intentional torts include assault, battery, false imprisonment, invasion of privacy, and the intentional infliction of emotional distress. In other situations, the activity is so dangerous that it is public policy to demand absolute responsibility of the tort-feasor. These cases are known as strict liability torts.

Negligence

The most common tort is the tort of negligence. When a person or property is injured or damaged as a result of the actions of another person, an allegation of negligence is often made. Negligence is often divided into two degrees: ordinary negligence (the failure to perform as a reasonably prudent person would perform under similar circumstances) and gross negligence (the intentional or wanton disregard of care).

Forms of Negligence

Several forms of negligence exist:

- Malfeasance is an unlawful or improper act.
- Misfeasance is the incorrect performance of a permitted act.
- Nonfeasance is the failure to act when an act is required by law or when there is a duty to act.
- Malpractice is the negligent or careless action of a person who is held to a professional standard of care.
- Criminal negligence is the willful indifference to the potential for injury or the reckless disregard for the safety of another.

Standards of Care

Professionals are held to a higher standard of care than nonprofessionals. A nonprofessional is judged by a "reasonable person" standard: What would a reasonable person do in this situation? A professional is held to a higher standard: What would a reasonably prudent person with this type of specialized training do in this type of situation?

How Is Negligence Proven in a Court of Law?

Usually, a jury will decide, based on facts presented at trial, if a person acted reasonably or negligently. Custom and common sense often determine what standard of care the jury will apply.

Sometimes the standard of care is defined by statute. If someone acted in violation of law, he or she is usually presumed to have acted negligently and is held liable for any damages that result.

Res ipsa loquitur means "the thing speaks for itself." The doctrine of res ipsa loquitur applies when the defendant had exclusive control of the item or instrument or "thing" that caused the harm, when the plaintiff did not in any way contribute to the accident, and when the accident would not have occurred unless someone was negligent. For example, if an X ray clearly shows that a surgical instrument was left in the chest cavity of a man who underwent heart surgery, the plaintiff could allege that the doctrine of res ipsa loquitur applies. In this case, the mere fact that the accident happened is enough to infer that someone (the doctor, nurse, or hospital) was negligent and will be held liable for damages.

Standards of care applicable to medical professional activities can also be found in government regulations and in accreditation manuals for hospitals and other institutions. Sometimes the standard of care changes based on changes in statutes, rules, and court cases.

For example, in the case of *Darling v. Charleston Community Memorial Hospital*, 33 Ill. 2d 326, 211 N.E. 2d 253 (1965), the Illinois Supreme Court held that a hospital is liable for the improper review of the credentials of its staff, and that a hospital cannot limit its liability as a charitable corporation to the amount of its liability insurance. In this case, because the evidence supported the verdict for the plaintiff, the hospital was found liable for damages.

In the *Darling* case, a college football player was injured while playing. He was taken to the emergency room and was treated by a general practitioner who had not treated a leg fracture in recent years. X rays were taken and the doctor set the fracture and applied a cast. The patient complained of pain, but the doctor did not call in a specialist. After two weeks, the plaintiff was transferred to a larger hospital under the care of an orthopedic surgeon. The surgeon found a considerable amount of dead tissue that, in his opinion, was caused by swelling of the leg against the cast. The surgeon attempted several operations to save the leg, but ultimately it was amputated 8 inches below the knee.

The Illinois court held that the hospital was liable based on the evidence that the nurses at the hospital did not test the leg for circulation as often as necessary, that skilled nurses would have promptly recognized conditions that signaled impaired circulation, and that the nurses knew that the situation would become irreversible. In those circumstances, it became the "nurses' duty to inform the attending physician and if he failed to act, to advise the hospital authorities so that appropriate action might be taken."[7]

The court also held that the hospital negligently failed to review the doctor's work and negligently failed to require a consultation with a specialist. In addition, it held that the doctrine of charitable immunity did not apply and that the defendant was liable for the full judgment, even that which was in excess of its insurance coverage.

Defenses Against Negligence

A defendant may be relieved from having to pay damages, even if he or she is found to be negligent. The possible defenses are contributory negligence, comparative negligence, assumption of the risk, and release.

Contributory Negligence

The doctrine of contributory negligence provides that if a person was negligent at all, he or she cannot recover against another person, even if that person was far more negligent. This rule is still the law in some states, but most states have now changed to a comparative law standard. Contributory negligence was the law in all states at one time.

Comparative Negligence

Since abandoning the doctrine of contributory negligence, most states have adopted a comparative negligence rule. Under this rule, one party's negligence is "compared" with the other party's negligence. Recovery of damages will be limited to an amount reduced by the percentage of fault assessed to that party. For example, if the defendant car driver was held to be 80% at fault but the plaintiff was held to be 20% at fault, the most the plaintiff could recover would be 80% of his or her claim.

Releases

Many times businesses will try to limit their liability by printing a release on the back of a ticket claiming they cannot be sued if there is an injury. Sometimes this measure will preclude a person from suing the business—but sometimes it will not. If the release is written in very fine print and was not noticed, the person signing will not be held to it. If it is written in a complicated way and was not understood, the person signing will not be held to it. Also, that person's right to sue will not be waived if the injuries were caused by an act of gross negligence or if the act was intentional.

Equitable Relief

In some cases involving nuisance or trespass, a plaintiff may ask the court to issue an injunction to order the defendant to stop doing something tortious.

Money Damages

As mentioned previously, a tort is not considered a crime. Rather, in a tort action, the plaintiff has somehow been injured. The plaintiff seeks damages (monetary compensation) for these injuries in his or her own name in a civil (not criminal) court. By contrast, in criminal law, it is "the people" as a whole who seek justice. In a criminal case, the state brings the case, not the wronged individual. A victim of theft or rape cannot bring a criminal action against a person; rather, the complaint is filed in the name of the state.

Tort law compensates a person with money. The person responsible for the injury is required to pay to make the harmed person whole again. Criminal law punishes the criminal who violated a law. The penalty can be a fine or imprisonment, or both.

Sometimes a Tort Is Also a Crime

Confusing the issue, some crimes are also torts. For example, battery is both a crime and a tort. If one person strikes another person, the victim can sue to recover damages. This suit would be brought in a civil court, and if the plaintiff (the person who was hit) could prove that he or she was injured and those injuries were caused by the defendant (the person who did the hitting), the plaintiff could be compensated for the injuries. The state can also prosecute the defendant for the crime of battery, in which case the defendant might go to jail.

■ Restraint of Trade

Antitrust litigation is an important legal issue for healthcare providers. The competition in the healthcare industry creates an arena for many kinds of possibly illegal actions involving the restraint of trade.

In 1890, the U.S. Congress passed the Sherman Antitrust Act (15 U.S.C. § 1). Section 1 provides that "Every contract, combination in form of trust or otherwise, or conspiracy, in restraint of trade or commerce among the several States, or with foreign nations, is hereby declared to be illegal." Thus, any time there is an action to reduce market competition, fix prices, bar or limit members, or provide a preferred provider system, or when there is an exclusive contract, there is the possibility of restraint of trade.

Antitrust problems may potentially arise when a hospital limits its medical staff. For this reason, the process that a hospital uses to determine who may have staff privileges and who may not must be based on objective criteria and not on the financial advantages that may be realized by granting or denying the right to practice at the hospital. Of course, a hospital may deny privileges to certain individuals, but the decision must be made for cause (for instance, the doctor involved has been cited for improper actions or does not possess the qualifications required for all doctors) and not merely to limit competition.

Sometimes a hospital will enter an exclusive contract with specialty groups to provide services to the hospital. For example, it may contract with a pathology, radiology, emergency medicine, or anesthesiology group. If these contracts are reasonable and are not made to limit competition, they are usually permitted. In several cases in which hospitals were sued, the courts held that the contracts were not against public policy.[8]

Hospitals and other healthcare facilities must be sure that any action or proposed action to limit access or to close their medical staff is based on objective criteria. In many states, government agencies review hospital actions regarding the granting or the denying of hospital privileges. Individual physicians and medical groups will continue to challenge hospital actions, and if objective standards are not the basis for the action, the challengers will prevail—as Chapter 16 describes in more detail.

■ Notes

1. In any case, the title of the case is always written *Plaintiff v. Defendant*. The plaintiff (or plaintiffs)—that is, the party bringing the action—will always be listed first. Also, each case will have a citation. Using the citation, the case can be looked up and the complete decision read. For example, in the citation 220 F. 2d 118, the "F. 2d" refers to the *Federal Reporter*, Second Series. The "220" refers to the volume, and "118" refers to the page number of that volume. The citation can also be used to learn if the case has been upheld or overturned by a higher court, and to determine if there are other cases with similar results.
2. The highest court in New York State is called the Court of Appeals.
3. In some states, a summons may only be served by a person who is older than 21 years of age and who is not a party to the action.
4. United States Constitution, Art. VI.
5. *Bishop v. United States*, 334 F. Supp. 415 (S.D. Tx. 1971), cert. denied 414 U.S. 911 (1973).
6. *Neff v. George*, 364 Ill. 306, 4 N.E. 2d 388 (1986).
7. 211 N.E. 2d at 258.
8. *Jefferson Parish Hospital v. Hyde*, 466 U.S. 2 (1984). See also *Belmar v. Cipolla*, 96 N.J. 199, 475 A. 2d 533 (1984).

Medical Staff Law and Important Legal Cases

CHAPTER 16

Joanne P. Hopkins, JD, BSN, MSN

The relationship between a hospital and its medical staff, as well as the relationship between the medical staff and practitioners seeking access to the medical staff, is the subject of state and federal legislation and case law. The medical staff services professional (MSSP) should be familiar with the law applicable to the jurisdiction in which he or she practices. This chapter provides a general discussion of legal issues that are usually common among the states and alerts the professional to situations when legal counsel should be consulted.

■ The Medical Staff

Relationship Between the Hospital and the Medical Staff

The hospital's medical staff is generally composed of licensed independent practitioners who provide healthcare services within the hospital. The hospital's governing board groups these practitioners together as a medical staff to comply with legal and accreditation requirements and to perform certain functions for and on behalf of the governing board. For example, accreditation and licensure requirements compel a hospital to credential practitioners seeking to provide services in the hospital. The hospital's governing board utilizes the services of the medical staff, generally operating through medical staff officers and committees, to perform this credentialing and provide recommendations to the governing board for final decision.

Whether the medical staff is a separate legal entity has not been addressed conclusively in all jurisdictions. Self-governance by the medical staff may support a finding of a separate entity. Some medical staffs find it in their best interests not to be construed as a separate legal entity, but rather to serve as an integral component of the hospital. Generally, this arrangement enables the medical staff members, when performing functions on behalf of the hospital and its governing board, to be protected under the hospital's liability insurance as an agent of the hospital. In contrast, medical staffs that charge membership dues or carry other attributes of separateness may find in a particular court case that they are held to be a separate legal entity capable of being sued independently and capable of conspiring with the hospital for purposes of antitrust liability.

Medical Staff Bylaws

To satisfy accreditation and licensure requirements, the hospital must have medical staff bylaws that establish the method or manner by which the practitioners comprising the medical staff perform the functions assigned to them. The medical staff bylaws also establish the relationship between the medical staff and its members and the medical staff and the governing board. There is no specific structure required of medical staff bylaws, but certain elements must be included in the bylaws as set forth in accreditation[1] and state hospital licensure standards. Additionally, for those hospitals that are Medicare providers, the Medicare Conditions of Participation[2] address requirements for the medical staff and medical staff bylaws.

Generally, medical staff bylaws contain the following key components:

1. Responsibilities of the medical staff and duties of members
2. Organization of the medical staff, such as staff categories and specialty departments, sections, and/or services
3. Qualifications and procedures for medical staff appointment and reappointment
4. Qualifications and procedures for granting clinical privileges
5. Medical staff officers
6. Structure and function of the medical executive committee (and other medical staff committees if any)
7. Meetings, quorum, and voting of the medical staff and other organizational components
8. Corrective action, and hearing and appellate review procedures
9. Peer review confidentiality and immunity
10. Amendment and adoption of bylaws and related manuals

Medical staff bylaws also generally include, as a separate manual, a set of rules and regulations. Although the bylaws contain general principles on the organization and operation of the medical staff, documents such as the rules and regulations provide significant detail on operational requirements and procedures. Many hospitals have developed separate manuals on credentialing, corrective action, and hearing and appellate review procedures to set out the particular details for those respective areas. A separate manual may also address allied health professionals or healthcare practitioners who are not eligible for medical staff appointment (see Chapter 8). The process for amending a manual may differ from the process of amending the medical staff bylaws, which almost always requires approval by the voting members of the medical staff and the governing board. A manual, in contrast, may require approval of only the medical executive committee and the governing board, enabling changes to be made more easily, provided those changes do not conflict with the medical staff bylaws. Therefore, the medical staff needs to be comfortable with the content of any manual, as changes to it are not subject to approval of the entire medical staff.[3]

Just as issues may arise regarding whether the medical staff is a separate legal entity from the hospital, so there have been court cases addressing whether the medical staff bylaws constitute a contract between the hospital or the medical staff and each member of the medical staff.[4] Some hospitals and their medical staffs prefer that the medical staff bylaws not constitute a contract with each member of the medical staff, as that arrangement may open up the hospital and its medical staff to litigation by an individual practitioner based on breach of contract in connection with a medical staff privileging dispute. Hospitals and medical staffs wishing to negate the existence of a contract may provide statements to that effect in the bylaws or, alternatively, avoid statements in the bylaws that support the allegation of the existence of a contract.

Sources of Law

State statutes and regulations may address any or all of the following issues pertinent in the medical staff setting and should be reviewed by the MSSP:

1. Who can access the medical staff? Are podiatrists, dentists, or other licensed independent practitioners eligible for medical staff appointment, or is appointment limited to physicians?
2. Which procedures must be followed if medical staff appointment or reappointment is denied or if the hospital attempts to terminate or limit a practitioner's appointment or clinical privileges (e.g., procedural due process or notice and opportunity to be heard)?
3. Are the medical staff bylaws a contract between the practitioner and the hospital and its medical staff? Are the bylaws of the governing board a contract between the governing board and the practitioner?
4. What may be required as a condition of medical staff appointment, and what are permissible bases upon which to deny or terminate appointment or clinical privileges (e.g., completion of a residency, board certification)?
5. Which privileges of confidentiality and immunity are available for peer review actions and participants in peer review?

Case law (or court cases) in the medical staff area generally deals with either the reasons a hospital may use to exclude or terminate a practitioner from the medical staff or the procedures used to accomplish the exclusion or termination. Cases also address whether the hospital may be liable for credentialing of practitioners or for the actions of medical staff members. Depending on state law, there may be immunity for hospitals and medical staffs for credentialing and other peer review activities. Generally, this immunity is limited to authorized actions taken in the course of peer review and requires that the actions have been taken in good faith, in the absence of malice. (See the "Peer Review Privileges of Confidentiality and Immunity" section later in this chapter.)

At the federal level, the primary law dealing with peer review is the Health Care Quality Improvement Act (HCQIA).[5] This law was intended to provide immunity for participants in peer review provided that the peer review met certain standards (discussed later in this chapter). HCQIA also established the National Practitioner Data Bank (NPDB), along with required reporting by hospitals and other healthcare entities of professional review actions involving physicians as well as periodic mandatory querying by hospitals of the NPDB.

The other primary federal law that affects the medical staff is the Medicare Conditions of Participation for hospitals that are Medicare providers.[6] These federal regulations address duties and responsibilities of the medical staff, as well as operational requirements applicable to physicians and other practitioners.

■ Medical Staff Liability Issues

Hospital Liability for the Practitioner

A hospital may be held liable for the actions of a practitioner who is providing services in the hospital setting. There are three primary ways this may occur.

Respondeat Superior/Vicarious Liability

This type of liability occurs when the practitioner is an employee of the hospital. Most states impose liability on the employer for the actions of the employee, even if the employer itself did not engage in any direct negligence. Rather, the employer is held vicariously liable for the actions of the employee simply by virtue of the existence of the employer–employee relationship. This liability is premised on the assumption that the employer is in the best position to control the employee and will do so to minimize the employer's liability.

Ostensible Agency

In this situation, a hospital may be liable for the actions of a member of the medical staff even though the practitioner is not an employee of the hospital but rather an independent contractor. Depending on the type of services provided by the practitioner, the court may find that the practitioner is an agent of the hospital. For example, an emergency department physician may be an independent contractor of the hospital, but appears to be a hospital-employee to the patient who presents to the emergency department for treatment. In such a case, depending on the facts, the court may find that the patient had a reasonable expectation that the physician was an employee or authorized agent of the hospital. Therefore, the patient may look to the hospital for recovery of damages in the event the patient is injured by the emergency department physician's negligence. Ostensible agency liability is most frequently seen with hospital-based practitioners because the patient is less likely to select the practitioner and "relies" on the hospital or the primary practitioner for the selection.

Independent Liability/Corporate Negligence

In addition to liability a hospital may have for the actions of the medical staff member because of its relationship to the practitioner, many states have held that the hospital has independent duties to patients that may include a duty to supervise the care provided by the medical staff and to perform proper credentialing and, therefore, liability for its own "corporate" negligence in that regard.[7] The hallmark decision in this regard is *Darling v. Charleston Community Memorial Hospital*, an Illinois State Supreme Court case from 1965.[8] In the *Darling* case, there were allegations that the attending physician was not responsive to the hospitalized orthopedic patient's complaints of pain and other possible complications in his treatment of the patient. Ultimately, the patient had to be transferred to another facility and undergo a leg amputation. The hospital defended against the patient's allegation of negligence by stating that only the physician could practice medicine, not the hospital. The Illinois State Supreme Court, however, held that hospitals are independently responsible for monitoring, supervising, and controlling care where necessary to protect the patient. The *Darling* case decision has since been used as a precedent by courts in many other states.[9]

Hospital Liability to the Practitioner

A practitioner may seek to hold a hospital liable for denying the practitioner access to the medical staff or for a hospital's decision to terminate or limit the practitioner's medical staff appointment and/or clinical privileges. The practitioner's complaints may focus on the reason for the hospital's action, the manner in which the action was taken or the procedures used, or both. Lawsuits between a hospital and a practitioner most commonly involve allegations of failure to afford procedural due process, antitrust, violations of federal or state civil rights laws, breach of contract, libel, slander or defamation, and tortious interference with business or contractual relationships. Because of the importance to a practitioner of medical staff appointment to the hospital and requirements to disclose peer review or professional review actions when seeking appointment at other hospitals or managed care contracts, litigation by denied practitioners against hospitals is not uncommon despite the state and federal law provisions on peer review immunity.

Appointment and Clinical Privileges

The medical staff bylaws should contain two critical elements regarding appointment and clinical privileges:

- The criteria or requirements, such as education, training, and competence
- The process for making the decisions

The first element deals with the basis or reason for the decision, and the second deals with the mechanism and procedures used to make the decision. Although a court may be inclined to defer to the hospital and the medical staff as to the basis or reason for a decision to exclude or discipline a practitioner, it will likely scrutinize the procedures used to take the action. A key point is whether the procedures in the medical staff bylaws or manuals have been substantially complied with in making the decision and whether these procedures are fair to the practitioner.

The bylaws should include requirements for appointment as well as requirements for clinical privileges, which obviously will differ by privilege and specialty. Some hospitals group clinical privileges into categories or have a core set of privileges associated with completion of a residency in the particular specialty, along with a second category of special privileges that may require additional education or training. Separate procedures may be established for the appointment decision as compared to the clinical privileges decision, although many hospitals use the same process but simply apply different criteria when making these decisions.

In challenging the basis for a credentialing or peer review action, the practitioner may allege that the action was arbitrary or capricious or was applied in a discriminatory manner. The Joint Commission's medical staff standards require that professional criteria be specified in the bylaws.[10] The criteria are designed to ensure that patients will receive quality care. Therefore, criteria for appointment and clinical privileges should be clear and specific and applied equally to all practitioners unless otherwise provided in the bylaws.

Issues and Criteria

The following subsections describe some of the substantive issues that arise in credentialing and that are usually addressed in the medical staff bylaws.

Categories of Eligible Practitioners

The medical staff bylaws should clearly define which categories of practitioners are eligible to be considered for medical staff appointment and/or clinical privileges. This is most commonly done by defining the term "practitioner" or including a statement on this issue in the opening provisions of the bylaws. The hospital's governing board should be the decision maker when it comes to developing these categories, after consulting with the medical staff, so as to limit the involvement of direct economic competitors on the medical staff in the decision. State law should also be consulted, particularly hospital licensing statutes that may address access to the medical staff.

Medical staff applications should be provided only to those practitioners who are eligible to be considered. If an application is received from a practitioner who is not eligible, it should not be processed until the governing board makes a decision on whether that category of practitioners will be afforded access to the medical staff. Note that there may be some practitioners who are eligible for clinical privileges but are not eligible for medical staff membership.

Residency Training

Residency training may be more logically associated with clinical privileges rather than with appointment itself; however, it is frequently listed as a requirement for appointment. Some state laws specifically authorize a hospital to require that a practitioner have completed appropriate residency training to be a medical staff member.[11] In *Hay v. Scripps Memorial Hospital* (a 1986 California case), the appellate court held that it was permissible to require obstetrics residency training for obstetrical clinical privileges and, therefore, to deny those privileges to a family practitioner who lacked such training.[12] If the bylaws require residency training, it is recommended that the type of residency be specified, particularly if the requirement is tied to clinical privileges rather than appointment (e.g., a radiology residency may not be appropriate for internal medicine privileges). If tied to privileges, consideration should be given to whether several types of residencies may be appropriate for the particular specialty or clinical privileges. Finally, state law should be checked on permissible distinctions between residencies approved by the Accreditation Council on Graduate Medical Education and the American Osteopathic Association. Distinctions or discrimination between the two in a residency requirement may be prohibited by state law or found by a court to be arbitrary.

Board Certification

Whether board certification may be a requirement for appointment or clinical privileges may also be addressed by state law. To date, the court cases on this issue that have upheld exclusion of a practitioner for this reason have dealt with requirements that there be board certification or eligibility or compliance with some other alternative, not an "absolute" board certification requirement.[13] The theory often advanced in these cases is that the requirement is arbitrary in that it assumes that a practitioner who is board certified is competent, while one who is not board certified is incompetent.

Until recently, many hospitals avoided an absolute board certification requirement because the Medicare Conditions of Participation provided that "the accordance of staff membership or professional privileges...[may not be] dependent solely upon certification, fellowship, or membership in a specialty body or society."[14]

In 1997, the interpretive guidelines for the conditions were amended to clarify that board certification may be required, but may not be the only criteria used (e.g., the practitioner may not be automatically appointed to the medical staff because of being board certified).[15] If other criteria are included and the practitioner meets all those criteria except for board certification, the interpretive guidelines provide that the hospital may deny appointment based on lack of board certification.

As with residency requirements, if board certification is required, the governing board must consider whether any type of board certification is acceptable or whether the certification should be appropriate to the clinical privileges being sought by the practitioner. State law may not permit distinctions between programs approved by the American Board of Medical Specialties and the Bureau of Osteopathic Specialists.

Another point to be considered is whether recertification should be required if available. If board certification is an appropriate measure of competence, presumably it should be maintained.

Current Competence

The Joint Commission requires verification of "current competence" to perform the requested clinical privileges, necessitating a process for assessing this qualification for both new applicants and practitioners seeking reappointment.[16] On reappointment, the hospital should have its own internal practitioner-specific data on the practitioner's current competence available as a result of ongoing professional practice evaluation (OPPE). It may be more difficult to obtain this information at the time of initial appointment. Specific queries to other hospitals or healthcare entities at which the practitioner has provided services and peer recommendations may yield this information. Additionally, this is one of the primary reasons for a time-limited period of focused professional practice evaluation (FPPE) for all initially requested clinical privileges: to evaluate and determine the practitioner's current competence and performance through proctoring, chart review, observation by other members of the medical staff, or other processes.[17] To assess current competence at the time of reappointment, the medical staff may require that certain minimum numbers of procedures be performed either at the hospital or at other hospitals to maintain the specific clinical privilege.

Professional Liability Insurance

Case law has consistently upheld the hospital's authority to require that the practitioner maintain professional liability insurance for his or her actions in the hospital, because it helps ensure recovery by a patient injured by a practitioner's negligence and protects the hospital's assets.[18] Insurance requirements should be included in the medical staff bylaws with reference to minimum limits of liability, which may vary by specialty (if appropriate) and should be consistently enforced. The bylaws may reference limits to be set by the governing board by resolution; alternatively, the limits may be set out in a manual so that they may more easily be changed. Insurance requirements may also address the type of insurance or the type of carriers that are acceptable to ensure that the coverage will be there when needed. Additionally, the practitioner may be required to purchase prior acts or tail coverage if the insurance is claims made (or covers only claims filed during the term of the policy), thereby ensuring coverage if the practitioner changes policies or allows the policy to terminate after he or she leaves the medical staff. Insurance that is occurrence based usually covers only claims dealing with incidents that occur during the term of the policy.

Peer References

Information provided by the practitioner's peers related to current competence and other qualifications should be required as a part of the appointment and privileging process.[19] Many hospitals obtain references from residency or fellowship supervisors and department or section chiefs at other hospitals, as well as from other peers. Inquiries to peers should be specific and request detailed information, rather than just setting out a blanket question as to whether the practitioner should be appointed to the medical staff or granted requested clinical privileges. The Joint Commission requires that peer recommendations address six elements: medical/clinical knowledge, technical and clinical skills, clinical judgment, interpersonal skills, communications skills, and professionalism.[20]

In some states, peer references provided for purposes of peer review will be confidential under applicable peer review laws. This information, however, may need to be disclosed to the practitioner if it becomes the basis for an exclusion or termination of medical staff appointment and/or clinical privileges; therefore, the hospital should be careful about promising the peer reference strict confidentiality. Peer references should be marked as generated for purposes of peer review and obtained in a manner that maximizes the application of state peer review privileges to the information to the extent possible.

Health Status

The Joint Commission requires hospitals to verify the practitioner's ability to perform the clinical privileges requested.[21] This duty may need to be balanced with the limitations on discrimination based on disability, as set forth in the federal Americans with Disabilities Act (ADA).[22] In essence, the ADA prohibits discrimination in certain settings against a "qualified individual with a disability" solely based on the disability. A disability is defined as a physical or mental impairment that substantially limits one or more of the major life activities of such individual, a record of the impairment, or being regarded as having an impairment. To be a "qualified individual with a disability," the individual must be able to perform the essential functions of the job in question with or without reasonable accommodation. If the disabled individual can perform the essential functions of the job or task with reasonable accommodation, the ADA imposes a duty to provide that reasonable accommodation.

The ADA prohibits discrimination by employers of more than 15 employees, public entities, and private entities of public accommodation. Hospitals that employ practitioners will need to be cognizant of the provisions of Title I of the ADA dealing with employment. Title I's provisions relate to discrimination during the job application process, employment, and termination. When the medical staff is composed of independent contractors and not employees, hospitals may be subject to Title III of the ADA, which addresses places of "public accommodation," but not the employment provisions in Title I. Under Title I of the ADA, employers may not ask an applicant questions eliciting information about a disability during the pre-offer stage. Instead, these questions should be reserved until a decision has been made to make an offer (or condition an offer) of employment, as must a requirement to undergo a physical examination.

The ADA also prohibits discrimination based on past drug addiction or alcoholism. Questions about current illegal drug use are permissible; otherwise, the employer may address drug or alcohol abuse only as it affects the individual's ability to perform the job functions.

Some have raised concerns that the prohibition applied in the employment setting might also be applicable to providers of public accommodation under Title III, which protects individuals who are denied the full and equal enjoyment of the goods, services, facilities, privileges, advantages, or accommodations of a place of public accommodation such as a hospital. A few reported court cases have allowed independent contractor physicians to proceed with Title III claims against hospitals for actions against their medical staff appointment and/or clinical privileges.[23]

Because of some uncertainty regarding application of the ADA mandates, hospitals with nonemployed medical staffs may attempt to comply with the ADA's employment provisions even though they are dealing with independent contractors, rather than employees. The following is a question designed to track the ADA prohibitions for purposes of assessing the health status of applicants to and members of the medical staff:

Do you have the necessary health status or ability to perform the essential functions of medical staff appointment and exercise the clinical privileges requested, with or without reasonable accommodation, without posing a significant health or safety risk to your patients?

Some hospitals have taken an even more conservative approach and ask about health status only after a decision has been made that the applicant meets all other criteria for appointment and clinical privileges. The offer of medical staff appointment and clinical privileges is then made conditional upon verification that the applicant possesses the necessary health status to perform the essential functions of medical staff appointment and exercise the requested clinical privileges.

AIDS and HIV status are protected as disabilities under the ADA.[24] Using the reasoning set forth in the ADA, if a practitioner were HIV positive but could perform the essential functions of medical staff appointment and exercise the clinical privileges requested without posing a significant health or safety risk, discrimination based on HIV status alone would be problematic. With reasonable accommodation, a physician who is HIV positive may be able to meet the health status requirement. Generally, with regard to practitioners or other healthcare providers who are involved in surgery, or who come in contact with the patient's blood or bodily fluids, the courts have held that the provider cannot perform his or her clinical duties without presenting a significant threat to the health and safety of others and, therefore, have permitted exclusion from that practice.[25] Hospitals addressing this issue are strongly encouraged to seek legal counsel.

The medical staff bylaws should provide a mechanism to verify an applicant's or member's health status at the time of initial appointment and reappointment, as well as at other times, if concerns are raised regarding the individual's health status in the interim. Verification of health status may include documentation through a physical examination as well as drug or alcohol testing and/or testing for communicable diseases. In structuring these policies, hospitals should consult with legal counsel, as both the federal ADA provisions and state laws on discrimination may affect this analysis.

Ability to Work Cooperatively with Others

The courts have generally upheld the right of a hospital or medical staff to limit a practitioner's clinical privileges or appointment because of conduct that is disruptive to hospital operations and that has an adverse impact on overall patient care.[26] Professional review actions based on professional conduct are reportable to the National Practitioner Data Bank, just as are those based on professional competence.[27] For this reason, most hospitals include a requirement that the practitioner document his or her ability to work cooperatively with others as a condition of medical staff appointment. Information related to this issue is usually obtained through queries to other hospitals or healthcare entities where the practitioner has practiced, as well as via peer references.

In addition to addressing the ability to work cooperatively with others, the bylaws should require that the practitioner cooperate and participate in peer review. Although not required, medical staffs usually look for evidence of a pattern of unprofessional conduct before implementing corrective action, unless a particular incident is extremely serious in nature.

Conduct or Actions at Other Hospitals

Sometimes the medical staff may be advised of an incident at another hospital involving a practitioner, who is either applying to become or is already a member of the medical staff, that has potential implications for the practitioner's actions within the hospital. Although it may be difficult to obtain sufficient information about the incident, the medical staff should be able to act on that information when indicated. The bylaws should require the practitioner to advise the hospital within a stated time period of any corrective action taken by another hospital or healthcare entity as to medical staff appointment or clinical privileges. If the practitioner fails to do so, corrective action may be indicated based on the failure to comply with the requirement to disclose the corrective action (*not* what occurred at the other hospital). If the practitioner advises the hospital that he or she has been the subject of corrective action elsewhere, the practitioner should be required to ensure that the hospital obtains detailed information about the incident so that it can determine whether the event has implications for the practitioner's participation at the hospital.

Distance from Hospital

The Joint Commission requires that the management and coordination of each patient's care, treatment, and services be the responsibility of a licensed independent practitioner during the entire hospitalization.[28] Many hospitals require that active members of the medical staff reside within a certain distance or travel time of the hospital, so as to be available for care of hospitalized patients and, when on call, for the emergency department. Proximity requirements must be carefully structured and not used as a means of limiting competition with other practitioners on the medical staff. Proximity requirements may vary by specialty based on patient care considerations. Generally, it is best to avoid general or vague requirements such as a requirement to be "close enough to the hospital," and to set objective requirements that deal with mileage or travel time. If the specialty departments are involved in establishing these requirements, approval of the requirements should be required of a medical staff committee that is not composed of direct economic competitors to verify the reasonableness of the requirement.

Economic Considerations

True economic credentialing is used to refer to appointment or privileging criteria (and even contracting decisions) that deal with economic or cost issues only, as compared to the competence of the practitioner or the quality of the care that he or she provides. Some cost factors such as overutilization of hospital resources may relate to the quality of care provided by the practitioner as well. Recent developments in the area of economic credentialing address whether a hospital may limit a practitioner's participation on the medical staff based solely on the practitioner's ownership or investment interest in a competing hospital or other healthcare facility. Legal counsel should be consulted on the use of economic considerations or economic credentialing, as this is an emerging area and not all issues related to this practice have been definitively settled. (See the "Contract Practitioners" section later in this chapter.)

Hospital Utilization

Medical staffs are increasingly examining the appropriateness of requiring minimum levels of hospital utilization as a condition for appointment to the staff. Most commonly, this practice is seen in conjunction with active staff appointment. Hospital medical staffs may also consider the appropriateness of limitations on utilization for courtesy staff or other nonactive staff categories. In such cases, the purpose may be to prevent practitioners from utilizing the full services of the hospital for their patients while escaping the emergency department or on-call coverage obligations commonly imposed on active staff members. Utilization requirements that have a reasonable basis in patient care considerations or hospital operations may be justifiable, whereas requirements that are designed to increase use of the facility or require referrals should be questioned. As with any professional criteria, utilization requirements should be applied consistently and uniformly to all members of the medical staff category.

Malpractice History

Practitioners should be required to disclose their malpractice or professional liability claims history at the time of initial appointment and to update that information at the time of reappointment (if not more frequently). Although the fact of having malpractice claims alone may not be a basis for exclusion or termination of a practitioner, the hospital and its medical staff should examine the nature of the claims to determine whether there is a basis for further inquiry and possible professional review action. In *Purcell v. Zimbelman,* the Arizona appellate court held that a hospital had failed to adequately fulfill its duty to review the qualifications of medical staff members and ensure that they were properly trained and qualified for the privileges being exercised.[29] The physician in this case had been the defendant in previous malpractice lawsuits, some of which involved the procedure that allegedly injured the plaintiff.

Some hospitals query the court system to determine whether a practitioner has been named as a defendant in lawsuits or has properly disclosed all claims. The difficulty with these types of queries is the scope: depending on state law, claims may have been filed in many jurisdictions, making a query of just the local court system inadequate.

Burden of Proof and Duty to Provide Information

The medical staff bylaws should place the duty of documenting current competence and satisfaction of requirements of appointment and clinical privileges on the practitioner. With this approach, rather than the hospital's medical staff being responsible for showing that the applicant *is not* competent, it is the duty of the practitioner to show that he or she *is* competent and meets the requirements for appointment and the requested clinical privileges. In some cases, the medical staff may receive inadequate or incomplete information about the practitioner, making a decision as to competence or the satisfaction of other qualifications difficult. In such cases, rather than finding that the practitioner is incompetent or denial of the application, consideration should be given to whether the more appropriate finding is that there is inadequate information to document competence or make a decision. If the medical staff has inadequate or incomplete information, it may be appropriate to consider not processing the application, rather than denying it, because a denial implies a finding of incompetence.

The medical staff bylaws or credentialing manual should provide a clear process for identifying when additional information is needed, notifying the practitioner of the information that is needed (whether from the practitioner or a third party), providing the practitioner with a specific time frame within which the information must be received, and notifying the practitioner that the application (whether it be for appointment or reappointment) will be withdrawn from processing if the information is not received within the stated time period.

Use of Institutional Criteria

Hospital medical staffs are increasingly moving toward the development of specific objective criteria for clinical privileges whenever possible. These criteria, which are often referred to as minimum or threshold criteria, must be met before the practitioner's application for a particular clinical privilege is considered. When objective criteria are applied equally to all practitioners seeking the specific clinical privilege, even if a denial for failure to meet the criteria were to result, it would not be classified as a professional review action that is reportable to the NPDB.[30] An example would be a requirement that practitioners seeking cardiac catheterization privileges document successful completion of a residency in cardiology and performance of at least 50 cardiac catheterizations within the prior two-year period. Only those practitioners who document satisfaction of the two criteria would be considered for the clinical privilege. Compliance with the criteria, however, would not guarantee that the privilege will be granted. As noted earlier, these criteria are only minimum or threshold requirements; a medical staff may still examine other issues or consider other factors in making the final decision about whether to grant the clinical privilege.

The use of minimum or threshold criteria decreases the element of subjectivity that may be associated with the granting of clinical privileges. The criteria selected should have a reasonable basis and be approved by a medical staff committee that is not composed of direct economic competitors, to avoid the use of such criteria in an anticompetitive manner. Resources that may be helpful in establishing minimal or threshold criteria include state and national professional standards, board certification requirements, and requirements for specialty residencies.

Provisional Period and Proctors

Although the Joint Commission medical staff standards do not specifically require a provisional period, such a period is an excellent time for the medical staff to verify information they have received on new practitioners regarding their current competence to exercise the clinical privileges requested through the use of the required FPPE.[31] This review should be a formal process whereby competence can be evaluated in accordance with medical staff policy. If used, proctors should be required to prepare written reports, preferably using a standardized form. Documentation should prove that information generated during the provisional period was considered by the appropriate committees.

If a practitioner has difficulty with the designated proctors, the process should include provisions to appoint alternative proctors. Because the proctor must hold the clinical privilege that is being reviewed, situations may sometimes arise in which none of the medical staff members can serve as proctors. In these cases, it may be appropriate to permit proctorship at other facilities or proctoring by a practitioner who is not a member of the medical staff.

In terms of reporting to the NPDB, the imposition of proctoring or other limitations during the provisional period are not reportable to the NPDB if those requirements are imposed on all practitioners seeking those clinical privileges during the provisional period.[32] In contrast, limitations during the provisional period that exceed those routinely imposed on practitioners may be reportable.

Cross-Privileging

Although a particular clinical privilege is usually available in only one specialty department or service and is reviewed by that department or service, a hospital may make certain clinical privileges available to practitioners in multiple specialties; therefore, several specialties may be credentialing for the same privilege.

One option for dealing with this issue is to have each specialty department or service grant credentials for the same privilege, but this approach may result in inconsistent criteria or judgments as to the qualifications and competence of practitioners between the different departments or services. Medical staffs that encounter this issue may find it helpful to utilize a joint or ad hoc committee to review the criteria established by the different departments or services, thereby ensuring consistency across the hospital. The requirements, however, need not be exactly the same. For example, where a clinical privilege will be exercised by both gastroenterologists and general surgeons, it may be appropriate to require that the gastroenterologists provide additional documentation of specific surgical training or skill, whereas the additional requirements placed on the general surgeon may deal more with diagnosis or pathology recognition.[33] Criteria of this type acknowledge the specific skills of the different specialties, but are designed to provide for consistency regardless of the specialty.

The other option is to only allow one department or service to offer the clinical privilege and require that all practitioners be reviewed by that department or service, even though some will be assigned elsewhere. Unfortunately, this approach frequently is open to criticism based on the potential anticompetitive implications and the potential for turf battles.

Contract Practitioners

In some cases, hospitals have contracted with practitioners for the delivery of professional services. Examples include emergency medical services, anesthesia, radiology, and pathology. Hospitals may also contract for the services of intensivists or hospitalists or for the staffing of outpatient clinics. The courts have generally upheld the right of a hospital to contract for professional services, including on an exclusive basis.[34] Exclusive arrangements should be justified by documented patient care or hospital operational considerations, such as the need to ensure a single standard of care, facilitate scheduling of procedures, or provide 24-hour coverage for the professional services. A practitioner who provides professional services pursuant to a contractual arrangement is often credentialed in the same manner as any other member of the medical staff.

A significant issue that must be addressed when this type of arrangement is in place is the relationship between the contract for professional services and the practitioner's hearing and appeal rights pursuant to the medical staff bylaws. By contract, the hospital and practitioner can agree to different rights or procedures for terminating clinical privileges or terminating a practitioner's authority to provide services in the hospital. In the absence of a contractual provision to this effect, however, the practitioner would be entitled to the rights set forth in the medical staff bylaws. Some hospitals include a provision in the medical staff bylaws providing that contract practitioners are entitled to the same rights as other members of the medical staff, in the absence of a contrary provision in the contract. In the event of a conflict between a contract and the medical staff bylaws, many professional services contracts provide that the terms of the contract control.

In the area of exclusive contracting for professional services, the governing board, in consultation with the medical staff, should address the following issues:

- How are medical staff applications handled when the applicant requests privileges in an area that is subject to an exclusive contract?
- What happens to the clinical privileges of the practitioners providing services under an exclusive contract when that contract terminates or, in the case of an exclusive contract with a professional association or group, when the practitioner's relationship with the association or group ends?
- How does the hospital move from a situation in which there is no exclusive contract (and numerous practitioners hold clinical privileges in the particular area) to an exclusive contract (e.g., what is the effect on the clinical privileges of those practitioners who are not subject to the exclusive contract), and must procedural rights of review be afforded to any excluded practitioners?

Although the hospital's governing board maintains final authority over decisions related to contracts and other business decisions, to the extent these issues can be addressed in advance in the medical staff bylaws, conflict between the hospital, the medical staff, and individual practitioners may be lessened.

Allied Health Professionals

Hospitals should have a mechanism in place to verify the qualifications and competence of all individuals who provide patient care services in the hospital setting. For members of the medical staff, this concern underlies the entire medical staff credentialing and the peer review process. For hospital employees, this evaluation is done pursuant to the human resources process, with the scope of each employee's practice set forth in a written job description. Allied health professionals (AHPs) should refer to those healthcare professionals who are not eligible for appointment to the medical staff and who are not employed by the hospital. For these individuals, a method of credentialing or evaluating their qualifications and competence must be established to ensure that they are also qualified and competent to provide patient care services.

Particularly for AHPs who are permitted by the hospital to function independently, or without direction or supervision from another practitioner, the hospital and medical staff often utilize the same credentialing and clinical privileging processes that are applied to the medical staff (the Joint Commission requires that "licensed independent practitioners" be privileged through the medical staff process).[35] For AHPs who require direction or supervision, the hospital may use the medical staff credentialing process or may opt to use another process, such as a hospital multidisciplinary committee (see the discussion of the Joint Commission requirements later in this chapter). If the latter approach is used, the hospital committee should include representation from both the hospital administration and the medical staff, as well as other practice areas affected by the AHP's practice, such as nursing, pharmacy, and surgical services. The hospital committee might issue recommendations to one or more of the medical staff committees, which then report to the governing board, or it might issue its recommendations directly to the governing board or its designee. Whenever a system is used other than the medical staff credentialing process, there should be clear mechanisms for obtaining medical staff input into the scope of practice for AHPs and particularly in relation to practitioner supervision when required either by the AHP's licensing statutes or by hospital policy.

One of the most controversial areas in today's hospitals is the determination of which types of AHPs should be permitted to provide services in the facility. This decision should be made by the governing board, as the AHPs may be direct economic competitors of the practitioners on the medical staff. Even so, a mechanism should be established for obtaining medical staff input. If a request is received from an AHP in a category for which the governing board has not made a decision regarding access, the request should be tabled until the governing board can decide whether that particular category of AHP should be permitted access and, if so, under which conditions. Only if the governing board has granted access should an application be considered.

Finally, in establishing procedures to credential AHPs, the procedures should address the following concerns:

- Whether the AHP will be afforded clinical privileges or functions pursuant to a task description (the Joint Commission requires that the former be used for physician assistants and advanced practice registered nurses and that either the medical staff process or an equivalent process be used)[36]
- How the services provided by the AHP will be monitored and incorporated into the hospital's quality improvement program
- How complaints or concerns will be addressed regarding the AHP's practice
- How the AHP's authorization to provide services may be limited or terminated
- Whether the AHP is entitled to any procedural rights of review in the event of denial, limitation, or termination of authority to practice

State statutes may address the procedural rights of review to which an AHP may be entitled. The Joint Commission requires that the medical staff have a fair hearing and appeal process for adverse decisions dealing with privileges "that may differ for members and nonmembers of the medical staff."[37] When using the medical staff credentialing procedures to credential AHPs, the medical staff bylaws should be very specific as to whether the AHP is entitled to the same procedural rights of review as members of the medical staff, given that the credentialing procedures usually incorporate those rights.

■ Quality Improvement and Corrective Action

As discussed earlier, a hospital's governing board has certain responsibilities for monitoring and maintaining the quality of patient care in the hospital. The governing board uses the medical staff to assist in fulfilling this responsibility through peer review and quality improvement programs. It is through the ongoing monitoring of patient care services delivered in the hospital that concerns and problems are identified. The Joint Commission refers to this process as ongoing professional practice evaluation (OPPE) as to the medical staff.[38] Given that the hospital's governing board has overall responsibility for the quality of care, these concerns and problems involving a member of the medical staff must be addressed, if necessary, with corrective action affecting the practitioner's clinical privileges and/or medical staff appointment.

Role of Quality Improvement Data

Ideally, problems or concerns regarding the quality of services provided by a member of the medical staff are addressed through the quality improvement process, rather than by corrective action. The quality improvement process may be implemented through medical staff departments or committees or by hospital committees with medical staff representation, or through some combination of the two approaches. Some mention of the quality improvement process should be included in the medical staff bylaws, particularly as to the relationship between the quality improvement process and the corrective action process.

The department or committee responsible for quality improvement should have the authority to collect data related to the practitioner and to meet with the practitioner if problems or concerns are identified. The department or committee should also have the authority to work with the practitioner to implement voluntary practice changes, if possible, to address quality improvement problems that are confirmed. The medical executive committee should be kept apprised of quality improvement activities, including the implementation of voluntary practice changes when indicated. When a practitioner is unwilling or unable to address documented quality improvement concerns on a voluntary basis, the medical staff should consider the need for corrective action.

Grounds for Corrective Action

Corrective action or discipline against a member of the medical staff should be taken when actions or conduct by the practitioner have or may have a detrimental effect on the delivery of patient care services or operation of the hospital. Some common examples of situations in which corrective action is taken include the following:

- Failure to practice in accordance with customary or accepted professional standards
- Failure to comply with medical staff or hospital bylaws, rules and regulations, or policies (e.g., failure to cooperate in peer review or to provide required emergency services)
- Unprofessional conduct
- Violation of professional ethics
- Commission of crimes

Impairment of health status affecting the ability to exercise clinical privileges may also lead to corrective action. This usually follows attempts to address the impairment voluntarily and in a nonpunitive manner pursuant to a practitioner health policy.[39]

The authority to monitor the practitioner's hospital practice and to implement corrective action, including reasons for taking corrective action, should be specified in the medical staff bylaws as well as in the governing board bylaws (albeit in less detail).

Types of Corrective Action

The medical staff bylaws usually provide for three types of corrective action: standard, summary or emergency, and automatic. What distinguishes the different types of corrective action is whether the action is taken before the practitioner is given a right to a hearing, after a hearing takes place, or without the benefit of a hearing at all, respectively.

Standard corrective action is the most common type of action taken. In this situation, the affected practitioner is given notice of the allegations and procedural rights of review prior to the corrective action being imposed if the proposed action will adversely affect the practitioner's exercise of clinical privileges in the hospital (see the "Procedural Rights of Review" section later in this chapter).

Summary or emergency corrective action is action taken before affording the practitioner any procedural rights of review; therefore, it is usually reserved for situations in which failure to take an action may result in imminent danger to the health of an individual.[40] This form of corrective action is used in extreme situations in which it would be inappropriate to allow the practitioner to continue to practice until a full investigation has been completed and hearing held. Rather, the action is taken, and the practitioner is given the right to a hearing after the fact (generally on an expedited basis). Depending on the provisions in the medical staff bylaws, summary or emergency action may involve a suspension of all of a practitioner's privileges or imposition of more limited action such as a mandatory coadmission requirement or consultation requirement. Only the action necessary to address the immediate problem should be taken on a summary or emergency basis.

Automatic action is usually imposed in cases where there is no dispute as to the facts. For example, automatic action in the form of termination of medical staff appointment would be taken if the practitioner loses his or her professional license. Because a practitioner cannot practice without a license, there would be no issues to be addressed in a hearing—the practitioner either does or does not have a license. Some medical staff bylaws also provide for automatic action in the case of exclusion from participation in the Medicare program, loss of required professional liability insurance, loss of prescribing authority, and repeated or continued delinquency in completion of medical records. The key point with automatic action is that there is no dispute regarding whether the event or action that is the basis for automatic action has occurred. Otherwise, the practitioner may be entitled to a hearing to determine whether there is a reasonable basis for the action.

Corrective Action Procedures

Corrective action procedures (and related procedural rights of review) should be clearly specified in the medical staff bylaws. Generally, standard corrective action proceedings begin with the filing of a written request for corrective action. The bylaws should specify which individuals or committees may file a request. The request is usually directed to the medical executive committee. Upon receipt of a written request, this committee may initiate an investigation of the events or concerns that prompted the request. Most medical staff bylaws require that the practitioner be notified of the request for corrective action and of initiation of the investigation. The investigation may be conducted by a standing medical staff committee or an ad hoc investigating committee, and will likely involve at least an interview with the affected practitioner. The results of the investigation are then reviewed by the medical executive committee, which issues a recommendation indicating whether corrective action is appropriate and, if so, which type of corrective action should be taken. The practitioner is notified of the recommended action in writing and, if the action is adverse (see the "Procedural Rights of Review" section), is given procedural rights of review or an opportunity to address the concerns through a hearing before the matter is referred to the governing board for a final decision.

When summary or emergency action is imposed, the practitioner is immediately notified and the appropriateness of the action may be reviewed by the medical executive committee or the practitioner's department as soon as possible. If the reviewing committee determines that the summary or emergency action was indicated and is adverse to the practitioner, then the practitioner is afforded a hearing while the action remains in effect. Automatic action, by definition, requires no decision by the medical staff and is imposed immediately, without a hearing.

The purpose of corrective action should be the furtherance of the delivery of quality patient care within the hospital and proper operation and functioning of the hospital. Corrective action should be taken after a reasonable effort to obtain information about the questionable conduct or activities and upon the reasonable belief that corrective action is warranted by the facts. The type of corrective action taken will depend on the severity of the problem and should be tailored to the specific circumstances.

Collegial or Informal Intervention

A practitioner for whom minor deficiencies have been identified initially might be approached by the department chair or chief of staff for informal counseling and resolution, rather than resorting to corrective action. The chair or chief should point out the deficiency (or deficiencies); discuss alternative methods of patient care or professional conduct, depending on the nature of the problem; and encourage the affected practitioner to take the necessary steps to improve his or her practice. Collegial or informal intervention is often used initially when problems are caused by a practitioner's unprofessional conduct or disruptive behavior.

Although this intervention may be informal in nature, a dated written record should be made by the department chair or chief of staff, including a general description of the problem and the essence of the intervention or counseling, and placed in the affected practitioner's confidential peer review file. It is always important to document these kinds of interventions, because the problem may continue or recur in a more serious manner, necessitating corrective action. Documentation that prior attempts have been made to address the problem may be important to support corrective action later.

One drawback of collegial or informal intervention is that the intervention may not be eligible for or covered by statutory immunities or protections that exist for actions by peer review committees. To the extent possible under state peer review law, these interventions should be structured to fall within available protections, such as by having the individual involved in the intervention act on behalf of or as agent for a peer review committee.

Additional Education or Training

In some cases, a problem with variations in patient care may best be addressed by corrective action that requires the affected practitioner to obtain further education or training. For example, a practitioner might be misusing a category of drugs due to lack of knowledge about the indications and effects of the drugs. To correct this knowledge deficit, the individual might be required to attend a continuing medical education program on the use of that category of drugs. Likewise, a practitioner whose technical skill in performing a procedure is deficient might be required to attend a "hands-on" formal course to sharpen his or her skills.

Supervision and Retrospective Chart Review

A practitioner who performs a procedure with less skill than is consistent with professional standards may benefit from performing the procedure under supervision by a qualified practitioner for a stated period of time or for a stated number of procedures. Supervision or observation may also be used to obtain additional information about a practitioner, such as to confirm whether the practitioner possesses the necessary technical skill to perform a procedure in cases where concerns have been raised. Mandatory second consultations, for example, may be appropriate where a practitioner's documentation of clinical indications for admission or a surgical procedure have been questioned. A peer could also be asked to review a practitioner's medical records to determine whether there is documentation that appropriate standards of patient care are being maintained. A record should be created of each procedure or patient whose care was observed, supervised, or reviewed, with the record being maintained in the affected practitioner's peer review file.

Letter of Warning

In some cases, the action needed is to formally warn the practitioner of the identified problem and advise that the problematic actions or conduct must cease.

Particularly when dealing with conduct issues, the letter of warning should set out exactly what is expected of the practitioner or which conduct is unacceptable and will not be tolerated.

Limitation of Privileges

A practitioner who has serious problems or complications, for whom a lesser form of corrective action has been undertaken and failed (e.g., observation) or is inappropriate, may require an actual limitation or restriction of clinical privileges. This type of corrective action may be necessary when it has been determined that a practitioner is performing a procedure or treating cases that go beyond his or her skill or knowledge base or has an unacceptable rate of complications from a particular procedure.

For example, the patients of a cardiologist who performed permanent pacemaker implantation experienced several complications, followed by a death while a patient was undergoing the procedure. Having noted the complications earlier, the department chair had required the affected practitioner to perform at least five procedures under supervision. The fifth patient expired while undergoing the procedure due to actions by the practitioner. The department chair then initiated corrective action, recommending that the practitioner's privilege to perform pacemaker implantation be suspended.

Revocation of Privileges and/or Appointment

A practitioner who has serious problems, beyond normal or expected complications, deaths, or infractions of hospital policies or rules, may be subject to a revocation of privileges or a recommendation that all of the practitioner's privileges be removed. This step, in effect, removes the practitioner from the medical staff. Such corrective action usually follows other unsuccessful attempts to address the practitioner's problem, but it may also be the first type of corrective action if the problem is particularly serious or significant.

■ Procedural Rights of Review

Entitlement

Recommendations or actions by the medical executive committee and/or governing board that will entitle a practitioner to procedural rights of review, or a hearing and appellate review, should be clearly delineated in the medical staff bylaws following review of the federal and state law requirements. Because medical staff appointment and the right to exercise clinical privileges are often essential for the practitioner to be able to engage in his or her profession, the law usually affords the practitioner certain procedural rights of review before medical staff appointment or clinical privileges can be taken away. Procedural rights of review may arise in connection with initial appointment, reappointment, or corrective action. They may also arise in connection with the provisional period or a practitioner's request to increase clinical privileges during the term of appointment. A hearing should be afforded for any actions that are considered "adverse" or "adversely affecting" a practitioner's clinical privileges or medical staff appointment based on the practitioner's competence or professional conduct. Health care quality improvement act (HCQIA) defines "adversely affecting" to include "reducing, restricting, suspending, revoking, denying, or failing to renew clinical privileges or membership."[41] The Joint Commission's medical staff standards require a fair hearing and appeal process for adverse decisions regarding reappointment, denial, reduction, suspension, or revocation of clinical privileges that may relate to quality of care, treatment, and services issues.[42]

If the proposed action will limit or restrict the practitioner's exercise of clinical privileges, the practitioner will usually be afforded the right to a hearing prior to imposing the adverse action (except in the case of summary or emergency action).[43] Conversely, if the proposed action does not interfere with the practitioner's right to practice, a right to a hearing may not be required or provided by the medical staff bylaws. For example, the imposition of retrospective chart review does not limit the practitioner's right to practice or exercise clinical privileges. Requiring a practitioner to obtain the approval of another practitioner before performing surgery, however, may limit the practitioner's ability to exercise his or her surgical privileges and require that the practitioner have procedural rights of review depending on the provisions in the bylaws. The bottom line is that the decision of whether to provide for a hearing should not be addressed on a case-by-case basis, but rather should be specified in advance in the medical staff bylaws.

The procedural requirements for the hearing will be based on both state and federal law and should be clearly delineated in the medical staff bylaws or a related manual. Many bylaws offer more hearing procedures than are actually required by law. The purpose of a hearing is to provide the practitioner a fair opportunity to be heard, and reasonable procedures that facilitate this process should be included in the medical staff bylaws or the related manual. The reason for mandating the right to a hearing or procedural rights of review is to allow the practitioner an opportunity to address the specific concerns that have been raised about his or her delivery of patient care services or conduct and to demonstrate that the proposed adverse action is not warranted.

Health Care Quality Improvement Act (HCQIA)

The federal Health Care Quality Improvement Act, enacted in 1986, was intended to promote effective professional peer review for physicians. HCQIA was enacted in the aftermath of *Patrick v. Burget*, a successful antitrust lawsuit brought by an excluded physician in Oregon, to encourage effective and professional peer review by limiting liability for monetary damages of healthcare entities and participants in good faith peer review.[44] HCQIA establishes certain standards for professional review actions and provides that entities and individuals who comply with those standards will be entitled to certain limited immunities if sued by the affected physician.[45] HCQIA defines a physician as an MD or DO physician or dentist; podiatrists and other types of independent practitioners are not mentioned.[46]

A professional review action is defined as follows:

> [an] action or recommendation of a professional review body . . . in the conduct of professional review activity, which is based on the competence or professional conduct of an individual physician (which conduct affects or could affect adversely the health or welfare of a patient or patients), and which affects (or may affect) adversely the clinical privileges, or membership in a professional society, of the physician.[47]

"Professional review activity" is defined as a healthcare entity's activity with respect to an individual physician's clinical privileges or membership in the entity, the scope or conditions of the privileges or membership, or charging or modifying the privileges or membership.[47]

The standards established for a professional review action that would qualify for limited immunity are that the action be taken in the following manner:

1. In the reasonable belief that the action was in the furtherance of quality health care
2. After a reasonable effort to obtain the facts of the matter
3. After adequate notice and hearing procedures are afforded to the physician involved or after such other procedures as are fair to the physician under the circumstances
4. In the reasonable belief that the action was warranted by the facts known after reasonable effort to obtain facts and after meeting the notice and hearing requirements[49]

Compliance with the standards is not required by HCQIA. Compliance is necessary, however, to invoke the immunity afforded by the statute.

With regard to the third standard, which provides for "adequate notice and hearing," HCQIA sets out procedures that will be deemed to meet this standard.[50] The specific procedures are described in Appendix B of this chapter and include the following measures: (1) providing notice to the practitioner of the proposed action and a list of witnesses expected to testify against the practitioner, (2) affording the practitioner the right to representation by an attorney or other person of the practitioner's choice, and (3) providing the practitioner with the written recommendation of the hearing panel.

Immunity may be available even if a hospital or medical staff does not provide all of the specific "adequate notice and hearing" procedures set out in HCQIA, as HCQIA also allows the use of "such other procedures as are fair to the physician under the circumstances."[51] Many hospitals and medical staffs, however, have not wanted to gamble with whether other procedures might be considered fair and have incorporated all of the HCQIA procedures in their medical staff bylaws or fair hearing manual unless they find them to be particularly burdensome. Some believe that it will be easier, in the event of litigation, for the hospital and participating medical staff members to assert immunity if the HCQIA procedures have been precisely followed. Others believe that immunity will be available even if the actual procedures in the HCQIA are not complied with, if the peer review is conducted in good faith, and basic hearing procedures are followed in accordance with the medical staff bylaws. Those hospitals that have followed the HCQIA procedures should have an easier time documenting that the practitioner has been afforded procedural due process in the event of litigation. In any event, the ultimate objective is to further quality patient care through the use of effective peer review—not just to avoid litigation by affected practitioners.

A hospital and medical staff may use a single set of fair hearing procedures both for denial of appointment or reappointment and for corrective action. A hospital may vary these procedures somewhat if it is determined that different obligations are owed to an existing member of the medical staff as compared to an initial applicant. For example, the burden of proof may differ, with a greater burden being placed on the applicant as compared to the member. This will ultimately be a matter for the hospital and medical staff to address in consultation with legal counsel. The objective—whether there is one fair hearing plan or two—is that the plan be comprehensive, clear, and fair.

■ Legal Issues in Corrective Action and Hearings

Legal challenges to medical staff privileging decisions generally fall into two categories: substantive and procedural. A substantive challenge focuses on the reason for the adverse action: Was there a reasonable basis for limiting or terminating the practitioner's clinical privileges or medical staff appointment? Each case is evaluated on its own merits in this area, and the courts most often defer to the medical staff and hospital governing board in this regard.

A procedural challenge focuses on the procedures followed in imposing the adverse action or affording the procedural rights of review: Were the procedures fair, and did they comply with the requirements in the medical staff bylaws? As previously mentioned, the HCQIA procedures for adequate notice and hearing are an example of what are regarded as fair. The key for the hospital is to make sure that three criteria are met: (1) know the procedures and requirements in the medical staff bylaws (or related manuals) on adverse actions and hearings/appellate review; (2) ensure they comply with legal requirements; and (3) follow them to the fullest extent possible. Failure to follow the procedures in one's own bylaws is a common reason for litigation, yet can often easily be avoided.

The following subsections highlight some of the legal considerations that may arise in connection with adverse action and affording procedural rights of review.

Documentation of the Problem

One of the most difficult aspects of adverse action, whether on appointment or reappointment, or in corrective action, is actually documenting the problem. Sometimes there may be a concern regarding a practitioner, but either individuals are not willing to put the concern in writing or the time is not taken to examine the relevant information so as to be able to appropriately document the problem. There must always be a basis for adverse action, and the basis should be documented. Concerns, problems, or complaints should be put in writing, and both that information and the practitioner's practice should be subjected to an objective evaluation. For example, if a practitioner's complication rates for a certain surgical procedure are particularly high, a retrospective review of the practitioner's cases could be performed to ascertain the actual frequency of complications and identify whether unique factors related to the patient population might explain the complication rate.

Equal Application of Requirements

Another problem area is that requirements or standards imposed on a practitioner may not be applied equally to other practitioners. Continuing with the surgical complication rate example, it is entirely appropriate to intervene if a practitioner's complication rate exceeds accepted professional standards. Sometimes, however, several practitioners have similar or worse complication rates, yet action is taken against only one practitioner.

In other situations, requirements or standards are rarely or inconsistently enforced. As an example, suppose a bylaws provision allows for termination of a practitioner's active staff appointment for failure to attend medical staff meetings. If the provision is never enforced until suddenly there is a practitioner who is not liked or whose practice is "borderline," the adverse action may be subject to a challenge of arbitrariness or application in a discriminatory manner. Requirements or standards should be applied consistently.

Practitioner Involvement in Corrective Action

The medical staff bylaws should include specific procedures to be followed once a request for corrective action is filed. Frequently, the bylaws will require that the affected practitioner be advised of the filing of the complaint, and they may allow the practitioner to participate in the investigative process or meet with the investigating committee. These requirements are often overlooked in the corrective action process. The bylaws should be consulted immediately when adverse action looks likely, and legal counsel should be involved in the matter as appropriate. An error in the early stages can create problems with later aspects of the action and even the hearing process. If an error is made, an attempt should be made to correct it, even if a procedure or step in the process must be repeated.

Investigation

Two issues deserve mention as to investigations. First, certain professional review action reporting requirements are triggered depending on whether the affected practitioner is then under "investigation."[52] For this reason, the medical staff bylaws should clearly define when an investigation commences. The *National Practitioner Data Bank Guidebook* (*NPDB Guidebook*) contains helpful information on what constitutes an investigation and should be reviewed in addressing this issue.[53] An investigation for purposes of imposing a professional review action (e.g., corrective action) should be distinguished from reviews that occur on a periodic or ongoing basis for purposes of quality improvement.

Second, more often than hospitals and medical staffs like to admit, a complete investigation takes place *after* a hearing has been scheduled and the practitioner has retained an attorney. The proper time for the investigation is *before* any recommendation for adverse action is made. Once a recommendation for adverse action has been made, there should be no need for further investigation, but merely preparation for the hearing itself. The practitioner should be advised of the reasons for the adverse action at the time he or she is notified that adverse action is being recommended. If all information is not available when that notice letter is written or if additional information is identified later, the notice will need to be supplemented prior to the hearing. The hearing may need to be postponed to allow the practitioner adequate time to address the new information in advance of the hearing.

Right to a Hearing

Sometimes a question may arise regarding whether an action entitles the practitioner to request a hearing. Both state law and the HCQIA provisions must be consulted to make this determination, and entitlement should be specifically addressed in the bylaws. Generally, hospitals and medical staffs opt to afford hearing rights for those actions that will be reportable to the NPDB if subject to a final decision by the governing board. Examples of particular actions that may be overlooked in the bylaws are whether probation, consultation requirements, or supervision requirements entitle the practitioner to request a hearing. Another matter that should be addressed is whether termination of a practitioner's clinical privileges because of termination of a professional services contract with the hospital entitles the practitioner to a hearing. Some find it beneficial, in drafting the bylaws provision or fair hearing manual, to list those actions that are adverse (and, consequently, that entitle the practitioner to procedural rights of review) as well as those that are not adverse.

Notice of Charges

Under HCQIA's recommended procedures, the first notice to the practitioner advising that a professional review action has been proposed must include the reasons for the proposed action.[54] This notice requirement is one of the most essential elements of procedural due process. The practitioner must be given adequate notice of the charges and must be informed of the reasons for the proposed action, so as to be able to adequately defend himself or herself at the time of the hearing. Failure to properly advise the practitioner of the allegations or basis for the proposed adverse action may jeopardize the entire proceeding.

The notice to the practitioner should include a list of the hospital or patient records that support each of the allegations and that will be presented in the hearing.[55] The practitioner should be given reasonable access to these records and documents upon request. Withholding information from the practitioner that he or she reasonably needs to prepare for the hearing raises the possibility of a procedural challenge. Questions pertaining to access to documents in the prehearing period and during the hearing should be discussed with legal counsel and addressed in the bylaws or fair hearing manual.

Discovery and Deposition Rights

Although few legal cases have addressed this issue, practitioners are generally not given the right to pretrial discovery, such as depositions or interrogatories, unless otherwise provided for by state law or in the medical staff bylaws.[56] Despite appearances to the contrary, the hearing is not intended to be a mini-trial. Any rights that the practitioner has in this regard should be specifically identified in the bylaws or the fair hearing manual. This is an area where the use of an attorney as a presiding officer to advise the hearing panel and handle procedural matters and objections will be helpful. Frequently the attorney presiding officer will conduct prehearing conferences in an attempt to address these issues prior to the actual hearing.

Waiver of Procedural Rights

Occasionally there are procedures, either in the medical staff bylaws or required by law, that both the practitioner and the hospital or medical staff want to modify. For example, a practitioner may be willing to waive the 30-day time period recommended by HCQIA between the notice of the date of the hearing and the hearing itself so as to start the hearing as soon as possible. If a waiver is being obtained and the practitioner is represented by counsel, both the practitioner and counsel should sign the waiver.

Hearing Panel Bias

HCQIA limits the inclusion of direct economic competitors of the affected practitioner on the hearing panel.[57] Even before the federal statute was enacted, efforts were made to ensure that the hearing panel members could be fair and were unbiased as a key component of procedural due process. The hospital should be able to document that the individuals who will judge the practitioner in the hearing meet any requirements or qualifications set in the bylaws. In particular, individuals who have participated in the investigation leading to or the issuance of the adverse action, or who may be witnesses, should be excluded from the panel.

Hospitals may find it helpful to send a preliminary questionnaire to the prospective hearing panel members requesting information necessary to determine whether the individual is qualified to serve, so that there will be adequate time to secure replacements if any problems are detected. Alternate hearing panel members should be designated in the event that a member is later disqualified or cannot attend the hearing at the last minute. In addition, the practitioner may be allowed to question the members of the hearing panel regarding bias or conflicts of interest. Objections to the hearing panel members may be handled by the attorney presiding officer or as otherwise provided in the bylaws.

Role of Attorneys

HCQIA's recommended hearing procedures afford the practitioner the right to "representation by an attorney or other person of the physician's choice."[58] This language raises a question as to whether the use of the word "or" means that the hospital and medical staff can choose between affording the right to an attorney or the right to another person of the physician's choice, or whether it must allow both options. Another question is whether there is any reasonable alternative to representation by an attorney that would still entitle the hospital and medical staff to the qualified immunity available under HCQIA. As mentioned earlier, HCQIA provides that, to be eligible for the qualified immunity, either the procedures detailed in the statute must be used or "such other procedures as are fair to the physician under the circumstances." But can there be any substitute for representation by an attorney—and is representation by someone who is not an attorney fair?

Some hospitals and medical staffs wishing to limit the role of attorneys allow the attorney to be present during the hearing, but do not allow the attorney to question parties or witnesses or address the hearing panel. This practice of limiting what the attorney may do has been upheld under HCQIA in at least one federal circuit.[59] Public hospitals particularly should examine applicable legal requirements, as the right to representation by an attorney without limitations may be an essential element of procedural due process. If the practitioner is permitted to be represented by an attorney, the committee that issued the adverse action or recommendation is usually afforded the same right.

Right of Cross-Examination

The right of the practitioner to cross-examine any witnesses or evidence presented against the practitioner is another essential element of the hearing. The use of written statements from witnesses in the hearing may be challenged by the practitioner unless the witnesses are also available to be questioned by the practitioner at the time of the hearing. For example, use of a consulting expert's report in the hearing may be challenged if the expert is not available to be cross-examined by the practitioner. The right of cross-examination also may limit the use of anonymous complaints or written statements in the hearing. In some cases, if the witness cannot be available to testify at the hearing, it may be possible to submit written questions in advance to the witness and have them answered, with the answers then being presented at the time of the hearing.

New or Additional Information

The initial notice of charges containing reasons for the proposed adverse action is important because it defines for the practitioner which issues or allegations the practitioner must address in the hearing. If, during a hearing, additional allegations or reasons for the proposed adverse action come to light, it may be appropriate to recess the hearing (if the practitioner so desires) for a reasonable amount of time to allow the practitioner to prepare to address the additional matters. HCQIA procedures may even require issuance of a new and amended notice of charges and waiting at least 30 days before resuming the hearing.

All evidence to be considered by the hearing panel must be presented to the practitioner at the time of the hearing. The hearing panel should not conduct its own private investigation. If it relies on information learned other than that presented at the hearing, the practitioner may be denied the right of cross-examination. If the hearing panel decides during the hearing that it needs additional information, a request to obtain that information should be made by the panel to the parties in open session and the hearing recessed until that information can be presented.

Hearing Report

The hearing panel should issue a written report setting out its findings and recommendation according to what is required by the bylaws. This report needs to be sufficiently detailed to indicate the basis for the recommendation and may reference pertinent provisions in the hearing transcript or documents presented during the hearing. Under the HCQIA-recommended procedures, the affected practitioner must be given a copy of the report; most bylaws and fair hearing manuals also require this step.[60]

Standard of Review in Appeal

The appeal or appellate review is not intended to be a "second hearing." Rather, it is a limited review, and the bylaws should specify those limits or the standard of review to be used. The purpose of an appeal is twofold: (1) to determine if the adverse recommendation is arbitrary, capricious, or unreasonable or not supported by evidence in the record, and (2) to determine if there has been substantial compliance with the procedures set out in the bylaws or fair hearing manual. The appeal may also verify compliance with the four immunity standards set out in HCQIA.

The appeal may be conducted by the full governing board of the hospital or by a committee appointed by the board to serve as an appellate review committee. The committee reviews the hearing record, the hearing panel's report, and any information considered since the hearing. If the practitioner is permitted to submit a written statement or make an oral presentation at the time of the appeal, this information would also be considered by the appellate review committee, and the committee that originally issued the adverse recommendation or action would be afforded these same rights. New or additional evidence should be received and considered by the appellate review committee only if the evidence was not reasonably available at the time of the hearing. In some cases, new evidence may necessitate reopening the hearing and sending the issue back to the hearing panel for a revised recommendation.

Composition of the Appellate Review Committee

Although there generally are limitations on who may serve as members of the hearing panel, it is not so clear whether the same restrictions apply to the individuals who conduct the appellate review. HCQIA does not require or address appeals or appellate review procedures. Even if this separation of responsibilities is not legally required, it is still recommended that individuals who have been involved in the investigation or the hearing not serve on the appellate review committee. (If nothing else, this approach may lessen the risk of their becoming individual defendants in case of subsequent litigation.) If a hospital has a joint conference committee, composed of members of both the medical staff and the governing board, this committee often serves as the appellate review committee. As with the hearing, the appellate review committee should issue a written report setting out its findings, as required by the bylaws or fair hearing manual.

Final Decision

Unless otherwise provided in the bylaws, the governing board must issue a final decision on the adverse recommendation or action. Under the HCQIA-recommended procedures, the decision must be stated in writing and include the basis or reason for the decision, and a copy must be provided to the affected practitioner.[61]

■ Peer Review Privileges of Confidentiality and Immunity

Privilege of Confidentiality

Many states afford a statutory privilege of confidentiality to records and proceedings generated in the course of peer review in a hospital setting, as well as in other healthcare settings.[62] State statutes may be limited to those records and proceedings generated by peer review committees or may also include information provided by individuals to peer review committees for purposes of peer review. Confidentiality privileges generally prevent discovery or access to the records or proceedings of peer review in a lawsuit such as a professional liability action by a patient or a lawsuit by an excluded practitioner. The purpose of this special protection is to encourage appropriate and effective peer review and candor in the process, without fear of creating information or documents that will be used against the hospital or the affected practitioner. In some states, the confidentiality privilege applies even if there is evidence of bad faith or malice.[63]

To be protected as peer review records and proceedings, it must be demonstrated that the information or documents were, in fact, generated in the course of peer review. Hospitals and medical staffs should examine the manner in which certain information and documents are created to determine whether they would be protected under their state's peer review privilege of confidentiality. Generally, routine administrative or business records will not fall within the category of peer review records and proceedings, even if they were forwarded to a peer review committee. In contrast, if a particular document or report is generated at the specific request of a peer review committee or is generated in the course of the peer review committee's fulfillment of its responsibilities, the document or report may be privileged.

Privileges may be waived, either by an intentional act or sometimes by an unintentional act, such as unauthorized disclosure to a third party. Any provisions in the medical staff bylaws or credentialing procedures addressing the confidentiality of peer review information should also identify the procedures required to actually waive the privilege. Because of the seriousness of a waiver of the privilege, it should occur only with the approval of appropriate medical staff officers and hospital administration. Peer review privileges protect not just the hospital and medical staff participants in the peer review, but also the affected practitioner who is the subject of the peer review.

Because they are created by state law, most state privileges of confidentiality apply only to lawsuits involving causes of action under state law such as professional liability. If a lawsuit is filed in federal court and involves federal causes of action, there is usually no obligation of the federal courts to honor the state privileges of confidentiality.[64] For this reason, it should never be assumed that particular records or proceedings will always be protected from discovery, nor should promises be made to those persons who participate in peer review or provide peer review information that confidentiality is absolute or guaranteed.

Privilege of Immunity

The same state laws that afford a privilege of confidentiality to peer review records and proceedings may also extend a privilege of immunity, or freedom from liability if sued, to those persons who perform peer review or participate in the process. Grants of immunity are limited to actions taken in good faith or without malice; therefore, these privileges may be more limited in application than privileges of confidentiality.

HCQIA also provides for qualified immunity in the peer review process at the federal level. Under this legislation, the following entities and individuals are not liable for monetary damages with respect to a professional review action that meets the four standards specified in HCQIA:

- The professional review body
- Any person acting as a member or staff to the body
- Any person under a contract or other formal agreement with the body
- Any person who participates with or assists the body with respect to the action[65]

The limitation on liability does not apply to damages involving civil rights violations or to an action by the United States or any state attorney general. A "professional review body" is defined as a healthcare entity or a governing body or any committee of a healthcare entity that conducts professional review activity; it includes any committee of the medical staff of the healthcare entity when assisting the governing body in a professional review activity.[66] "Professional review activity" is an activity to determine whether a physician may have clinical privileges or membership in the entity, to determine the scope or conditions of the privileges or membership, or to change or modify the privileges or membership.[67]

HCQIA also extends a second grant of immunity to those individuals who provide information to a professional review body. Under the first grant of immunity, the professional review action must meet all four standards in HCQIA, but the immunity afforded to those providing information is not so limited. A person providing information to a professional review body regarding the competence or professional conduct of a physician may not be liable for monetary damages unless two requirements are met: (1) the information provided was false and (2) the person providing it knew that the information was false.[68]

HCQIA Reporting Requirements

The HCQIA immunity for a professional review body may be lost for a three-year period under certain circumstances if the healthcare entity fails to report professional review actions as required by HCQIA.[69] Under this statute, three levels of reporting are required, though only the third level affects the grant of immunity to a healthcare entity for professional review actions.

The first level of required reporting deals with medical malpractice payments. Each entity (including an insurance company) that makes payment under a policy of insurance, self-insurance, or otherwise in settlement or satisfaction of a judgment in a medical malpractice action or claim is required to report information regarding the payment as set forth in HCQIA.[70] Failure to report under this provision exposes the entity to civil monetary penalties.

The second level of reporting requirement applies to state boards of medical examiners. Each board that revokes or suspends (or otherwise restricts) a physician's license or censures, reprimands, or places on probation a physician for reasons relating to competence or professional conduct is required to report this information to the NPDB.[71]

The third level of reporting requirement is imposed on healthcare entities and requires a report from each healthcare entity that meets any of the following criteria:

- Takes a professional review action that adversely affects the clinical privileges of a physician for a period longer than 30 days
- Accepts the surrender of clinical privileges of a physician while the physician is under investigation by the entity relating the possible incompetence or improper professional conduct (or in return for not conducting such an investigation or proceeding)
- In the case of a professional society, takes a professional review action that adversely affects the membership of the physician in the society[72]

These reports of professional review actions are also provided to the state board of medical examiners.

Permissive reporting of a professional review action is permitted for other licensed healthcare practitioners.[73] The information that must be reported on the professional review action includes the name of the physician and a description of the acts or omissions or reasons for the action, or if known, for the surrender. For significant detail and information on reporting, refer to the *NPDB Guidebook*.

Recommendations

The following are some general recommendations to maximize the availability of applicable privileges of confidentiality and immunity in the peer review setting:

1. Mark all documents generated or received by a peer review committee as "Privileged and Confidential—for Purposes of Peer Review" or "Privileged and Confidential—Records and Proceedings of Peer Review Committee," depending on the precise language of the applicable state statute.
2. Ensure that the medical staff bylaws authorize medical staff committees to conduct peer review and function as peer review committees, using the precise language set forth in applicable state statutes of confidentiality and immunity in peer review, as well as set forth in HCQIA. If hospital or governing board committees conduct peer review, examine the governing board bylaws as well to ensure proper authorization.
3. Ensure that the actions of individuals in the course of peer review are taken as agents for or on behalf of peer review committees, if applicable. For example, the authority given to a chief of staff or CEO to impose summary or emergency corrective action should be taken as agent for or on behalf of the medical executive committee or the governing board. This approach should facilitate application of any privileges of immunity afforded to the peer review committee.
4. Limit distribution of peer review records and proceedings to those people who have a need to know. When appropriate, retrieve original documents at the close of meetings. Limit copying of peer review records and proceedings to designated persons.
5. Establish policies and procedures regarding access to peer review records and proceedings, including access by the affected practitioner and other members of the medical staff. Committee records and proceedings should be made available only to members and agents of the committee for purposes of carrying out committee responsibilities, medical staff committees to which that committee reports, and the governing board.
6. Identify those provisions in state statutes on confidentiality that permit disclosures to third parties. For example, the state statute on confidentiality of

peer review records and proceedings may permit disclosure to licensing and accreditation agencies of the healthcare entity, without such disclosure resulting in a waiver of the privilege. The state statute may permit disclosure to any governmental agency that is permitted by law to access records, such as the state board of medical examiners or the licensing agency for the hospital or healthcare entity. These provisions should be reflected in the medical staff bylaws or applicable policies and procedures regarding disclosure of peer review records and proceedings. These documents should also set out the requirements for waiver of the privilege.

7. In responding to requests for information from other hospitals engaged in credentialing or peer review, written authorization from the affected practitioner should be obtained (although state law may not require it). Verify that the authorization contains appropriate language both authorizing the disclosure of information by the hospital and releasing the hospital from liability for any disclosure pursuant to the authorization.

8. Verify that a requested disclosure is permitted by applicable state law and will not result in a waiver of the privilege. If the disclosure is permitted by state law, structure the disclosure to fit within any provisions in the statute. For example, if the statute authorizes disclosure from one peer review committee to another peer review committee, require that queries from other hospitals come from their peer review committees and that the responses be provided by your own hospital's peer review committee. Mark the response as "Privileged and Confidential—Records and Proceedings of Peer Review Committee."

9. In providing information in response to a query, rely on information that is available in the credentials file; avoid inclusion of opinions and recommendations, as those items are more properly covered through peer references or recommendations. Provide factual and accurate information that answers the questions. Avoid volunteering information except under special circumstances. Avoid general requests for information, such as "Tell us anything you think might be important," and instead require specific questions.

10. Most applications for medical staff appointment or reappointment contain language requiring the applicant to release the hospital, the medical staff, and any individuals or committees participating in peer review from liability related to peer review actions or recommendations. When drafting these releases of liability, make sure that they are not more limited than the immunity afforded by state or federal law. Additionally, the medical staff bylaws should ensure that operation of the release of liability is not contingent on the practitioner's signature on the document, but rather is activated by the submission of the application itself.

Credentialing in the Managed Care Setting

Comparison to Hospital Medical Staff Credentialing

Credentialing and peer review is no longer exclusive to the hospital medical staff setting, owing to the proliferation of managed care organizations, provider networks, and integrated healthcare delivery systems. As new methods develop for the delivery of healthcare services, these entities need to credential their care providers. To do so, they often delegate credentialing to hospitals or other healthcare entities that already have significant expertise and credentialing processes already in place.

Although many parallels exist between credentialing in the hospital medical staff setting and credentialing in the managed care setting, several interesting differences are also apparent. For example, credentialing in the managed care setting usually addresses the practitioner's office practice standards rather than just hospital practice. The geographic location and numbers of practitioners for a managed care organization or provider network may different in significant ways from the composition of a hospital's medical staff. In addition, managed care organizations may require a different ratio of primary care practitioners to specialists than do hospitals. Economic and efficiency-based criteria may be utilized by the managed care organization to a greater extent than hospitals. Finally, there may be different relationships (and consequently legal requirements) between the medical staff member and the hospital, as compared to the participating provider and a managed care organization.

Particularly in the managed care setting, factors related to economics or business may be pertinent in deciding whether to terminate a provider's participation. Examples include the provider's agreement to provide 24-hour availability and coverage to enrollees, conduct of office staff or office conditions, and compliance with utilization review appeal procedures. Often these factors do not have any relationship to the clinical competence of the provider. For these reasons, different processes may be established to deal with disciplinary action or termination of participating provider status for quality of care issues as compared to economic or business reasons.

Credentialing in both hospital and managed care organization settings has tended to focus on independent practitioners, such as physicians, dentists, podiatrists, and chiropractors. State legal requirements for managed care organizations may, however, require access and credentialing of other types of providers that will need to be handled by managed care organizations. State law has increased some providers' scope of practice over the last few years in many states, and managed care organizations' financial arrangements with physicians and other practitioners may create incentives for the use of physician extenders or allied health professionals. Increasing interest in the incorporation of allied health professionals into managed care organizations will necessitate credentialing of those professionals as well.

Duty to Credential

As with hospitals, the managed care organization's duty to credential is controlled by both accreditation and state licensure standards as well as by case law. Several agencies offer accreditation or certification for managed care organizations, with two of the most prominent being the National Committee for Quality Assurance (NCQA) and URAC (formerly the Utilization Review Accreditation Commission).[74]

Just as the courts have extended various forms of liability to hospitals related to the actions of practitioners and negligent credentialing, so the courts have applied these theories to managed care organizations. In *Harrell v. Total Health Care, Inc.*[75] (a 1989 Missouri case), a patient was injured by a health service organization urologist to whom she was referred by the organization's primary care practitioner. The appellate court found that, like hospitals, health service organizations have a common-law duty to their members to conduct a reasonable investigation to ensure that practitioners are competent and capable of providing care that meets community standards. In this case, the health service organization had credentialed the urologist, a process that consisted of verifying licensure, admitting privileges to hospitals, and authority to prescribe controlled substances. No other credentialing procedures were required or performed.

In a 1992 Pennsylvania case, *McClellan v. HMO of Pennsylvania*,[76] the court ruled that the enrollee could maintain an action for negligent selection of a practitioner against the health maintenance organization (HMO). In this case, Ms. McClellan had sought treatment for a mole on her back. The HMO primary care practitioner failed to order a biopsy or histological examination of the mole tissue.

Legal Issues

Although there may be different implications in the managed care setting, many of the legal issues related to credentialing are the same for both managed care organizations and hospitals. Managed care organizations, however, must also address the issue of access to a provider network or the managed care organization. Many states have enacted legislation referred to as "any willing provider" laws that require HMOs and other types of managed care organizations to permit their enrollees access to all practitioners who meet the requirements established by the managed care organization or health care network or to permit access to certain disciplines or professions.

Managed care organizations must also decide which procedural rights of review must be provided if a practitioner is excluded from participation in the provider network or if a decision is made to terminate the practitioner's current participation. This issue is increasingly being addressed by state laws, some of which require a minimum of written notice to the practitioner of the basis for denial or termination and, in some cases, an opportunity for review by a panel of peers. To some extent, the decision as to whether to extend procedural rights of review may depend on whether the managed care organization is subject to the HCQIA reporting obligations to the NPDB. HMOs are included in the HCQIA definition of a healthcare entity and must report their professional review actions to the NPDB; therefore, these types of managed care organizations may decide that the immunity benefits of affording adequate notice and hearing as set forth under HCQIA outweigh the burden of affording this process.[77] Managed care organizations, in contrast, are more likely to make decisions regarding practitioner participation based on factors other than quality of care, such as costs or compliance with utilization review procedures. The only actions that must be reported under HCQIA and to which the limited immunity will apply are those relating to the practitioner's competence or professional conduct, when that conduct affects or could affect adversely the health or welfare of a patient.[78]

A final issue deals with whether managed care organizations are entitled to invoke state privileges of confidentiality or immunity for peer review. In some states, these laws may be drafted broadly enough to apply to HMOs and other types of managed care organizations. Under those circumstances, credentialing and peer review by these organizations should be structured to comply with applicable privileges. In other states, where the laws have been focused only on hospitals, this area may be targeted by future legislation as managed care organizations increasingly engage in credentialing and the litigation potential increases.

Delegated Credentialing

Frequently, the managed care organization delegates either the entire credentialing function or a portion of credentialing responsibility to a hospital or healthcare entity that also has established credentialing policies and procedures in place. Generally, the network or managed care organization will maintain authority over final decisions, such as approval of new practitioners and termination of practitioners. In addition, there must be evidence of oversight by the network or managed care organization and evaluation of the delegate's activities.

Delegation may involve outsourcing of the information gathering and primary source verification function and the actual evaluation of the qualifications of the practitioner, or it may involve outsourcing of only one portion of the function. In some cases, a credentials verification organization (CVO) handles these tasks. The CVO gathers information and conducts primary source verification, but does not evaluate the qualifications of the practitioner or make recommendations on whether the practitioner should be granted access to the provider network.

Several key legal issues arise when an organization is contemplating any arrangement for delegated credentialing. The first is that the arrangement should be structured to maintain the confidentiality of any peer review information generated by the delegate. If the managed care organization or network is itself eligible for privileges of confidentiality and immunity for peer review actions, state law may permit the delegate to be eligible for those same privileges when providing services on behalf of the managed care organization or network. There should be a written agreement between the two entities, clearly setting out the delegate's status as to the delegating entity. The written agreement should also specify the precise scope of duties, access to original information by the delegating entity, the means by which confidentiality of the information will be maintained by the delegate, and ownership and access to the delegate's information, particularly when the delegation arrangement ends. The agreement and any disclosure of information should include statements that the information generated as a consequence of the delegation is privileged under applicable state law and that disclosure is not intended to waive any applicable privileges of confidentiality.

A second legal issue involves final decision-making authority. In delegated credentialing arrangements involving more than just information gathering and primary source verification, the managed care organization or network needs to ensure that it has not given so much authority to the delegate as to compromise its own responsibilities for purposes of accreditation or licensure. Generally, any form of delegated credentialing provides for the managed care organization or network to retain final authority over decisions regarding practitioner participation.

Uniform or Centralized Credentialing

One variation on delegated credentialing is the move toward uniform or centralized credentialing. In this situation, several organizations (which are often related or components of an integrated healthcare delivery system including one or more hospitals) conduct credentialing together, rather than having one organization conduct credentialing on behalf of another, as occurs in delegated credentialing. Uniform or centralized credentialing may be limited to use of a joint application for practitioner participation in affiliated hospitals and managed care organizations, may extend to shared or joint credentialing committees that evaluate and issue recommendations on practitioner participation to the respective governing boards of the participating healthcare entities, or may involve joint decision making as to a practitioner's participation in all of the entities in the integrated healthcare delivery system.

The main benefits of uniformed or centralized credentialing are the reduced duplication, time, and expense for the various entities of the integrated healthcare delivery system as well as the practitioners. The use of a uniform or centralized system also promotes consistent standards among related organizations—an important consideration because criteria for participation will likely be consistent among the components. As with delegated credentialing, the primary legal issues with this approach to credentialing involve application of state peer review laws on confidentiality and immunity as well as assuring that each entity maintains sufficient final decision-making authority so as not to jeopardize each entity's separate accreditation or licensure status.

Queries for Managed Care Organizations

Given that credentialing is equally important in the managed care setting as in the hospital setting, managed care organizations and networks frequently seek information from hospitals and other healthcare entities about practitioners wanting to participate with the organizations and networks. Although state peer review laws on confidentiality may permit the exchange of confidential peer review information between hospitals, these laws need to be carefully examined to determine whether peer review information may be disclosed to managed care organizations or networks without risking loss of that same privilege. In some states, managed care organizations such as HMOs are included in the statutes on privileges of confidentiality for peer review. In other states, this may not be the case, making it difficult to disclose privileged and confidential peer review information. CVOs and preferred provider organizations may or may not be addressed by state peer review laws.

■ Conclusion

Although the law significantly influences the field of medical staff credentialing and will likely continue to do so, the medical staff services professional need not be an attorney to be successful. The most important factors to success are to have medical staff bylaws that reflect current legal and accreditation requirements and actual practice at the hospital, to know and consult those bylaws frequently (and always as a first step when there is a question), and to follow the provisions in the bylaws to the fullest extent possible.

■ Notes

1. See, for example, the Joint Commission. *2009 Hospital Accreditation Standards.* Oakbrook Terrace, IL: Author; 2009. Accreditation by the Joint Commission results in "deemed status" for purposes of compliance with the Medicare Conditions of Participation for Hospitals. Other voluntary accreditation programs approved for deemed status are the American Osteopathic Association's program and (most recently) Det Norske Veritas (DNV) Healthcare Inc.'s program, National Integrated Accreditation for Healthcare Organizations. For purposes of this chapter, references here are limited to the Joint Commission standards.
2. Conditions of Participation for Hospitals, Centers for Medicare and Medicaid Services, 42 C.F.R. Part 482.
3. This has been a controversial issue with the Joint Commission and hospital attorneys over the past few years. Revisions to former JCAHO MS.1.20 (now MS.01.01.01) approved by the Joint Commission in June 2007 for implementation July 1, 2009, were suspended by the Joint Commission's Board of Commissioners after significant concerns were raised by hospitals. According to the hospitals, the revised standard would have required many hospitals to revise medical staff bylaws to incorporate information traditionally addressed in rules and regulations, manuals, and/or policies, because it required more to be included in the bylaws proper (and subject to medical staff approval, rather than just approval by the medical executive committee in some cases). The

current version of MS.01.01.01 sets out in Elements of Performance (EP) 1–18 what must be listed in the bylaws. EP 19 (not currently in effect) would allow "administrative procedures" to be addressed in supplemental or governance documents other than the medical staff bylaws, such as rules and regulations, manuals, and policies, albeit only under certain conditions. In comparison, "processes" must be addressed in the bylaws and, therefore, are subject to approval of the medical staff and the governing board.
4. See, for example, *East Texas Medical Center Cancer Institute v. Anderson*, 991 S.W.2d 55 (Tex. App.—Tyler 1998, pet. denied) (finding medical staff bylaws are a contract); *Gianetti v. Norwalk Hosp.*, 557 A.2d 1249 (Conn. 1989) (holding that bylaws are not a contract).
5. HCQIA, 42 U.S.C. §11101 et seq.
6. See Conditions of Participation for Hospitals, note 2.
7. But see *Agbor v. St. Luke's Episcopal Hospital*, 952 S.W.2d 503 (Tex. 1997) (holding that state peer review immunity statute applied to patient's cause of action against hospital for negligent credentialing).
8. 211 N.E.2d 253 (Ill. 1965). (See Appendix A.)
9. See Appendix A for discussion of additional cases dealing with corporate negligence (e.g., *Purcell, Johnson, Elam*).
10. The Joint Commission, note 1, MS.01.01.01, Elements of Performance (EP) 7.
11. See, for example, Tex. Health & Safety Code §241.101.
12. *Hay v. Scripps Memorial Hospital*, 228 Cal. Rptr. 413 (Ct. App. 1986).
13. *Kahn v. Suburban Community Hospital*, 340 N.E.2d 398 (Ohio 1976); *Hull v. Board of Commissioners of Halifax Hospital*, 453 So. 2d 519 (Fla. Dist. Ct. App. 1984); *Cameron v. New Hanover Memorial Hospital, Inc.*, 293 S.E.2d 901 (N.C. Ct. App. 1982); *Sarasota County Public Hospital Board v. Shahawy*, 408 So. 2d 644 (Fla. Dist. Ct. App. 1981); *Armstrong v. Board of Directors of Fayette County General Hospital*, 553 S.W.2d 77 (Tenn. Ct. App. 1976).
14. Conditions of Participation for Hospitals, note 2, §482.12(a)(7).
15. "State Operations Manual: Appendix A Survey Protocol, Regulations, and Interpretive Guidelines for Hospitals, Interpretive Guidelines for §482.12(a)." Available at: http://cms.hhs.gov/manuals/Downloads/som107ap_a_hospitals.pdf. Accessed July 2009.
16. The Joint Commission, note 1, MS.06.01.03.
17. The Joint Commission, note 1, MS.08.01.01.
18. See, for example, *Stein v. Tri-City Hosp. Auth.*, 384 S.E.2d 430 (Ga. App. 1989); *Kling v. St. Paul Fire & Marine Ins. Co.*, 626 F. Supp. 1285 (C.D. Ill. 1986); *Backlund v. Board of Commissioners*, 724 P.2d 981 (Wash 1986), appeal dismissed, 481 U.S. 1034 (1987); *Holmes v. Holmako Hosp.*, 573 P.2d 477 (Ariz. 1977).
19. The Joint Commission, note 1, MS.06.01.05, EP 2, MS.07.01.03.
20. The Joint Commission, note 1, MS.06.01.05, EP 8.
21. The Joint Commission, note 1, MS.06.01.03; MS.06.01.07; MS.06.01.05, EP 6.
22. Americans with Disabilities Act of 1990, 42 U.S.C. Chap. 126 (§12182(a) for Title I and §12112(a) for Title III).
23. The primary issue with Title III is whether its protection is limited to "clients and customers" of the place of public accommodation (and, if so, whether medical staff members and applicants fall within that group) or whether it applies to all individuals. The U.S. Supreme Court ruled in connection with a professional golf tournament that the Title III protection extended not only to the public attending the tournament but also to the professional golfers competing in the tournament. *PGA Tour, Inc. v. Martin*, 532 U.S. 661 (2001). The few federal courts that have addressed this issue have taken both positions. See, for example, *Menkowitz v. Pottstown Medical Center*, 154 F. 3d 113 (3rd Cir. 1998) (physician allowed to proceed with Title III claim for summary suspension allegedly based on attention deficit disorder); *Hetz v. Aurora Medical Center*, No. 06-C-636

(E.D.Wis. June 18, 2007) (court allowed the physician's claim under Title III for denial of medical staff appointment allegedly based on bipolar disorder and sleep apnea to proceed). But see *Wojewski v. Rapid City Regional Hospital*, 394 F.Supp. 2d 1134 (D.S.D. 2005) (a physician with bipolar disorder whose privileges were terminated not entitled to Title III protection).
24. See, for example, *Bragdon v. Abbott*, 524 U.S. 624 (1998).
25. See, for example, *Estate of William C. Mauro v. Borgess Medical Center*, 137 F.3d 398 (6th Cir. 1998).
26. See the cases in Appendix A of this chapter.
27. HCQIA, note 5, §11133(a), 11151(9).
28. The Joint Commission, note 1, MS.03.01.03, EP 1.
29. 500 P.2d 335 (Ariz. Ct. App. 1972). (See Appendix A.)
30. Health Resources and Services Administration (HRSA). *National Practitioner Data Bank Guidebook*. DHHS Pub. No. HRSA 95-255. Washington, DC: Author; 2001:E-18, E-22.
31. The Joint Commission, note 1, MS.08.01.01.
32. HRSA, note 30, E-21.
33. Joint Commission on Accreditation of Healthcare Organizations. *Medical Staff Credentialing*. Oakbrook Terrace, IL: Author; 1993:28–29.
34. See, for example, *Jefferson Parish Hosp. Dist. No. 2 v. Hyde*, 466 U.S. 2 (1984); *Dutta v. St. Francis Regional Medical Center*, 867 P.2d 1057 (Kan. 1994); *Bartley v. Eastern Maine Medical Center*, 617 A.2d 1020 (Me. 1992). (See Appendix A of this chapter regarding the *Jefferson Parish* case.)
35. The Joint Commission, note 1, Overview to Medical Staff Standards.
36. The Joint Commission, note 1, Overview to Medical Staff Standards; see also HR.01.02.05, EP 10–15.
37. The Joint Commission, note 1, MS.10.01.01, EP 1.
38. The Joint Commission, note 1, MS.08.01.03.
39. The Joint Commission, note 1, MS.11.01.01. The Joint Commission requires that medical staffs have a process to identify and manage health issues that is separate from the corrective action process.
40. The standard for imposing a summary or emergency corrective action here is taken from HCQIA, note 5, §11112(c)(2).
41. HCQIA, note 5, § 11151(1).
42. The Joint Commission, note 1, MS.10.01.01.
43. See the exception in HCQIA, note 40.
44. 486 U.S. 94 (1988). (See Appendix A.)
45. HCQIA, note 5, §11111(a).
46. HCQIA, note 5, §11151(8).
47. HCQIA, note 5, §11151(9).
48. HCQIA, note 5, §11151(10).
49. HCQIA, note 5, §11112(a).
50. HCQIA, note 5, §11112(b).
51. HCQIA, note 5, §11112(a)(3).
52. HCQIA, note 5, §11133(a)(1)(B).
53. HRSA, note 30, E-19.
54. HCQIA, note 5, §11112(b)(1)(A).
55. See *Rosenblit v. Fountain Valley Regional Hospital and Medical Center*, 282 Cal. Rptr. 819 (Cal. App. 1991) for excellent discussion of notice issues.
56. See, for example, *Huntsville Memorial Hospital v. Honorable Erwin G. Ernst*, 763 S.W.2d 856 (Tex. App.—Hous. [14th Dist.] 1998, no writ history).

57. HCQIA, note 5, §11112(b)(3)(A)(iii).
58. HCQIA, note 5, §11112(b)(3)(C)(i).
59. *Smith v. Ricks*, 31 F.3d 1478 (9th Cir. 1994).
60. HCQIA, note 5, §11112(b)(3)(D)(i).
61. HCQIA, note 5, §11112(b)(3)(D)(ii).
62. Florida significantly altered its peer review privileges with the November 2004 enactment of state constitution Amendment 7, the "Patient's Right to Know About Adverse Medical Incidents." A recent Florida Supreme Court opinion held that Amendment 7 preempts state statutory peer review privileges, allowing patient access to previously confidential medical provider information. *Florida Hospital Waterman, Inc. v. Buster*, 984 So.2d 478 (Fla 2008).
63. See, for example, *Irving Healthcare System v. Honorable David Brooks*, 927 S.W.2d 12 (Tex. 1995).
64. See, for example, *Memorial Hosp. v. Shadur*, 664 F.2d 1058 (7th Cir. 1981); *Viramani v. Novant Health Inc.*, 259 F.3d 284 (4th Cir. 2001); *Adkins v. Christie* (11th Cir. 2007). HCQIA addresses confidentiality, but only regarding information provided to the National Practitioner Data Bank. HCQIA, note 5, § 11137(b). HCQIA does not afford the same confidentiality to peer review records and proceedings that most state laws do.
65. HCQIA, note 5, §11111(a)(1). Keep in mind that HCQIA's immunity only applies to actions involving a physician defined as a medical doctor, doctor of osteopathic medicine, or doctor of dental surgery or medical dentistry. HCQIA, note 5, §11151(8).
66. HCQIA, note 5, §11151(11).
67. HCQIA, note 5, §11151(10).
68. HCQIA, note 5, §11111(a)(2).
69. HCQIA, note 5, §11111(b).
70. HCQIA, note 5, §11131.
71. HCQIA, note 5, §11132.
72. HCQIA, note 5, §11133.
73. HCQIA, note 5, §11133(a)(2).
74. National Committee for Quality Assurance (NCQA), www.ncqa.org. URAC, www.urac.org.
75. 1989 WL 153066 (Mo. App.), affirmed, 781 S.W.2d 58 (Mo. 1989) (en banc). (See Appendix A.)
76. 604 A.2d 1053 (Pa. Super. Ct. 1992), appeal denied, 616 A.2d 985 (Pa. 1992). (See Appendix A.)
77. HCQIA, note 5, §11133, §11151(4).
78. HCQIA, note 5, §11133(a)(1), 11151(9).

■ Appendix A

Significant Case Law Summary

■ *Darling v. Charleston Community Hospital*, 211 N.E.2d 253 (Ill. 1965)—Hospital's Duty to Supervise Physicians

This lawsuit was brought by a patient against a hospital for acts of nurses and negligence on the part of the attending physician that caused a patient's orthopedic injury to result in amputation. The patient alleged that the hospital was negligent in permitting the physician to treat orthopedic injuries and not requiring him to update operative procedures, in failing through the medical staff to exercise adequate supervision, and in not requiring consultation especially after complications set in. The hospital's defense was that only a physician may practice medicine; therefore, the hospital cannot be liable for the acts of a physician where reasonable care was exercised in selecting the physician originally. The Illinois Supreme Court upheld the verdict for the patient, noting that hospitals do more than just provide facilities for treatment; they also assume certain responsibilities for the care of the patient.

■ *Purcell v. Zimbelman*, 500 P.2d 335 (Ariz. Ct. App. 1972)–Improper Review of Clinical Competence

This lawsuit was brought by a patient against a hospital for failing to take action against the attending surgeon when it knew or should have known that he lacked the skill to treat the condition in question. The hospital's defense was that it could not be held liable for acts of an independent contractor physician where it had no reason to believe a specific act of malpractice would occur. The jury found in favor of the patient. Evidence showed that two prior cases involving similar questions about the treatment of diverticulitis had been presented to the hospital's department of surgery, but no action was taken. A total of four malpractice cases had been filed against the physician and hospital prior to his treatment of Mr. Zimbelman.

After describing accreditation standards and the custom at hospitals regarding the medical staff, the Arizona appellate court found that the hospital had assumed the duty of supervising the competence of its staff physicians. It also found that the hospital was responsible for the actions of the department of surgery because it acted on its behalf and, if the department was negligent in not intervening after the first two cases, then the hospital would also be negligent. Evidence of the filing of the four lawsuits was admissible against the hospital to show it had notice not only of concerns of Dr. Purcell's competence regarding the particular condition, but also regarding his general competence, and should have reviewed his records.

■ *Gonzalez v. Nork*, 131 Cal. Rptr. 717 (Cal. App. 1976)–Failure of Peer Review Process

This lawsuit was brought by a patient against a physician and a hospital for damages resulting from an operation in which the physician did not inform the patient that more conservative treatment was available. The physician had a history of unnecessary or negligent surgery in years prior to the laminectomy on the patient. The jury found for the patient. The court affirmed the hospital's duty to create a mechanism by which it may discover inadequacies of its staff members.

■ *Johnson v. Misericordia*, 294 N.W.2d 501 (Ct. App. 1980), *affirmed*, 301 N.W.2d 156 (Wisc. 1981)—Failure of Initial Credentialing Process

This lawsuit was brought by a patient against a hospital for negligently granting orthopedic surgical privileges to the physician who had settled prior to trial. The patient had suffered damage following the physician's removal of a pin fragment from the hip. Despite provisions in the medical staff bylaws, no investigation was made of any of the information provided on the application form (which was incomplete). Contrary to the physician's representations on the application, he had experienced denial and restriction of privileges elsewhere (involving his orthopedic surgical privileges) and had not been granted privileges at some of the hospitals listed on the form. Expert testimony stated that a hospital exercising ordinary care would not have appointed him to the medical staff.

The Wisconsin Supreme Court held that a hospital has a duty to exercise due care in the selection of its medical staff: "[T]he promotion of quality care and treatment of patients requires hospitals to perform a thorough evaluation of medical staff applicants . . . and further, to periodically review the qualifications of its staff through a peer review or medical audit mechanism." Delegation of the responsibility to the medical staff does not relieve the governing body of its duty to appoint only qualified practitioners and to periodically monitor and review their competence. On the initial application, at a minimum, the hospital should require that the application be complete and verify the applicant's statements especially regarding education, training, and experience. Additionally, it should solicit information from peers, including those not referenced in the application; determine current licensure and identify whether licensure has been subject to challenge; and inquire as to malpractice history.

■ *Elam v. College Park Hospital*, 183 Cal. Rptr. 156 (Cal. App. 1982)—Failure to Have Proper Supervision

This lawsuit was brought by a patient against a group of podiatrists, the coadmitting physician, and the hospital as a result of injuries following podiatric surgery. The podiatrists were independent contractors, not employees of the hospital. The hospital was granted summary judgment, and the California appellate court reversed this decision, finding that the hospital had a duty to ensure the competence of its medical staff and to evaluate the quality of medical treatment rendered on its premises. In reaching its decision, the court examined the hospital's general duty to protect patients from harm; the statutory requirements for hospitals and accreditation standards regarding appointment, reappointment, and peer review; and the public's perception that the hospital is a healthcare facility responsible for the quality of medical care and treatment rendered.

■ *Mitchell County Hospital Authority v. Joiner*, 189 S.E.2d 412 (Ga. 1972)—Governing Body Is Ultimate Authority

This lawsuit was brought by a deceased patient's wife against a physician and hospital from which the patient had been sent home from the emergency room after experiencing chest pain and died later at home. The patient's wife alleged that the hospital was negligent in failing to require satisfactory proof of the professional qualifications of the physician; failing to investigate his qualifications, character, or background; and failing to exercise ordinary care in determining competence and character. The hospital's defense was that it had delegated screening of applicants to the medical staff. The Georgia Supreme Court held that the fact that the medical staff had recommended appointment did not relieve the hospital of liability if the appointment was negligent, because the medical staff acts as an agent for the hospital.

■ *Patrick v. Burget*, 486 U.S. 94 (1988)—Medical Staff Peer Review and Antitrust

This antitrust lawsuit was brought by Dr. Patrick against the physicians of the Astoria Clinic, alleging that they caused him to lose his hospital medical staff privileges as a result of his decision not to join the clinic and instead compete against it. Although the jury found in Dr. Patrick's favor, the appellate court held that the physicians were immune from antitrust liability for even bad faith under the state action exemption. (The state action exemption applies if the action—here peer review—is articulated and affirmatively expressed as state policy and if the state actively supervises the activity.) The U.S. Supreme Court held that, although the state mandates that hospitals engage in peer review, the state is neither involved in nor supervises the actual peer review decisions; therefore, the state action exemption did not apply and the physicians participating in the peer review could be held liable under antitrust theory.

■ *Miller v. Eisenhower Medical Center*, 614 P.2d 258 (Cal. 1980)—Disruptive Behavior

This lawsuit was brought by a physician against the hospital for denial of medical staff membership based on inability to work with others, as required by the medical staff bylaws. The physician argued that the standards for medical staff membership were so vague and uncertain as to allow for arbitrary or discriminatory application. The California Supreme Court held that even a private hospital may not permit exclusion from the medical staff on an arbitrary or irrational basis. The requirement to be able to work with others was permissible if there is a showing that the inability presents a real and substantial danger that patients might receive other than a high quality of medical care. In other words, there must be a link between the conduct and the potential effect on patient care. The court reversed the trial court's judgment which had been in favor of the hospital.

■ *Rao v. Auburn General Hospital*, 573 P.2d 834 (Wash. Ct. App. 1978)–Disruptive Behavior

This lawsuit was brought by a physician against a hospital for denying privileges. After a trial court held the physician was not entitled to recover damages, the physician appealed. The Washington appellate court affirmed the trial court, holding that a hospital has a discretionary right to exclude physicians whether based on lack of proficiency or a personality that will be detrimental to the working of the hospital. Additionally, the court should not substitute its evaluation of such matters for that of the hospital's governing board.

■ *Robinson v. Magovern*, 521 F.Supp. 842 (W.D. Pa. 1981), *affirmed without opinion*, 688 F.2d 824 (3rd Cir.), *cert. denied*, 459 U.S. 971 (1982)–Denial of Application Not a Restraint of Trade

This lawsuit was brought against a hospital's board members and certain thoracic surgeons by a physician whose application for staff privileges was rejected. Allegations included violations of the antitrust law (Sherman Act) by agreements to limit thoracic surgery privileges to one group, of which the department chief was a member, as well as denial of due process and breach of contract. The court found that no hospital or surgical group had a monopoly; found a lack of evidence of specific anticompetitive intent, conspiracy, or agreement to take joint action; and rejected Dr. Robinson's allegation that the hospital was an "essential facility" (in which denial of access creates a severe handicap for market entrants). The court stated that (1) the hospital's policy of encouraging its medical staff to concentrate their practices at that hospital, (2) the concern regarding Dr. Robinson's contribution to the residency program, and (3) the concerns regarding his alleged inability to work harmoniously with others advanced the hospital's institutional objectives of providing quality patient care and did not reasonably restrain trade. Because Dr. Robinson had open-heart surgery privileges at other hospitals, the denial did not prevent cardiologists from referring to him or patients selecting him.

■ *Jefferson Parish Hospital District No. 2 v. Hyde*, 466 U.S. 2 (1984)–Upholding a Hospital's Exclusive Contract

This lawsuit was brought by an anesthesiologist who was denied admission to the medical staff based on the hospital's exclusive anesthesia contract; the plaintiff alleged that the contract violated antitrust law. The U.S. Supreme Court reversed the decision of the Fifth Circuit, which held that the contract was illegal per se because it involved a "tying arrangement" by which the patient buying the operating room service also had to buy the anesthesia service. The Supreme Court found that the contract did not constitute an illegal tying arrangement because patients were not forced to purchase the anesthesia service, but could enter a competing hospital and use another anesthesia group. Tying arrangements are condemned if they restrain competition by forcing purchases that would otherwise not be made. In the absence of an impermissible tying arrangement, the plaintiff must show that the challenged contract unreasonably restrained trade. In this case, there was no evidence that the price, quality, or supply or demand for either the operating room service or the anesthesia service had been adversely affected by the exclusive contract or that the market as a whole had been affected by the contract.

■ *Boyd v. Albert Einstein Medical Center*, 547 A.2d 1229 (Pa. Super. Ct. 1988)–Managed Care Organization Liable for the Practitioner's Actions

This lawsuit was brought against a HMO and its participating physicians following the death of a patient after an alleged misdiagnosis. The patient's estate sought to recover damages against the HMO, which had represented that the participating physicians were competent and evaluated for up to six months prior to being accepted into the HMO, on the theory that the physicians were ostensible agents of the HMO and, therefore, the HMO was liable for their actions. The Pennsylvania Superior Court found that the policy reasons for holding hospitals liable for medical staff members under the ostensible agency theory applied equally to HMOs, based on the limited provider list from which patients can select, the selection of the participating physicians by the HMO, the role of the gatekeeper in accessing a specialist, the fact that the patient does not contract directly with the physician but with the HMO, and the mechanics of payment for services. The court reversed the summary judgment granted for the HMO and remanded the case to the trial court.

■ *Harrell v. Total Health Care, Inc.*, 781 S.W.2d 58 (Mo. 1989)—Failure to Credential

This lawsuit was brought by a patient against Total Health Care, Inc. (Total), for injuries that occurred as a result of malpractice during surgery, where the claims were based on corporate negligence and negligence in the selection of the surgeon. The court examined the relationship between Total and the physician, and noted the limited choice of physicians available to the patient. The court, finding an unreasonable risk of harm to subscribers if the physician is incompetent, held there was a common law duty owed to conduct a reasonable investigation to ascertain the physician's reputation for competence. The court left the extent of the investigation to be determined on a case-by-case basis, but said failure to conduct an investigation means the duty has not been met. By statute, a health service corporation was immune from liability for any negligence of a person or entity rendering health services to the corporation's members and beneficiaries; therefore, the Missouri Supreme Court affirmed the summary judgment granted for Total. The court also stated it saw no reason that a HMO might not also be a health service corporation and, therefore, eligible for the same immunity.

■ *McClellan v. Health Maintenance Organization of Pennsylvania*, 604 A.2d 1053 (Pa. Super. Ct. 1992)—Duty to Select and Monitor Providers

This lawsuit was brought by a patient against a HMO based on corporate negligence and ostensible agency theory; the claim dealt with negligence of a participating physician in not submitting a mole tissue sample for testing. The Pennsylvania Superior Court held that there was sufficient evidence to submit to the jury the issue of whether the physician was an ostensible agent of the HMO based on the representations of the HMO as to the quality of the physicians and other factors. Although the court did not extend the theory of corporate negligence used with hospitals to HMOs, it held that HMOs have a nondelegable duty to select and retain only competent physicians, allowing that issue also to be submitted to a jury for decision.

■ *Kadlec Medical Center v. Lakeview Anesthesia Associates*, 527 F.3d 412 (5th Cir. 2008)—Duty of a Hospital to Avoid Affirmative Misrepresentation in Disclosure to Another Hospital

This lawsuit was brought by Kadlec Medical Center against Lakeview Regional Medical Center for negligence and misrepresentation. Kadlec had settled a $7.5

million medical malpractice lawsuit that resulted from the actions of a former member of Lakeview's medical staff. In the course of the litigation, Kadlec learned that Lakeview had been aware of substance abuse concerns regarding the involved physician, which it did not disclose to Kadlec. Kadlec also sued Lakeview Anesthesia Associates, the physician's former employer, and, as individuals, its partners who had provided favorable references for the physician. Lakeview did not answer Kadlec's specific questions about the physician and, citing the large number of inquiries, advised Kadlec only of the years of the physician's medical staff membership (this was different from Lakeview's customary response for physicians who had no adverse information "that there is no information of a derogatory nature contained in Dr. [X]'s file").

The federal district court found that, under Louisiana law, Lakeview had a duty to disclose information to Kadlec. It denied Lakeview's motion for summary judgment, allowing the case to proceed to trial on the claims of intentional and negligent misrepresentation and negligence. The jury then awarded Kadlec and its insurer $8.24 million in damages.

On appeal, the Fifth Circuit reversed the judgment against Lakeview Regional Medical Center, finding there was no duty to disclose. The court did find that once the defendants chose to make a disclosure, they assumed the duty not to make affirmative misrepresentations in the disclosure letters. The hospital had not made an affirmative misrepresentation because it failed to answer the specific questions; in contrast, the physician's employer's letters were "false on their face and materially misleading" and they had violated their duty to Kadlec. The judgment as to the other defendants was vacated and remanded to the trial court for proper apportionment of damages in line with the Fifth Circuit's ruling.

■ *Poliner v. Texas Health Systems*, 537 F.3d 368 (5th Cir. 2008), *cert. denied*, 129 S. Ct. 1002 (Jan. 21, 2009)– Upholding HCQIA Immunity for Voluntary Abeyance/Summary Suspension

This lawsuit was brought by Dr. Poliner against the hospital and several physicians for damages resulting from a 29-day restriction of his cardiac catheterization privileges. After alleged quality concerns, Dr. Poliner had been asked to agree to a 14-day voluntary abeyance of his privileges and then an extension. After an ad hoc investigation, the privileges were summarily suspended, though they were ultimately reinstated by the governing board following a favorable hearing. The litigation involved only the voluntary abeyance and extension, because the trial court judge found that all defendants involved in the summary suspension that followed were entitled to HCQIA immunity.

As stated in the appellate court's opinion, Dr. Poliner's theory was that he was forced to agree to the voluntary abeyance; therefore, the corrective action was a summary suspension that failed to meet the criteria in the medical staff bylaws. At trial, the jury awarded approximately $366 million to Dr. Poliner, which was later reduced to a $33 million judgment and then reversed by the Fifth Circuit on appeal. The Fifth Circuit found that the first 14-day action qualified under HCQIA's provision allowing for a suspension or restriction of clinical privileges not to exceed 14 days during which an investigation is conducted to determine the need for a professional review action (42 U.S.C.A. §11112(c)(1)(B)). The extension, which followed initial findings by the ad hoc committee of substandard care, qualified under the HCQIA provision allowing for an immediate suspension or restriction, subject to subsequent notice and hearing or other adequate procedures, when failure to act may result in imminent danger to an individual's health (42 U.S.C.A. §11112(c)(2)). Both actions were professional review actions protected by the HCQIA immunity, and the good or bad faith of the reviewers (or individual physician defendants) was irrelevant.

■ *Brown v. Presbyterian Healthcare Services*, 101 F. 3d 1324 (10th Cir. 1996)—HCQIA Immunity Does Not Protect Defamation Liability for Incorrect Data Bank Report

This lawsuit was brought by a family practice physician against a hospital for revocation of her privileges, as well as against the hospital administrator, a competing physician, and other parties for antitrust violations, intentional interference with contract, and defamation. Following peer review at the hospital, Dr. Brown had agreed to consult with an obstetrician/gynecologist in treating high-risk patients. Thereafter, Dr. Williams, an obstetrician/gynecologist, initiated corrective action proceedings against Dr. Brown for failure to abide by the consultation agreement. After a hearing, the governing board revoked Dr. Brown's obstetrical privileges on that basis. The hospital then submitted an NPDB report on the revocation using the adverse action code "Incompetence/Malpractice/Negligence."

At trial, the jury found for Dr. Brown, but the trial judge set aside the damages awards on some of the claims, leading all parties to appeal. On the defamation claim, the appellate court held that the hospital administrator was not entitled to HCQIA immunity because there was sufficient evidence for a jury to conclude that the NPDB report was false and the reporting party knew it was false. The record showed that neither the hearing panel nor the governing board ever found Dr. Brown negligent, incompetent, or guilty of malpractice—only that she breached her agreement to obtain consultation. On the antitrust claims, the appellate court found that even though the hospital administrator and Dr. Williams did not participate in the actual decision to revoke privileges, they were in a position to control the decision-making process, or coerce or unduly influence the decision, and, therefore, could be held liable for antitrust violations.

■ Appendix B

Practitioner's Hearing Rights Under the Health Care Quality Improvement Act

(1) Notice of proposed action
   The physician has been given notice stating—
   (A) (i) that a professional review action has been proposed to be taken against the physician,
      (ii) reasons for the proposed action;
   (B) (i) that the physician has the right to request a hearing on the proposed action,
      (ii) any time limit (of not less than 30 days) within which to request such a hearing; and
   (C) a summary of the rights in the hearing under paragraph (3).
(2) Notice of hearing
   If a hearing is requested on a timely basis under paragraph (1)(B), the physician involved must be given notice stating—
   (A) the place, time, and date of the hearing, which date shall not be less than 30 days after the date of the notice, and
   (B) a list of the witnesses (if any) expected to testify at the hearing on behalf of the professional review body.
(3) Conduct of hearing and notice
   If a hearing is requested on a timely basis under paragraph (1)(B)—
   (A) subject to subparagraph (B), the hearing shall be held (as determined by the health care entity)—
      (i) before an arbitrator mutually acceptable to the physician and the health care entity,
      (ii) before a hearing officer who is appointed by the entity and who is not in direct economic competition with the physician involved, or
      (iii) before a panel of individuals who are appointed by the entity and are not in direct economic competition with the physician involved;
   (B) the right to the hearing may be forfeited if the physician fails, without good cause, to appear;
   (C) in the hearing the physician involved has the right—
      (i) to representation by an attorney or other person of the physician's choice,

(ii) to have a record made of the proceedings, copies of which may be obtained by the physician upon payment of any reasonable charges associated with the preparation thereof,
  (iii) to call, examine, and cross-examine witnesses,
  (iv) to present evidence determined to be relevant by the hearing officer, regardless of its admissibility in a court of law, and
  (v) to submit a written statement at the close of the hearing; and
(D) upon completion of the hearing, the physician involved has the right—
  (i) to receive the written recommendation of the arbitrator, officer, or panel, including a statement of the basis for the recommendations, and
  (ii) to receive a written decision of the health care entity, including a statement of the basis for the decision.

■ Appendix C

Recommended References on Legal Issues

Health Care Quality Improvement Act, 42 U.S.C.A. §11111 et seq.

Health Resources and Services Administration (HRSA). *National Practitioner Data Bank Guidebook*. Pub. No. HRSA-95-255. Rockville, MD: Author; 2001. Available at: http://www.npdb-hipdb.hrsa.gov/pubs/gb/NPDB_Guidebook.pdf. Accessed July 2009.

Medicare Conditions of Participation for Governing Body and Medical Staff, 42 C.F.R. §482.11-.66.

"State Operations Manual: Appendix A. Survey Protocol, Regulations and Interpretive Guidelines for Hospitals. Interpretive Guidelines for Hospitals." Available at: http://cms.hhs.gov/manuals/Downloads/som107ap_a_hospitals.pdf. Accessed July 2009.

State laws on the following topics:

- Healthcare entity licensure as applicable to medical staff
- Peer review privileges of confidentiality and immunity, including governmental agency access to peer review information
- Reporting of professional review actions or other issues involving physicians or other practitioners on the medical staff

Supporting Corrective Action and Fair Hearing Procedures

CHAPTER 17

Cindy A. Gassiot, CPMSM, CPCS

As mentioned in an earlier chapter, the medical staff services professional (MSSP) often acts as the medical staff organization's conduit to the healthcare facility's legal counsel. There is no more critical time for the MSSP to contact the medical staff's attorney than when the medical staff organization is contemplating corrective action that may trigger the fair hearing process. Medical staff leaders are often unfamiliar with procedures for investigations, corrective actions, and fair hearings, and the legal and time frame requirements that are usually detailed in the medical staff bylaws or a fair hearing plan. It is of critical importance that the MSSP guides medical staff leaders toward exact adherence with bylaws provisions for these activities and ensures that legal advice is obtained early in the process. Should an adversely affected practitioner resort to litigation following exhaustion of due process rights, the courts will carefully scrutinize the process used by the healthcare facility. Good documentation supporting protection of the affected practitioner's rights is obviously the best defense in case of any action against the facility.

■ Role of the Medical Staff Services Professional

The MSSP plays an important role in supporting the corrective action and fair hearing processes. These responsibilities include planning, adherence to bylaws and legal requirements, documenting the process, and maintaining confidentiality. Making arrangements for a hearing can be very time-consuming and challenging. The MSSP must be prepared to spend many hours conferring with legal counsel, preparing correspondence and evidence notebooks, arranging dates with busy practitioners, arranging for a court reporter and hearing officer, contacting witnesses, and paying careful attention to numerous details.

■ Corrective Action

Keeping the medical staff leaders and committees on track during the corrective action process is crucial. When corrective action is contemplated, the MSSP should immediately review with all practitioners involved the bylaws provisions guiding this process. Typically, medical staff members are not familiar with every nuance and detail of the bylaws provisions—which means they can easily start down the wrong track. That is why the MSSP's role in these processes is so important.

■ Steps in the Corrective Action Process

Investigation

The corrective action process usually starts with an investigation into the allegations made or the results of performance improvement activities that may signify problems with a practitioner's clinical competence or behavior. Typically the medical executive committee (MEC) appoints a committee to conduct the investigation within a time frame that is specified by the bylaws or by the MEC. This committee is charged with reviewing medical records, aggregate performance evaluation data, any verbal or written reports, and other information available concerning the matter being investigated.

Notice to Affected Practitioner

The affected practitioner should have the right to notification that an investigation is being conducted and to meet with the committee conducting the investigation. It should be made clear to the affected practitioner that the meeting does not constitute a hearing and is informal in nature. Careful records of this meeting must be prepared and maintained by the MSSP.

Recommendation to the MEC

Upon completion of its investigation, the investigating committee recommends to the MEC either that corrective action is not warranted or that corrective action is warranted. Sometimes the action recommended consists of a letter of reprimand, need for continuing education to improve performance, or notice that future conduct or performance will be closely monitored and that there are expectations of improvement. In those cases, no hearing is held. If the recommendation will affect the practitioner's membership or clinical privileges, or if it involves a stipulation that there will be significant consultation requirements, the practitioner must be offered rights to a fair hearing and appeal. Remember that a hearing is always offered to the practitioner before the recommendation is forwarded to the governing body.

■ Planning for a Hearing

When an adverse recommendation has been made by the MEC and the fair hearing procedure has been triggered, meticulous attention must be given to the time frames

Table 17-1	Checklist for Steps in the Fair Hearing Process	
Procedural Steps Accomplished	**Date Required**	**Date**
1. Recommendation for adverse action		
2. Notification to practitioner, including reason for proposed action (30 days to request hearing)		
3. Request for hearing		
4. Hearing panel appointed		
5. Hearing scheduled		
6. Practitioner notified of hearing date, time, and place (not less than 30 days from date of notice)		
7. Medical staff representative designated		
8. Court reporter notified		
9. Hearing officer appointed		
10. Hearing panel orientation		
11. Hearing held		
12. Hearing panel report		
13. Notice to practitioner, and others required by fair hearing plan or bylaws, with basis for recommendation		
14. Appellate review, if applicable		
15. Final action by governing body		
16. Notice of final decision to affected practitioner with basis for action		
17. NPDB report to State Board of Medical Examiners, if indicated (within 30 days of final action)		

allowed for each step of the procedure. A checklist (see TABLE 17-1) outlining each step of the procedure and the time within which the step must be accomplished will be a helpful tool in adhering to the required procedure.

■ Correspondence

When the hearing process has been triggered, the MSSP usually prepares the correspondence to the affected practitioner. Again, careful attention should be given to required time frames when preparing correspondence to the affected practitioner. Also, to ensure that legal requirements have been met, all correspondence should be reviewed by legal counsel. A sample notice of an adverse recommendation letter to the practitioner and a sample notice of hearing are included in the CD that accompanies the book. When composing these letters, pay careful attention to the bylaws provisions and use the same language where appropriate.

■ Orientation of the Hearing Panel

Most practitioners are not familiar with a fair hearing procedure. If a hearing panel or committee is used for the hearing (rather than an arbitrator or a hearing officer), when the members have been identified, it is helpful to orient them to the procedure. Legal counsel should be engaged to provide this orientation session, which should describe the manner in which the hearing will be conducted. The facts or details of the matter under consideration are never discussed with the panel prior to the actual hearing; rather, the purpose of the orientation is to prepare panel members for what can be expected to occur in the actual proceeding. A copy of the fair hearing plan or bylaws article should always be provided to panel members and can be used as the basis for the orientation session.

Members of the hearing panel should be instructed to arrange for practice coverage during the hearing and advised to leave their pagers and cell phones turned off.

■ Evidence Notebook

Thorough, accurate documentation of all events leading up to a fair hearing procedure is critical. The written results of an investigation will typically be used as evidence in any hearing and play an important role in the outcome. Many healthcare facilities use an evidence notebook as a means of supporting the facility's case against the affected practitioner. The MSSP usually prepares this notebook, which must also be made available to the affected practitioner prior to the hearing, as he or she has a right to review all evidence so as to prepare a defense against the allegations made. Again, legal counsel should be consulted to assist in preparation of the evidence notebook and to advise about its release to the affected practitioner and his or her attorney.

■ Arranging the Hearing Room

Because the parties involved in a fair hearing will most likely spend many hours listening to the evidence presented, a comfortable setting is important. Comfortable

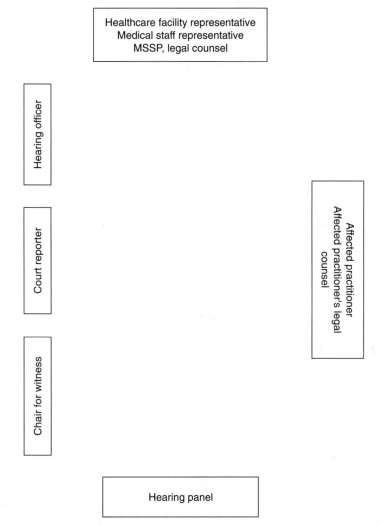

FIGURE 17-1 Room Arrangement for Fair Hearing Procedure

chairs should be at the top of the list when organizing the hearing room, even if they have to be brought from other locations in the facility. Food and drink should also be available, as hearings usually go on into the night. The room in which the hearing is held is typically arranged somewhat like a courtroom setting (see FIGURE 17-1).

■ The Hearing

The MSSP usually attends the hearing and sits alongside the organization's legal counsel, the medical staff representative, and other healthcare facility representatives, if present. The MSSP can assist with calling witnesses into the hearing room, referring to the medical staff bylaws, and performing other tasks as needed.

Hearings frequently cannot be completed in one session. As a consequence, the MSSP may be required to schedule subsequent sessions.

■ Follow-up

When the hearing panel has reached its decision, the MSSP assists in preparation of the report and assures that the report is forwarded through channels as outlined in the fair hearing plan or bylaws. Once a final decision is made, the MSSP will prepare the correspondence notifying the affected practitioner of that decision. Again, legal counsel should be consulted when preparing any correspondence or other documentation relating to the process (see EXHIBIT 17-1).

■ Reporting Adverse Decisions

When the final decision is adverse to the practitioner in question and an action is taken that will adversely affect membership or clinical priviledges for more than 30 days, this action must be reported within 30 days to the National Practitioner Data Bank (NPDB) via the state licensure board, in accordance with the Health Care Quality Improvement Act. The MSSP will be responsible for preparing the report on the specified NPDB reporting form. The report should be prepared in consultation with legal counsel. Authorized entities can locate reporting forms online on the NPDB Web site at www.npdb.com.

Fair hearings will test the ability of the MSSP to precisely follow the procedures outlined and to guide medical staff leaders and other participants in doing the same. Assisting with the fair hearing process is one of the most important and interesting functions the MSSP performs.

A sample notice of hearing, hearing committee recommendations, and notice of final decision by governing body are included in the CD that accompanies the book.

■ Examples of Language to Insert in Notice Letter

Examples of Language to Insert

A. The medical executive committee has recommended that your clinical privileges to perform hysterectomy be terminated for the following reasons:

Exhibit 17-1 — Notice of Adverse Recommendations and Sample Language to Insert in Letter

Privileged and Confidential Medical Peer
Review Committee Records and Proceedings
Certified Mail—Return Receipt Requested

Date

Name
Address
City, State, ZIP

Dear Doctor _____:

The Medical Executive Committee of _____ Hospital met on (date) to review the request for corrective action regarding (your conduct, your performance, or other reason).

The Committee has recommended to the Governing Board that (action recommended) because (findings and reasons for corrective action). This is based on (see attached examples).

The Medical Staff Bylaws, Article _____, afford you the right to a hearing pursuant to the Fair Hearing Plan before this recommendation is forwarded to the governing body for a final decision. If you wish to have a hearing, your written request (by messenger or certified mail) must be received within 30 days of your receipt of this letter. Following receipt of a timely request, you will be notified of the date, time, and place of the hearing.

If you fail to request a hearing within 30 days, you will waive your right to a hearing or to contest the adverse recommendation, and you will be deemed to have accepted the recommendation.

The following is a summary of your rights regarding the hearing, subject to the more comprehensive and detailed provisions in the medical staff bylaws.

- To have a hearing held before a panel or individuals appointed by the hospital who are not in direct economic competition with you (include an arbitrator mutually acceptable to you and the hospital or hearing officer appointed by the hospital and not in direct economic competition with you options if appropriate)
- To attend the hearing, but this right may be forfeited if you fail, without good cause, to appear
- To be represented by an attorney or other person of your choice
- To have a record made of the hearing and obtain a copy by paying any reasonable charges associated with its preparation
- To call, examine, and cross-examine witnesses

Exhibit 17-1 Notice of Adverse Recommendations and Sample Language to Insert in Letter (continued)

> - To present evidence determined to be relevant by the panel's chairman (or hearing officer if one is appointed), regardless of its admissibility in a court
> - To submit a written statement at the close of the hearing
> Upon completion of the hearing, you also have the right:
>   - To receive the written recommendation of the panel (arbitrator or hearing officer), including a statement of the basis for the recommendation
>   - To receive the governing body's written decision, including a statement of the basis for the decision
>
> A copy of the Medical Staff Bylaws and the Fair Hearing Plan is attached for your use. Please call me if you have any questions.
>
> Respectfully,
>
> CEO/Administrator

- Your failure to abide by the terms of the monitoring restrictions placed on your surgical procedures in the letter of reprimand, dated _____. (List all medical record numbers that are questioned.)
- Your performance of hysterectomy without documenting adequate diagnostic indications for the surgery. (List all medical record numbers that are questioned.)
- Your failure to follow the criteria developed by the Department of Obstetrics/Gynecology for performance of hysterectomy. (List all medical record numbers that are questioned.)
- Your failure to attempt appropriate conservative management of patients for a reasonable period of time prior to the performance of hysterectomy. (List all medical record numbers that are questioned.)

B. The credentials committee has recommended to the medical executive committee that you be required to obtain a concurring consultation from a child psychiatrist prior to admitting a minor younger than 13 years of age. This recommendation is based on your failure to identify and document the clinical indications for admission in the following cases (list medical record numbers):

C. The medical executive committee has recommended to the governing body that your clinical privileges to perform PTCAs be suspended until you have successfully completed a training program to be approved by the medical executive committee, because of failure to perform those procedures in accord with accepted professional standards of care. This recommendation is based on:

- Improper assessment of the severity of stenosis in evaluating indications for PTCAs (List medical record numbers.)
- Rate of complications exceeding accepted national professional standards (List medical record numbers.)
- Failure to perform and record appropriate pre-PTCA clinical workup (List medical record numbers.)

D. The medical executive committee has recommended to the governing board that your surgical privileges be suspended for a period of six months because of your inability to work cooperatively with other members of the hospital staff. This recommendation is based on:

- Your statements and behavior (describe statements and behavior) toward the nursing staff on (list dates) while performing surgery on (list medical record numbers)
- Your refusal to give verbal orders to registered nurses and continued use of licensed practical nurses in this regard who are not authorized to accept verbal orders
- Your repeated statements to hospital employees that you would sue them, with examples being the events occurring on (list dates), involving the staff on Unit 3B
- Your refusal to answer pages from Unit 4A unless the nurse manager places the calls, as occurred on (list dates)
- Your behavior (describe behavior) during the Surgery Department meetings on (list dates)

Instructions for Completion of the Continuing Education Quizzes

- Please circle the one best answer to each question.
- One (1) NAMSS-endorsed CEU will be granted for each quiz completed with a score of 80% or better (maximum 16 CEUs).
- Once your quiz has been scored with a score of 80% or better, you will receive a continuing education certificate from NAMSS.
- Please allow 4–6 weeks for processing.
- Submit the completed quiz(zes), along with your full contact information and appropriate fees to:*

NAMSS
Continuing Education
2025 M Street, Suite 800
Washington, DC 20036

*Quizzes will not be accepted after December 31, 2012

Fees:

SINGLE QUIZ
Member—$10.00 per chapter quiz
Non-NAMSS member—$25 per chapter quiz

QUIZ PACKAGE—You may submit all 16 quizzes at once for a discounted price:
Member—$129.00 for 16 quizzes
Non-NAMSS Member—$329.00 for 16 quizzes

Please note: Only original, hardcopy quizzes will be accepted by NAMSS. No photocopies or duplicates will be accepted. For additional questions regarding quiz submission, please contact education@namss.org.

Index

A

AAAASF (American Association for Accreditation of Ambulatory Surgery Facilities), 55
AAAHC (Accreditation Association for Ambulatory Health Care), 55–56
AAFP, on quota privileging, 197–198
ability to work cooperatively, 321–323, 379
ACGME (Accreditation Council for Graduate Medical Education), 307–308
ACCME (Accreditation Council for Continuing Medical Education), 305–306
accountability. *See* responsibility and accountability
accreditation, 39–62
   allied health professionals. *See* AHPs
   ambulatory care, 55–56
   assessing knowledge of, 11
   bylaws requirements and guidelines, 79–83
   cancer programs, 295–301
   CMS (Centers for Medicare and Medicaid Services), 40, 57–59
   continuing medical education programs, 303–306
   credentials review in survey, 60–61
   credentials verification organizations (CVOs), 52, 249–260
   Det Norske Veritas, *See also* NIAHO, 4–48
   graduate medical education, 306–308
   institutional review boards (IRBs), 293–297
   internationonal accreditation, 49–51
   ISO (International Organization for Standardization), 48, 59–60
   The Joint Commission (*see* The Joint Commission)
   knowledge of standards, 5–6
   long-term care, 51–52
   managed care, 52–54
      administration of credentialing operations, 234–236
      automation, 235–236
      contracting vs. credentialing, 233–234
      legal issues, 406–409
      NCQA 180-day rule, 231–232, 234, 237,
      organization of credentialing department, 238–239
      standards for, 227–232
      state and federal requirements, 239
   NIAHO (National Integrated Accreditation of Healthcare Organizations), 47–49
   rehabilitation facilities, 56–57
   support for, 34
   trauma centers, 301–303
   URAC, 54
ACGME (Accreditation Council for Graduate Medical Education), 191–192, 306–308
   moonlighting policy, 191–192
   multispecialty privileges, 274
   privileging and, 190–192
ACS-approved cancer programs, 297–301
ACS-approved trauma centers, 301–303
actions (meeting minutes), 344
actions at other hospitals, 379–380
active members of medical staff, 67
ADA (Americans with Disabilities Act), 319–320, 377–379
Administration, 19
   bylaws revision support, 91
   committee support, 32–33
   leadership development, 34–35
admissions department, 24
advanced practice registered nurses (APRNs)
   credentialing when not independent, 215
   reappointment of, 221
adverse effects on privileges, defined, 392
affiliate members of medical staff, 67, 141

435

affiliations with hospitals, verifying, 158, 191
agency sanctions, 164, 233, 250–251, 255
   conduct at other hospitals, 379–380
agendas for meetings, 331
   consent agendas, 332–333
   planning meetings for, 333
aging practitioners, 320–321
AHPs (allied health professionals), 213–223
   application for privileges, 217–219
   competency assessment, 221
   definition of, 213
   delineation of privileges, 219
   documentation maintenance, 221
   due process, 222
   legal issues, 385–386
   multidisciplinary AHP committees, 216–217
   performance evaluation, 221
   policy for, 217
   reappointment, 220–221
   scope of practice, 219
   Web resources, 223
AIDS, practitioners with, 378–379
alcohol use. *See* impaired practitioners
allied health professionals. *See* AHPs
AMA PRA certificates, 304–305
ambulatory care accreditation, 55–56
amending bylaws and related documents. *See* revision of bylaws and related documents
American Osteopathic Association. *See* HFAP
American Trauma Society, 303
Americans with Disabilities Act (ADA), 319–320, 377–379
announcements of meetings, 331
antitrust litigation, 366–367
AOA (American Osteopathic Association). *See* HFAP
appeals of professional review actions, 400–401
appellate courts, 358
appellate review rights, 400–401

under HCQIA, 392–394, 422–423
   waiver of, 398
application management services, 251
applications for CVO certification, 255
applications for membership and privileges, 170–175. *See also* clinical privileges; membership, staff
   allied health professionals (AHPs), 217–219
   reappointment, 147–149, 220–221
   delineation. *See* delineation of privileges
   managed care organizations (MCOs), 229–230
   preapplication, 149, 169
   processing, 122–134, 217
     allied health professionals (AHPs), 219–220
     credentials file, 120–121
     initial appointment recommendation form (example), 144–145
     potential problems (red flags), 133–141
     routine and critical information, 117–120
     routing, 142–143, 148–149
appointment privileges. *See* clinical privileges
appointment recommendation form, 208–209
approved cancer programs, 297–301
approved trauma centers, 301–303
APRNs (advanced practice registered nurses) credentialing, 215–216
arguer (meeting personality type), 340
arranging hearing room, 428–429
assistance for impaired practitioners, 323–324
attention to detail, 13
attorneys, 25
   bylaws revisions, 113–115
   medical staff attorney, 25
   role in dealing with disruptive physician, 320

   role in professional review actions, 398–399, 425, 428
audio recording devices in meetings, 350
authority, leadership, 98
authority of committee, 326
authority to practice. *See* clinical privileges; membership, staff
authorization for background check, 132, 306
authorization to prescribe drugs, 128–129, 219–220
   electronic verification, 122, 362
   restricted certificates, 134
automatic corrective action, 388, 389
automation of primary source verification, 122, 230–231

B
background investigations, 132–133
barriers to success of MSO, 71–72
behavior of group leaders, 327
behavior, practitioner. *See* practitioner health and behavior issues
bias on hearing panels, 398
Bioresearch Monitoring Program (FDA), 296–297
blood and blood components review, 270
board certification, 114–116, 123, 126–128
   verifying, 123, 126–128, 231
   verifying electronically, 235–236
board eligible, defined, 127
board investigations, as red flags, 138–139
board qualified, defined, 126
body fluid testing, 318
Boyd v. Einstein Medical Center, 418
Brown v. Presbyterian Healthcare Services, 421–422
budgeting, 9, *See also* finances
burden of proof, 381–382
business development and marketing, 23–24
bylaws, 63–77
   appointment and clinical privileges, 374–386

corrective action procedures, 388–391
for credentialing process, 107, 110
for impaired practitioners, 314
criteria for staff membership, 105–106, 114–116
definitions of terms, 80–81
disruptive behavior, 323
distribution of new documents, 91
fair hearing manuals, 81, 392, 394
legal requirements, 369–370
as living documents, 82
privileging and, 157–158, 217
proctoring programs, 162–176
revising, process of, 83–87, 90–92, 370–371
  amendment process, 86
  speeding up with multiple documents, 80–82
bylaws committee, 88–89

C
CAHPS surveys, 53–54
calendar of meetings, 328–329
cancer committees, 298
cancer programs, 297–301
CAQH (Council for Affordable Quality Healthcare), 230
care compliance. *See* compliance offices and programs
care financing. *See* finances
CARF (Commission on Accreditation of Rehabilitation Facilities), 57
case law, 371–372
case management department. *See* utilization management
case review, 287–291. *See also* quality improvement
category approach to privilege delineation, 152–153
Centers for Medicare and Medicaid Services. *See* CMS
centralized credentialing, 235, 241. *See also* CVOs; shared credentialing departments (SCDs)
  cooperative credentialing, 241–249

how to establish, 243–248
legal issues, 248, 405
operations manual for (example), 247–248
reasons for, 241–243
certification programs
  CVOs (credentials verification organizations), 401–405
  Health Care Staffing Services Certification, 184–185
  for physician executives, 99–100
  NAMSS, 1–2
  PRA (Physician's Recognition Award), 304–305
certified nurse-midwife, 221
CEUs. *See* CME (continuing medical education)
chairs of clinical departments, 82, 206
chairs of committees, 327, 340–341
change, physician executives and, 135
change of venue, 359
checklist, fair hearing process, 427
checklist, meeting, 336
chemical dependence. *See* impaired practitioners
chief of staff, 82
chiefs of clinical departments, 82, 206
circuit courts, 358
civil litigation, 355, 358–360. *See also* law
  as application red flag, 140
claims history verification, 130
  red flags with, 134, 139–140, 142
claims made policies, 130
classification scores for case reviews, 290
client access to CVO databases, 260
clinical departments, 69–70
  chairs (chiefs) of, 68–69, 206
  multispecialty privileges, 188–189, 274–276,
  proctoring programs, 160–176
  rules and regulations, 96, 148. *See also* policies and procedures
  for credentialing (example), 150–168
  turf battles over privileges, 189

clinical management requirements for cancer programs, 299
clinical performance. *See* quality improvement
clinical privileges, 142, 151–210, 214
  adding, process for, 163–165, 166
  allied health professionals. *See* AHPs
  applications for. *See* applications for membership and privileges
  competency requirements, 197–198
  cooperative credentialing, 199–210
  criteria for granting, 162–165, 382
  general surgery (example), 154–157
  temporarily, 182–183
  delineation of, 151–153
  general surgery (example), 154–157
  disaster and emergency privileges, 185–186
  documenting, 190–191
  impaired practitioners. *See* physician impairment
  The Joint Commission and CMS requirements, 157–158
  legal issues, 374–386
  limiting or withholding as corrective action, 391
  for economic reasons, 165, 380
  procedural rights of review, 391–394, 395, 422–423
  revocation, 391
  locum tenens, 183–185
  low-activity practitioners, 192
  multispecialty and turf battles, 188–189, 383
  provisional and proctoring, 80, 160–176, 383–384. *See also* FPPE
  quality improvement and, 274
  questions about, handling, 198–199
  reappointment and reprivileging, 28, 143, 146–149, 192–193

Index   437

clinical privileges (continued)
   allied health professionals (AHPs), 220
      competence requirements, 376
   standards for, 147
   surveying for, 60–61
   telemedicine, 186–188
   temporary, 182, 185–186
   during training, 190–192
CME (continuing medical education), 303–306
   verifying CME activity, 162–163
CMS (Centers for Medicare and Medicaid Services), 4, 40, 57–59, 264
   bylaws requirements and guidelines, 79–83, 105
   conditions of participation (COPs) 58
   bylaws requirements, 80–82, 370–371
   policies and procedures requirements, 80–82
   Hospital Quality Measures, 58–59
   MCO accreditation, 227
   never events, 5, 59, 264
   operative procedure quality requirements, 4, 267, 270–272
   quality initiatives, 58–59
   privileging requirements, 158
   sanctions, verifying, 164
CMSC examination, 2
collaboration. *See* communication
collecting data
   for credentialing, 142
   practitioner health status, 319
   for reappointment, 176–183, 192–193
columnar format for meeting minutes, 344–345
comfort with change, 135
committees, 70–71. *See also* meetings
   appellate review committees, 401
   bylaws committee, 88–89
   cancer committees, 298
   credentials committee, 144–145, 351
   evaluation tool for, 75
   hearing panel, 398, 428
   physician well being, 316
   multidisciplinary AHP committees, 216–217

physician impairment, 314–316
providing support for, 27–28
quality improvement, 272–273
role of, 326
understanding and evaluating, 75, 344
when to establish, 352
common law, 360–361
communication, 15
   ability to work cooperatively, 321–323, 379
   with applicants, 144
   bylaws revisions, 91
   with disruptive practitioners, 322–323
   with impaired practitioners, 319
   interdisciplinary quality improvement, 272–273
   meeting minutes as tool for, 338
   in meetings. *See* meetings
   new privileges, 163–166
   notices of meetings, 331
   patient relations, 29
   peer review, 287–289, 291
      ability to work cooperatively, 379
      evaluation of, 291
      hearing panel bias, 398
      legal issues, 392–394
      peer, defined, 288
      physician impairment and, 319
      policy for, 168–174, 177–181
   physician executives, 136
   physician relations, 37–38
   PR (public relations), 24
   relationships with other departments, 19–25
      bylaws language and, 84–86
      turf battles over privileges, 188–189
community outreach requirements for cancer programs, 299
comparison of hospital quality, 264–265
comparative negligence, 365
competency. *See also* performance improvement
   AHPs (allied health professionals), 221
   defined, 141
   establishing requirements for, 10–13
   evaluation of staff, 11–13

knowledge requirements, 3–7, 493
for effective leadership, 133
physician executives, 99–101
legal issues, 376
privileging and, 153–154, 197–198
self-assessment checklists, 8–12
skills requirements, 11–16, 493
competency assessment for AHPs, 221
managerial, 7, 133, 136
multispecialty privileges, 188–189, 383
complaints. *See* civil litigation; sanctions, monitoring and verifying
compliance offices and programs, 25, 38
computer literacy, 15–16. *See also* technology
computer operations. *See* information systems
conclusions (meeting minutes), 344
conditions of participation (COPs), CMS, 36, 71, 158, 372
   non-compliance with, 39–40
   policies and procedures requirements, 81
conduct at other hospitals, 379–380
conduction phase of meetings, 328, 331–334
confidentiality, 14
   applications for privileges, 121
   duty to provide information, 381–382
   meeting minutes, 345–346
   peer references, 131–132, 377
   peer reviews, 287–289, 291, 401–402, 404
   physician impairment, 315, 319
   practitioner data (CVO databases), 259–260
conflicts of interest, leaders with, 98
consent agendas, 332–333
consistency of credentialing process, 242
consulting members of medical staff, 67
continuing medical education (CME), 303–306
   verifying CME activity, 130–131
continuity of leadership, 97

438   Index

contract, bylaws as, 96, 371
contract practitioners, 233–234, 384–385
contracts with impaired physicians, 317–318
contributory negligence, 365
convictions, criminal. *See* criminal conduct history, verifying
cooperation with others, 321–324, 379
cooperative credentialing, 199–210
coordinator of meetings, 326
coordinator of monitoring (impaired practitioners), 319
COPs (conditions of participation), CMS, 39, 71, 158, 372
  bylaws requirements, 370–371
core privileging approach, 152–157
corporate negligence, 372–373
corrective action, 386–391
  appealing, 391–394
  investigation, 389
  challenges to, 394–398
  disruptive practitioners, 322–323
  responding to physician impairment, 317
  steps in process, 426–429
costs. *See* finances
court of appeals, 356
court records search, 132–133
court reporter in hearing, 425
court system, 356–358. *See also* law
courtesy members of medical staff, 67
courts of general jurisdiction, 358
CPCS examination, 2
CPMSM examination, 2
credentialing coordinators, 238
credentialing departments
  managed care, 238–239
  shared (SCDs), 241–249
  how to establish, 243–248
  operations manual for (example), 247–248
  reasons for, 241–243
  scope of services, 245
credentialing managers, 238
credentialing software systems, 247, 259–260
  See also information systems
credentialing specialists, 17, 238–239

credentials, reasons for, 103–105
credentials committee, 109–110, 351
credentials file, 120–121
credentials process, 103–150, 355, 401–405. *See also* accreditation
  allied health professionals. *See* AHPs
  applicable standards, 110
  applications. *See* applications for membership and privileges
  delegated arrangements, 36, 234–235, 408–409
  for documents, 110–120
  economic credentialing, 166, 380
  evaluation and decision-making, 143–144
  expedited credentialing, 143
  in health care systems, 241–249
  establishing centralized credentialing department, 243–248
  operations manual for (example), 247–248
  reasons for centralized credentialing, 241–243
  key definitions, 139–142
  key players, 106–110
  knowledge of, 5–6, 11
  managed care, 63–66, 225–239
    administration of credentialing operations, 234–235
    automation, 235–236
    contracting vs. credentialing, 233–234
    legal issues, 406–409
    NCQA 180-day rule, 231–232, 234, 237
    organization of credentialing department, 238–239
    standards for, 227–232
    state and federal requirements, 239
  preapplication, 113, 169
  reappointment and reprivileging, 28, 143, 146–149, 176–181, 192–197, 232
  allied health professionals (AHPs), 302, 324–327, 343–344
  competency checklist, 26

competence requirements, 376
credentials files, 121, 122
  paperless, 122, 248
credentials verification, 28–29, 121–134
  allied health professionals (AHPs), 219–220
  automating, 235–236
  difficulties with, 136
  organizations for. *See* CVOs
  potential problems (red flags), 134–142
  provisional period. *See* FPPE
  reappointment, 143, 144–149
  work flow management, 234, 235
crimes as torts, 366
criminal conduct history, verifying, 132–133, 141
criminal law, 355–356
criminal negligence, 364
criteria for granting privileges, 162–166, 382
  general surgery (example), 154–157
  multispecialty privileges, 188–189
  temporarily, 182, 185–186
criticism, physician executives and, 135
cross-examination, 360, 399
cross-privileging, 188–189, 383
  turf battles, 189
CTR (certified tumor registrar), 301
culture, bylaws language and, 84–86
customer satisfaction surveys, 32–33
customers of SCDs, 243
CAQH (Council for Affordable Quality Healthcare), 230
CVOs (credentials verification organizations), 37, 249–260. *See also* verification of credentials
  history and definitions, 249–250
  information systems of, 259–260
  The Joint Commission guidelines for, 257–258
  NCQA certification of, 53, 253–257
  operating models, 258–259

Index   439

CVOs (continued)
  services of, 250–252
  URAC certification of, 70–71, 257
  when to outsource to, 234, 252–253

D
Darling v. Charleston Community Hospital, 364–365, 413–414
dashboard reports, 282–286
data analysis. *See* quality improvement
data base manager (job title), 18
data collection
  for credentialing, 106–107
  practitioner health status, 319
  for reappointment, 146–148, 273–274
data evaluation in credentialing. *See* verification of credentials
data management
  cancer programs, 297–301
  for credentialing, 106–107
  information subject to expiration, 107, 221, 251–252
  role of QI data, 387
data security. *See* confidentiality
data verification. *See* verification of credentials
de novo reviews, 358
DEA registration, verifying, 129–130
  electronic verification, 235–236
  restricted or lost certificates, 134
decision making
  judgment, 14
  in meetings, 339–341
  corrective action (investigation), 396
  credentials process, 106–107
delegated credentialing, 36, 234, 244, 408–409. *See also* applications for membership and privileges
deemed status, 39–40, 57
  loss of, 40
defendant, defined, 358
delegation, 15, 78
  of credentialing, 36, 408–409

shared credentialing departments (SCDs), 234, 244
delineation of privileges, 151–210
  allied health professionals (AHPs), 219
  general surgery (example), 154–157
dental education, verifying, 122
department of medical staff services (MSSD), 25–31
  expanded roles for, 34–38
  functions of, 27–33
  quality improvement in, 31–35. *See also* quality improvement
  role in CME, 303
  roles in credentialing process, 107–109
departments, clinical, 68
  chairs (chiefs) of, 68, 206
  multispecialty privileges, 188–189
  peer review, 427
  proctoring programs, 160–176
  rules and regulations of, 96, 148. *See also* policies and procedures
  turf battles over privileges, 189
departments of credentialing
  managed care, 238–239
  shared (SCDs), 241–249
  how to establish, 243–248
  operations manual for (example), 247–248
  reasons for, 241–243
  scope of services, 245
depositions, 360, 397
development of new privileges, 159–162, 163–165
  multispecialty privileges, 188–189, 383
direct examination (civil litigation), 360
director of medical staff services (job title), 18
director of nursing, 19
disability discrimination law, 319–321, 377–379
disaster privileges, 185–186
disciplinary activity, 386–391. *See also* sanctions, monitoring and verifying
  appealing, 400–401
  challenges to, 394–398
disruptive practitioners, 321–323

history of, 140
responding to physician impairment, 314–319
disclosure, peer review, 404–405
discovery (in litigation), 360, 397
discrimination over practitioner health, 319, 321, 377–379
disruptive practitioners, 321–323
distance conferencing, 351–352
distance from hospital (practitioners), 380
distribution of new bylaws and P&Ps, 92
district courts, 356, 358
diversion program for physicians, 317
doctrine of *res ipsa loquitur*, 364
documentation,
  credentialing, 110, 112–113. *See also* credentials process
  allied health professionals (AHPs), 221
  of credentials verification, 122–134, 236
  hearing reports, 400
  HCQIA requirements, 403–404
  impaired practitioners, 322–323
  information subject to expiration, 107, 221, 251–252
  IRBs (institutional review boards), 293–297
  low-activity practitioners, 148, 192
  meeting minutes, 331–346
    agendas and, 331
    formats for, 332, 334–335
    recording and documenting, 339–344
    requirements for documentation, 343–344
  meetings schedule, 328–329
  peer review confidentiality, 345, 401–402, 404
  of policies. *See* policies and procedures
  privileging, 192
  of problems requiring corrective action, 395
  retrospective chart review, 290, 390
dominator (meeting personality type), 340

Drug Enforcement Agency registration, verifying, 128–129
   restricted certificates, 134
drug use by physicians. *See* impaired practitioners
dual roles of medical staff leaders, 97
due process for AHP credentialing, 222
duplication of effort, avoiding, 242
duplication of information, 110, 112
duty to credential, 369, 407
duty to provide information, 381–382

E
e-health privileges, 186–188
ECFMG (Educational Commission for Foreign Medical Graduates), 122–123
economic credentialing, 166, 380
education. *See* training and education
Elam v. College Park Hospital, 415
electronic meeting minute formats, 351
electronic services. *See* Web technologies
electronic transfer capabilities, 259–260. *See also* information systems
electronic verification of credentials, 235–236
eligible practitioners, categories of, 374–375
emergency corrective action, 389
emergency privileges, 185–186
emergency services, 23
employees. *See entries at* staff
employment discrimination, 377–379
entitlement to procedural rights of review, 391–392
equal application of requirements, 395
equitable relief, 358, 366
essential areas for accredited CME, 305–306
ethics, 7–8
   and proctoring, 174
evaluation
   of allied health professional competency, 221

certified nurse-midwives, 221
CRNAs, 221
of committees, 75–76
of credentialing data. *See* verification of credentials
customer satisfaction, 37, 41–43
dashboard reports, 282–286
meeting minutes, 341–342
peer review, 287–289, 291
   ability to work cooperatively, 379
   evaluation of, 291
   of peer review programs, 291
   of privileging applications, 134–142
   of quality. *See* quality improvement
   of staff performance, 10. *See also* quality improvement
   external, 289, 291
   hearing panel bias, 398
   legal issues, 392–394, 394–398
   peer, defined, 288
   physician impairment and, 319
   policy for, 321
   training director questionnaire (example), 123–124
executive committee (MEC), 32, 83, 326
credentials process, 106–112, 113–143
peer review responsibilities, 287–289, 291
reporting on quality (dashboard reports), 282–286
evidence notebook, 428
exclusive contracts, 367, 384
executives, physicians as, 95–102
expedited credentialing, 143
expiring data, management of, 107, 221, 251–252
external peer review, 289–291

F
facilitated meetings, 336, 338, 340
failure to respond (applications), 200
fair hearing manuals, 81, 394
fax machines and meetings, 351
FDA regulations for IRBs, 293–297

federal courts, 356
federal regulations, 361
Federation of State Medical Boards (FSMB), 133–134
fellowship, verifying, 122–125
felonies, 356
felony convictions, verifying, 132–133, 141
final decision (hearings), 401
finances
   benefits of CVOs, 252–253
   budgeting, 7, 11
   hearing panel bias, 398
   knowledge of, 4–5, 9, 11
   performance and, 264–265
   reimbursement systems, 4–5, 132
   utilization management, 4–5, 28, 380–381
   legal issues, 380
   withholding privileges (economic credentialing), 222, 380
flip charts, 349
focused peer review, 167–174, 273–274. *See also* FPPE
follow-up phase of meetings, 328, 346–348
foreign medical graduates, verifying information on, 122–123
form vs. function, 165–276
formal education programs, 2
format
   meeting agenda, 332
   meeting minutes, 344–345
Focused Professional Practice Evaluation. *See* FPPE
forms for clinical privileges. *See* clinical privileges
forms for recording meeting minutes, 348–349
four-column format for meeting minutes, 345
FPPE, 22, 160–176, 273–274
   policy, 168–174
frequency of meetings, 326
FSMB (Federation of State Medical Boards), 133–134, 251

G
general surgery privileges (example), 154–157
Gonzalez v. Nork, 414

governing body of hospital, 65–66.
    See also responsibility
    and accountability
credentials process, 145
government sanctions, 233, 391,
    250–251
    conduct at other hospitals,
        379–380
graduate medical education,
    306–308
granting privileges. *See* clinical
    privileges
ground rules for meetings, 337
group meetings. *See* committees;
    meetings
guiding principles. *See* bylaws

H
harassment. *See* disruptive
    practitioners
Harrell v. Total Health Care, Inc.,
    225
HCQIA (Health Care Quality
    Improvement Act), 372,
    392–394, 422–423
    hearing rights, 396–397, 422–423
    reporting requirements, 403–404
    roles of attorneys, 398–399
health care compliance. *See*
    compliance offices and
    programs
health care financing. *See* finances
health care organization
    affiliations, verifying,
    129
Health Care Staffing Services
    Certification, 184–185
health care systems, credentialing
    in, 241–249
    establishing centralized
        credentialing
        department, 243–248
    operations manual for
        (example), 247–248
    reasons for centralized
        credentialing, 241–243
    scope of services, 245
health information management
    department, 22
Health Facilities Accreditation
    Program. *See* HFAP
health of practitioner. *See*
    practitioner health and
    behavior issues
hearing panel bias, 398

hearing panels, 398, 428–430
    orienting, 428
    arranging room, 428, 429
hearing reports, 400, 430
hearing rights, 396–397, 422–423
    under HCQIA, 392–394,
        422–423
    waiver of, 398
HEDIS data, 53–54
HFAP (Health Facilities
    Accreditation Program),
    46–47, 56
HIM (health information
    management)
    department, 22
HIPDB (Healthcare Integrity and
    Protection Data Bank),
    251
historical record, minutes as, 338
HIV-positive practitioners,
    378–379
HMOs (health maintenance
    organizations), 226,
    406–407, accreditation,
    64
honorary members of medical
    staff, 68, 105
hospital, relationship with,
    369–370
hospital accreditation, 47–60
hospital-based programs for
    physician impairment,
    313–316
hospital compliance offices, 25, 32
hospital IRBs, 293–297
hospital liability. *See* liability issues
hospital privileges. *See* clinical
    privileges
Hospital Quality Measures, 44, 59
hospital utilization requirements,
    380–381
house staff privileges, 190–192
human resources, knowledge of,
    12

I
identification of speakers in
    meeting minutes, 341,
    343
identity protection. *See*
    confidentiality
identity verification, 133
immunity from liability (peer
    reviews), 402–403
impaired practitioners, 311–320

causes of impairment, 312
contracts with, 317–318
treatment programs and
    recovery plans, 141,
    142, 323–324
implementing new privilege forms,
    160–161
incomplete applications, 135
independent liability, 373
independent practitioners. *See*
    AHPs; contract
    practitioners
independent work, need for, 13
informal intervention, 389–390
information management, 7
information systems. *See also*
    technology
    role of, 7
    shared credentialing departments
        (SCDs), 244
    sold or licensed through CVOs,
        250
    within CVOs, 259–260
initial appointment
    recommendation form
    (example), 144–145
inspection of IRBs, 296–297
institutional criteria for privileges,
    382
institutional review boards (IRBs),
    293–297
insurance, verifying, 130
integrated delivery systems, 36
intent, organizational, 242
Interactive Survey System (ISS),
    227
internal credentialing, 235
international healthcare
    accreditation, 49–51
internships, verifying, 122
interpersonal skills, 15. *See also*
    communication
intervention (corrective action),
    389–390
    appealing, 400–401
    challenges to, 394–398
    disruptive practitioners, 316–317
    responding to physician
        impairment, 314–319
introvert (meeting personality
    type), 341
invasive and operative procedures
    review, 267, 270–272
investigations
    as application red flags, 137, 139

background investigations, 132–133
corrective action decisions, 396, 426
of disruptive behavior complains, 322
IRBs (institutional review boards), 293–297
ISO (International Organization for Standardization), 59–60
accreditation, 48–49
ISS (Interactive Survey System), 227

J
Jefferson Parish Hospital District No. 2 v. Hyde, 418
job titles, 16–18
Johnson v. Misericordia, 415
Joint Commission, The, 39–45
accreditation survey process, 44–45
AHP credentialing, 216
ambulatory care accreditation, 54–56
bylaws requirements and guidelines, 79–83
core measures, 44–45
credentialing standards, 145, 147
CVO guidelines, 257–258
description of medical staff organization, 64
disruptive behavior, 321
hearing rights, 392
history of, 40–43
Hospital Quality Measures, 59
impaired practitioners, 321
medical staff characterization, 64–66
meeting minutes requirements, 343
ORYX initiative, 43
patient safety 44, 43
privileging requirements, 157–158
disaster privileges, 185–186
reprivileging, 193–197, 324–327
sentinel events 44, 251, 343
student privileges, 190–192
telemedicine, 186–188
temporary privileges, 182, 185–186
quality improvement requirements, 267–272

blood and blood product use, 267, 270
FPPE, 160–176, 273–274
medication management, 267, 268–269
OPPE, 176–182, 273–274, 279–280,
operative and other procedures, 267, 270–272
Standards Manual, 43
judgment, 14
jurisdiction, 359
jury selection, 360

K
knowledge requirements, 4–9
effective leadership, 97–98
physician executives, 98–100

L
Kadlec Medical Center v. Lakeview Anesthesia Associates, 419–420
laptop computers in meetings, 350
late arriver (meeting personality type), 340
laundry list of clinical privileges, 151–152
law, 6, 355–367
appointment and clinical privileges, 374–386
bylaws as contract, 96
civil litigation, 358–360
compliance. *See* compliance offices and programs
corrective action, 386–391. *See also* hearing rights
appealing, 400–401
challenges to, 394–398
courts, 356–358
credentialing requirements 239, 369, 406–407
disruptive practitioners, 323
responding to physician impairment, 312–320
HMO accountability, 225
legal system, 355
medical staff, 369–373
meeting minutes requirements, 345
peer review privileges, 401–403
procedural rights of review, 391–394

recommended legal references, 423
restraint of trade, 366–367
SCD regulations, 243–244
significant case law, 413–422
statutes, laws, and regulations, 239
telemedicine, 186–188
tort law, 362–365
lawsuits as application red flags, 198
lawyers, 30–31
bylaws revisions, 83–87, 90–92
role in professional review actions, 398–399, 428
leadership
authority and accountability, 98
committee chairs and meeting leaders, 326
conflicts of interest, 98
developing and supporting, 34–35, 72
dual roles, 97
lack of managerial abilities, 98
role in credentialing process, 109
traditional, problems with, 73–7, 97–98
Leapfrog Group, 265
legal documents, minutes as, 338, 345–346
legal system, explained, 355–358. *See also* law
letter-writing for credentials verification, 236
letter-writing for hearings, 426–427, 430
letters of warning, 391
levels approach to privilege delineation, 151–152
liability issues, 372–373
insurance requirements, 376–377
insurance verification, 130
peer review immunity, 402–403
liaison to medical staff, 28
licensed independent practitioner, defined, 105
licenses, monitoring, 250–251
licenses, verifying, 128, 352
restricted licenses, 134
telemedicine, 186–188
limitations of privileges, as corrective action, 391
limiting privileges
as corrective action, 391
for economic reasons, 380

limiting privileges (continued)
  procedural rights of review, 391–394
  revocation, 391
  under HCQIA, 392–394, 422–423
  waiver of, 398
listening skills at meetings, 339, 341. *See also* communication
local courts, 358
location for meetings, 330–331
location of practitioners, 380
location of SCDs, 246
locum tenens privileges, 183–185
long-distance conferencing, 351
long-term care, accreditation for, 51–52
loss of hospital privileges, 134
low-activity practitioners privileges for, 192

M

malfeasance, 363
malpractice, defined, 364
malpractice documentation policy (example), 389–391
malpractice history, 135, 139–140, 142, 381
managed care credentialing, 225–239
  administration of credentialing operations, 234–239
  automation, 235–236
  contracting vs. credentialing, 233–234
  legal issues, 406–409
  NCQA standards, 227–228, 398
  180-day rule, 231–232, 234, 237
  organization of credentialing department, 238–239
  standards for, 227–228
  state and federal requirements, 239
management of credentialing operations, 234–236
management skills and knowledge, 8, 133, 136
management tool, meeting minutes as, 339
marketing and business development, 23–24

McClellan v. Health Maintenance Organization of Pennsylvania, 419
MCOs (managed care organizations). *See* managed care credentialing
MEC (medical executive committee), 27, 71, 326
  credentials process, 144–145, 206–207
  peer review responsibilities, 273, 287–289, 291
  reporting on quality (dashboard reports), 282–286
  sample agenda for, 335
medical education. *See* training and education
medical executive committee. *See* MEC
medical school, verifying, 152
medical staff assistant (job title), 17
medical staff attorneys. *See* attorneys
medical staff committees. *See* committees
medical staff coordinator (job title), 17–18
medical staff departments, 80–83
  chairs (chiefs) of, 82, 206
  multispecialty privileges, 274–276
  peer review, 427
  proctoring programs, 174–175. *See also* FPPE
  rules and regulations of, 96, 148. *See also* policies and procedures
  turf battles over privileges, 189
medical staff law. *See* law
medical staff leaders. *See* leadership
medical staff liaison, 28
medical staff membership
  applications for. *See* applications for membership and privileges
  categories of, 67–68, 105
  criteria for, 114–116
  privilege delineation and, 153
  provisional privileges, 80, 383–384. *See also* FPPE
  revoking, 391

utilization requirements, 380–381
medical staff officers, 80–82
medical staff organization, 4, 25–27, 64–77
  accountability, 65–66
  alternative models for, 74–77
  CMS, 65
  committee support, 27–28. *See also* committees
  functions of, 66
  leadership problems, 97–98
  membership categories, 67–68
  organizational chart, 69
  organizational effectiveness, 73, 74–77
  peer review, 427–430
  physician executives, 95–102.
  physician impairment response, 313–319
  purpose of, 66
  quality improvement and, 267–272
  relevance of, 73
  traditional model for, 66–71
  trauma centers, 301–303
medical staff policy. *See* policies and procedures
medical staff reappointment. *See* reappointment and reprivileging
medical staff roles in quality improvement, 267–278.
  See also quality improvement and OPPE
  form vs. function, 265–267
  peer review, 287–289, 291
  specific quality functions, 267–278
medical staff assistant (job title), 17
medical staff secretary (job title), 16
medical staff services clerk (job title), 16
medical staff coordinator (job title), 17–18
medical staff services department. *See* MSSD
medical staff services professionals. *See* MSSPs
medical students. *See* training and education
medical terminology, knowledge of, 9

Medicare and Medicaid. *See* CMS
medication management, 267, 268–269
meetings, 325–353. *See also* committees
  departmental, 70
  evaluating, 75
  keeping effective, 76, 325–338
    conducting phase, 328, 334–345
    follow-up phase, 328, 344–348
    preparation phase, 328, 331–334
  minutes of, 328, 338–348
    agendas and, 331
    formats for, 332, 334–335
    purpose of, 338
    recording and documenting, 339–340, 343
    requirements for documentation, 343–344
  tools for, 348–352
  rules for, 337
membership, staff applications for. *See* applications for membership and privileges
  categories of, 67–68, 141
  criteria for, 114–115
  managed care, 230–231
  privilege delineation and, 217
  provisional privileges, 67, 383–384
  revoking, 391
  standardized, 230
  utilization requirements, 380–381
Miller v. Eisenhower Medical Center, 416–417
minimum criteria for privileges, 382
minimum levels of hospital utilization, 380–381
Minimum Standard, 42
minutes of meetings, 328, 338–348
  agendas and, 331
  evaluating content of, 341–342
  formats for, 332, 334–335
  purpose of, 338
  recording and documenting, 339–340, 343
  requirements for documentation, 343–344
misdemeanors, 356

misfeasance, 363
Mitchell County Hospital Authority v. Joiner, 416
money damages (tort law), 366
monitoring licensing and sanctions, 250–251
monitoring practitioners. *See also* FPPE and OPPE
  in education (proctoring), 160–176
  physician impairment and, 319
  sample policy for, 168–174, 177–182
  for impairment, 319
moonlighting, 191–192
motion cards, 349
motions (civil litigation), 356
motions (in meetings), 349
MSSD (medical staff services department), 18–25
  expanded roles for, 33–38
  functions of, 27–31
  organization of, 25–27
  quality improvement in, 31–32. *See also* quality improvement
  role in credentialing process, 107–109
MSSPs (medical staff services professionals), 2–3
  evolution of role 2–3
  expanded roles, 33–38
  job titles, 3, 15–24
  knowledge requirements, 4–9, 493
    managerial, 8, 98
  role in CME, 303–304
  role in hearings, 425–430
  role in quality improvement, 263
  skills requirements, 9–16
multidisciplinary AHP committees, 216–217
multispecialty privileges, 188–189, 383
  structure of. *See* organization of medical staff
turf battles, 189

N
NAMSS (National Association Medical Staff Services), 1
  certification programs, 1–2

formal education, 2
National Association Medical Staff Services. *See* NAMSS
National Board of Certification for Training Administrators of Graduate Medical Education Programs, 308
National Integrated Accreditation of Healthcare Organizations. *See* NIAHO
National Committee for Quality Assurance. *See* NCQA
National Practitioner Data Bank (NPDB) queries, 133–134, 251
NCQA (National Committee for Quality Assurance) 52–54
  CVO accreditation, 69–70, 256–257
  data security guidelines, 260
  managed care accreditation, 52–54
  MCO accreditation process, 52–54
  180-day rule, 231–232, 234, 237
NCRA (National Cancer Registrar's Association), 301
negligence, 363–366, 372–373
never events of CMS, 5, 59
NIAHO (National Integrated Accreditation of Healthcare Organizations), 47–49
  ISO standards, 49–50
  survey, 48
nonadmitting members of medical staff, 68
nondepartmentalized medical staffs, 70
nonfeasance, 363
nonstructured committees on physician impairment, 314–315
notice of adverse recommendations, 430–433
notice of charges (corrective action), 426, 397
notices of meetings, 331
NPDB queries, 133–134, 396

Index 445

O
objective criteria for privileges, 161–162, 382
observing practitioners. *See also* FPPE and OPPE
  in education (proctoring), 160–176, 176–183
  physician impairment and, 317
  sample policies for, 1169–174, 177–182
  for impairment, 317
occurrence policies, 130
off-the-record reports, 135
office site surveys, 232, 252
office systems, knowledge of, 12
officers, 68
180-day rule (NCQA), 231–232, 234, 237
Ongoing Professional Practice Evaluation. *See* OPPE
online services. *See* Web technologies
OPPE (Ongoing Professional Practice Evaluation), 22, 176–182, 273–274, 279–280
  sources of information for, 275–278
operative and invasive procedures review, 267, 270–272
organization of credentialing department, 238–239, 243–248
organization of medical staff, 63–77
  accountability, 66–67
  alternative models for, 74–77
  committee support, 32–33. *See also* committees
  knowledge of, 4
  organizational effectiveness, 73, 74–77
  peer review, 287–289, 291
  physician executives, 95–102. *See also* delineation of privileges
  physician impairment response, 314–319
  quality improvement and, 267–272
  relevance of, 73–77
  scope of services and work products, 244–245
  traditional model for, 66–72
  leadership problems, 73–74, 97–98

trauma centers, 301–303
organizational intent, clarifying, 243
organizational skills, 13
organizational structure of MSSD 19, 20
orientation (hearing panel), 428
orientation (leaders), 72
orientation (new medical staff), 28
orientation (new MSSD staff), 10
  AHP credentialing, 301
ORYX initiative, 43–44
ostensible agency, 372–373
out-of-state telemedicine, 186–188
outreach requirements for cancer programs, 299
outsourcing to CVOs, reasons for, 252–253

P
paperless credentialing, 122, 248
P&Ps. *See* policies and procedures
parliamentary procedure, 336
participation in meetings, 334
PAs (physician assistants)
  credentialing, 296–297, 323
  delineation of privileges, 219
  reappointment of, 220
past behavior. *See* practitioner health and behavior issues
patient relations, 23
patient safety, 44, 278, 281
  credentialing and, 104
institutional review boards. *See* IRBs
telemedicine, 186–188
Patrick v. Burget, 416
pay-for-performance programs, 101, 198
peer references, 131–132
  allied health professionals (AHPs), 220
  requirements for, 220
peer review, 278–289, 291
  ability to work cooperatively, 379
  evaluation of, 291
  hearing panel bias, 398
  legal issues, 392–394, 394–398
  peer, defined, 288
  physician impairment and, 319–320
  policy for, 321

pending activity, as application red flags, 137–140
pending investigations, as application red flags, 137
performance and finance, 264–265
performance evaluation of staff, 9. *See also* performance improvement. *See* quality improvement
performance indicators, selecting, 289
periodic performance reviews (PPRs), 45
personal information. *See* confidentiality
personality, practitioner, 312–313. *See also* practitioner health and behavior issues
PGY1 (internship), verifying, 123
phone calls, applications and, 134, 142, 237
PHOs (physician-hospital organizations), 24, 226
physician assistants
  credentialing, 214–215, 222
physician executives, 95–102
  for effective leadership, 97
  qualifications of, 99–101
  role of, 101–102
physician-hospital organization (PHO), 24, 226
physician impairment, 311–320
  causes of impairment, 312
  contracts with, 317–318
  treatment programs and recovery plans, 141, 142, 319–320
physician office site surveys, 232, 252
physician organization certification (POC), 65
physician referral service, 37
physician relations, 37–38
Physician's Recognition Award (PRA), 304–305
plaintiff, defined, 358
planning agendas for meetings, 333
pledges from applicants, 119
podiatric education, verifying, 123
policies and procedures (P&Ps), 35. *See also* bylaws
  aging practitioners, 320–321

corrective action, 388–391
credentialing, 113
  of AHPs, 217
  of CVOs, 254
  definitions of terms, 95–96
  disruptive behavior, 321–323
  distribution of new documents, 92
  fair hearing manuals, 81, 394
  FPPE, 168–174
  IRBs (institutional review boards), 293–297
  as living documents, 106
  managed care credentialing, 227
  meetings and minutes, 346
  OPPE, 176–182
  peer reviews, 287–289, 291
  physician health and impairment, 321–323,
  privileging and, 246–250
    disaster privileges, 185–186
    FPPE, 169–174
    moonlighting, 190–192
    multispecialty privileges, 188–189
    quota privileging, 198
    telemedicine privileges, 188
    temporary privileges, 182
    proctoring programs, 174–175. *See also* FPPE
  revising, process of, 81, 370–371
    amendment process, 86–87, 90–92
    speeding up with multiple documents, 80–82
    sample language for rules and policy manuals, 84
  shared credentialing departments, 247–248
Poliner v. Texas Health Systems, 420–421
political skills, physician executives and, 100
postgraduate education, verifying, 123
PPOs (preferred provider organizations), 226. *See also* managed care credentialing
  accreditation, 65
PPRs (periodic performance reviews), 45
PR (public relations), 30
PRA (Physician's Recognition Award), 304–305

practitioner data security. *See* confidentiality
practitioner health and behavior issues, 311–324
  ADA (Americans with Disabilities Act), 319–320, 377–379
  aging practitioners, 320–321
  claims history, 130, 139–140
  conduct at other hospitals, 379–380
  criminal conduct history, 132–133, 141
  disciplinary activity, 134, 137–138, 139
  discrimination over practitioner health, 377–379
  disruptive practitioners, 321–322, 379
    impairment, 311–313
    causes of, 312–313
    definition of, 321
  malpractice history, 381
  sanctions. *See* sanctions, monitoring and verifying
  taking corrective action, 386–391
  appealing, 400–401
  challenges to, 394–398
  disruptive practitioners, 323
  responding to physician impairment, 311–320
  work history, 159–160, 231, 379–380
practitioner involvement in corrective action, 396
preapplication process, 113–114
precedents (in law), 361
preparation phase of meetings, 328, 331–334
prepared for evaluation, credentials file, 142
preparing for hearings, 426–430
preparing agendas for meetings, 331
preparing for accreditation surveys, 60–61
president of staff, 82
primary source verification, 120, 230–231
  automation of, 235–236
privacy. *See* confidentiality
privileges. *See* clinical privileges
privileges (legal) of peer review, 401–403

procedural challenges to corrective action, 395–396
procedural review of IRBs, 296–297
procedural rights of review, 391–394, 422–423
  under HCQIA, 392–394, 422–423
  waiver of, 398
procedures. *See* policies and procedures
process management (credentialing), 8–9, 237
processes, understanding of, 8–9
processing applications for membership and privileges, 175–199, 153. *See also* applications for membership and privileges
  allied health professionals (AHPs), 219–220
  credentials file, 120–121, 142
  initial appointment recommendation form (example), 144–145
  managed care, 228–234
  potential problems (red flags), 134–142
  process, understand, 8–9
  proctoring programs, 174–175, 169–174. *See also* FPPE
  physician impairment and, 319
  sample policy for, 169–174, 174–175
production-oriented work flow, 237
professional liability claims history, verifying, 130
  red flags with, 134, 139
professional liability insurance. *See also* liability issues
  requirements for, 376–377
  verification of, 130
professional references, verifying, 131–132
professional review actions, 379, 381, 382, 391. *See also* corrective action
  confidentiality, 401–402
  hearing panel bias, 398
  immunity from liability, 402–403

Index   447

reporting, 400
reporting requirements, 403–404
professional review actions (HCQIA), 391
professional training, verifying, 122–123
profiling performance, 192–197
program-specific accreditation, 293–308
  cancer programs, 297–301
  continuing medical education programs, 303–306
  graduate medical education, 306–308
  institutional review boards (IRBs), 293–297
  trauma centers, 201–303
protection of human subjects. *See* IRBs (institutional review boards)
protection of identity. *See* confidentiality
provisional privileges, 67, 383–384. *See also* FPPE
proximity requirements, 380
psychiatric problems, treatment for, 141, 142
public relations (PR), 24
Purcell v. Zimbelman, 414
purpose of committees, understanding, 326

Q

QA and QI. *See* quality improvement
quality improvement, 6, 22, 31–33, 37, 263–292
  AHPs (allied health professionals), 221
  cancer programs, 300
  comparing hospital quality, 263–264
  corrective actions, 386–391, 426
    appealing, 400–401
    challenges to, 392–398
    disruptive practitioners, 321–323
    responding to physician impairment, 312–319
  credentialing and, 140
  customer satisfaction surveys, 53–54
  CVOs (credentials verification organizations), 254

Department, 37
form vs. function, 414–416
The Joint Commission requirements, 267–272
  AHPs, 215
  blood and blood product use, 267, 270
  FPPE, 22, 160–176, 160–676, 273–274
  medication management, 267, 268–269
  OPPE, 22, 176–183, 279–280
  operative and other procedures, 267, 270–272
meeting minutes, 343–344
peer review, 287–289, 291
  evaluation of, 291
  FPPE, 160–176, 273–274
  hearing panel bias, 398
  legal issues, 392–394
  OPPE, 176–183, 279–280
  peer, defined, 288
  physician impairment and, 319
  policy for, 311
  profiling, reprivileging and, 192–197
transparent environment of health care, 263–264
quality department, collaborating with, 22, 28, 263
  role of QI data, 387
  specific quality functions, 267–272
questionnaires. *See* evaluation
quota privileging, 197–198

R

rambler (meeting personality type), 340
Rao v. Auburn General Hospital, 417
reappointment and reprivileging, 34, 143–149, 192–197,
  allied health professionals (AHPs), 220–221
  competence requirements, 376
  recommendation for initial appointment, 144–145
recommendations by peers. *See* references
recommendations for corrective action, 426

recommendations for action (meeting minutes), 344
recording meetings. *See* minutes of meetings
recording minutes at meetings, 339–340, 343. *See also* meetings
recovery plan, impaired physicians, 317
recredentialing in MCOs, 232
recruitment, 24
red flags in privileges applications, 134–142
reentry after physician impairment, 317, 319
references. *See* peer references
references on legal issues, 423
referral service for physicians, 37
regulations, 239, 293–297, 361. *See also* law
rehabilitation facilities accreditation, 56–57
reimbursement systems, 4–5, 96
relationship between staff and hospital, 369–370
relationships of MSSD with other departments, 19, 22–25
  bylaws language and, 107, 110
relationships with SCD customers, 243
release form for background check, 120, 218
releases from liability, 365
relevance of staff organization, 73–77
renewal of privileges. *See* reappointment and reprivileging
reporting
  adverse decisions, 430
  FPPE, 169
  OPPE, 273, 279–280
    examples of information for, 275–278
  physician impairment, 315
  professional review actions, 403–404
  quality functions, 282–286
res ipsa loquitur, 364
research monitoring. *See* IRBs (institutional review boards)
research requirements for cancer programs, 299
residency training, 190–192

moonlighting policy, 190–192
resignations, as application red flags, 137
resource center, establishing, 30–31
resource management, 8
respondeat superior, 372
responsibility and accountability. *See also* management skills and knowledge
　delegation, 15, 65–66
　of credentialing, 36, 234–235, 407
　shared credentialing departments (SCDs), 243–244
　HMOs, for provider actions, 225
　hospital trustees, 95–96
　managed care credentialing, 225
　nonemployed individuals. *See* AHPs (allied health professionals)
　organization of medical staff, 64–72
　peer review, 287–289
　student privileges, 190–192
restraint of trade, 366–367
restricting privileges
　as corrective action, 391
　for economic reasons, 166, 380
　procedural rights of review, 391–394, 422–423
　under HCQIA, 392–394, 422–423
　waiver of, 398
　revocation, 391
restructuring committees, 75–77. *See also* organization of medical staff
retrospective chart review, 390
review in appeal, 400–401
review of quality. *See* quality improvement
revising privileges, 159–161
revision of bylaws and related documents, 88, 90–92, 370–371
　amendment process, 84–87, 90–92
　speeding up with multiple documents, 80–82
revocation of privileges, 391
　hearing rights, 396–397, 422–423
right of cross-examination, 399

rights to review (hearing), 396–397, 397, 422–423
　under HCQIA, 392–394, 422–423
　waiver of, 398
risk and risk management, 8, 24–25
　credentialing and, 104
　temporary privileges, 182, 185–186
Robinson v. Magovern, 417
roles for MSSDs, 27–31, 107–109
roles for MSSPs
　expanded roles for, 33–38
　role in CME, 303–304
　role in hearings, 425–430
　role in quality improvement, 263
roles of committees, 326
roles of medical staff leaders, 133
room arrangement (for meetings), 330
routing applications for privileges, 143–144
reappointment, 148–149
rules and regulations. *See* policies and procedures

S
sales, 29–30
sanctions, monitoring and verifying, 233, 250–251
　conduct at other hospitals, 379–380
SCDs (shared credentialing departments), 24–249
　how to establish, 243–248
　operations manual for (example), 247–248
　reasons for, 241–243
　scope of services, 244–245
scheduling and time management, 13
　CVO turnaround time, 253
　meetings, 328–329
scope of practice for AHPs, 219
scope of services and work products, 244–245
scoring (peer review), 290
screening applicants for credentials, 113–114
　preapplication, 113–114
　reappointment of AHP, 220–221
screening for quality. *See* quality improvement
security, data. *See* confidentiality

self-assessment checklists, 11–12
self-governance by medical staff, 369
sensitive information. *See* confidentiality
sentinel events, 44, 321
separation of powers, 362
sequestering the jury, 360
setting-specific privileges, 162
sexual harassment. *See* disruptive practitioners
shared credentialing departments (SCDs), 241
　how to establish, 243–248
　operations manual for (example), 247–248
　reasons for, 241–243
　scope of services, 244–245
Sherman Antitrust Act, 366–367
shock jock (meeting personality type), 340
skills requirements, 9–16
　competency assessment for AHPs, 221
　managerial, 9–12, 133, 136
　multispecialty privileges, 188–189, 383
slips (impaired practitioners), 319
Social Security trace, 133
social work and social services, 23
software. *See* information systems
sources of medical staff law, 371–372
specialty lines, crossing, 188–189
sponsoring practitioners. *See* proctoring programs
staff committees. *See* committees
staff departments, 70
　chairs (chiefs) of, 68, 206
　multispecialty privileges, 188–189
　peer review, 288–289
　proctoring programs, 174–175
　rules and regulations of, 112–113. *See also* policies and procedures
　turf battles over privileges, 189
staff evaluation, 9. *See also* performance improvement
staff law. *See* law
staff leadership. *See* leadership
staff meetings. *See* meetings

Index　　449

staff membership
  applications for. *See* applications for membership and privileges
  categories of, 79–80, 105
  criteria for, 114–116
  privilege delineation and, 153
  provisional privileges, 80, 160–176, 383–384. *See also* FPPE
  revoking, 391
  utilization requirements, 380–381
staff organization. *See* organization of medical staff
staff policy. *See* policies and procedures
staff reappointment. *See* reappointment and reprivileging
staff roles in quality improvement, 263, 288–289. *See also* quality improvement
  form vs. function, 265–266
  peer review, 287–289, 291
  specific quality functions, 267–272
staff supervision, 9–13, 336
  as corrective action, 390
staffing and staffing analysis, 25–26
standard corrective action, 388
standard of review in appeal, 400–401
standardized meeting agendas, 335
standards, 401. *See also* accreditation; credentials process
standards of care, knowledge of, 364–365
stare decisis, 361
state courts, 356, 358
state license, verifying, 128
state medical association, CME accreditation through, 306
state medical board actions, as red flags, 138–139
state regulations, 239
statute of limitations, 362
statutory law, 361
stress, practitioner impairment and, 312
structure of medical staff. *See* organization of medical staff

structured committees on physician impairment, 314–315
student training. *See* training and education
substantive challenges to corrective action, 394
success. *See* quality improvement
summary corrective action, 388, 389
summons with the court, 359
supervision of staff, 9–13
  as corrective action, 390
Supreme Court (U.S.), 356
surveys for accreditation, 47. *See also* accreditation; certification programs
  Joint Commission, 60–61
  preparing for, 60–61
surveys for credentials. *See* credentials process
surveys for customer satisfaction, 37, 41–43
surveys of physician office sites, 232
symptom checklist for detecting physician impairment, 313
synthesizing conversation for meeting minutes, 340

T
tables for meetings, 330–331
table of contents from bylaws, 83
tail coverage, 130
tape recording devices in meetings, 350
teams. *See* committees
technology, 6
  information systems, 250, 259–260
  knowledge of, 6
  within CVOs, 250, 259–260
  role of, 6–7
  shared credentialing departments (SCDs), 244
  sold or licensed through CVOs, 250
  meetings, 350–351
teleconferences, 351–352
telemedicine, 186–188
telephone verification, 134, 142, 237
temporary privileges, 182, 185–186
termination policy. *See* policies and procedures

terminology (medical), knowledge of, 6–7
three-column format for meeting minutes, 345
threshold criteria for privileges, 382
time commitments of physicians, 97
time management and scheduling, 13
tort law, 362–366
traditional model of staff organization, 66–72
  leadership problems, 132–134
training and education
  cancer programs, 300
  CME programs, 303–306
  multispecialty privileges, 188–189
  privileges during, 190–192
  requiring as corrective action, 390
  residency training, 123, 306–308
  moonlighting policy, 190–192
  multispecialty privileges, 188–189
  privileging and, 190–192
  requirements for, 375
  verifying, 123
transitory actions, 359
transparent environment of health care, 263–265. *See also* quality improvement
trauma centers, 301–303
treatment for impaired physicians, 316–317
treatment program participation, 141, 142
trial courts, 356
trial preparation, 359
trust, 3
trustee accountability, 95–96
turf battles over privileges, 189
turnaround time with CVOs, 253
two-column format for meeting minutes, 345

U
unannounced accreditation surveys, 44
uniform credentialing. *See* centralized credentialing
United States Supreme Court, 356
updating privileges, 159–160
  CVO accreditation, 54, 257

URAC 54
    managed care accreditation, 54, 257
    utilization management, 8, 22–23
    legal issues, 380–381

V

validating identity of applicant, 139
venue (civil litigation), 359
verification of credentials, 29–30, 121–122
    allied health professionals (AHPs), 219–220
    automating, 122, 235, 236
    difficulties with, 136
    organizations for (CVOs), 249
    CAQH (Council for Affordable Quality Healthcare), 230
    The Joint Commission guidelines for CVOs, 257–258
    NCQA certification of, 69–70, 256–257
    operating models, 249
    services of, 250–252
    URAC certification of, 54, 257
    when to outsource to, 252–253
    potential problems (red flags), 134–142
    provisional period and, 383–384. *See also* FPPE
    reappointment, 143, 146–149, 192, 196, 220–221
    vicarious liability, 372
vice president (chief) of staff, 68
videoconferences, 351–352
virtual meetings, 347
voir dire, 360
voluntary accreditation. *See* accreditation
voluntary withdrawal of application, 180

W

waiver of procedural rights, 398
warning letters to practitioners, 391
Web technologies
    credentials verification, 259–260
withdrawal of application, 180
    as application red flag, 137
withholding privileges
    as corrective action, 391
    for economic reasons, 166, 380
    procedural rights of review, 391–394, 422–423
    revocation, 391
    under HCQIA, 392–394, 422–423
    waiver of, 398
work flow, 7
work history, verifying, 231, 379–380
workers. *See entries at* staff
working independently, 13–14

Chapter Quizzes

Quiz 1

Chapter 1: Introduction to Medical Staff Services

1. Which function does the medical staff services professional (MSSP) provide for the daily activities of the medical staff organization?
   - ☐ a. Facilitation
   - ☑ b. Coordination
   - ☐ c. Assignments
   - ☐ d. Advice

2. Through which function does the MSSP establish a unique relationship with an applicant for staff membership?
   - ☐ a. Committee assignments
   - ☐ b. Emergency room call assignments
   - ☑ c. Initial credentialing
   - ☐ d. Committee support

3. In the course of performance of his or her duties, the MSSP has access to sensitive information that must be maintained in what manner?
   - ☐ a. Openly
   - ☐ b. Secretly
   - ☐ c. Obscurely
   - ☑ d. Confidentially

453

4. With which of the following hospital departments should the MSSP have a strong link because of important information this department can provide related to legal issues?
    - ☐ a. Quality assurance/performance improvement
    - ☑ b. Risk management
    - ☐ c. Business office
    - ☐ d. Health information management

5. For which important service is the medical staff services department (MSSD) often the conduit for medical staff leaders?
    - ☐ a. Financial advice
    - ☐ b. Practice management
    - ☐ c. Office staff education
    - ☑ d. Legal counsel

6. Which management function in the medical staff services department is difficult to benchmark?
    - ☐ a. Budgeting
    - ☐ b. Planning
    - ☑ c. Staffing
    - ☐ d. Controlling

7. Which step must be performed before a staffing standard is established for the medical staff services department?
    - ☑ a. Staffing analysis
    - ☐ b. Hiring staff
    - ☐ c. Writing job descriptions
    - ☐ d. Reducing staff

8. What should the MSSP and the MSSD be responsible for providing with regard to the newly appointed medical staff member?
    - ☐ a. Delineation of privileges
    - ☐ b. Proctoring
    - ☑ c. Orientation
    - ☐ d. Committee appointments

9. Which individuals does the MSSD most frequently assist in a variety of ways?
   - ☐ a. New appointees
   - ☐ b. Courtesy staff members
   - ☐ c. Proctors
   - ☑ d. Medical staff leaders

10. Because elected medical staff leaders serve limited terms of office and come and go, what valuable role do the MSSP and the MSSD play in medical staff organization activities?
    - ☐ a. Documentation
    - ☑ b. Continuity
    - ☐ c. Coordination
    - ☐ d. Communication

Quiz 2

Chapter 2: Healthcare Organization Accreditation

1. Which of the following was one of the stated purposes of the American College of Surgeons (ACS) when it was founded in 1913?
   - ☒ a. Hospital standardization
   - ☐ b. Hospital accreditation
   - ☐ c. Hospital surveys
   - ☐ d. Hospital closures

2. When some of the most prestigious hospitals failed to meet the most basic standards, what did the ACS do in the Waldorf Astoria Hotel with the report of the hospital field survey?
   - ☐ a. Published it
   - ☐ b. Posted it
   - ☒ c. Burned it
   - ☐ d. Announced it

3. What were the five official hospital standards adopted by the ACS in 1919 called?
   - ☐ a. Optimal standard
   - ☐ b. Achievable standard
   - ☒ c. Minimum standard
   - ☐ d. Maximum standard

4. What modern process that continues today did adoption of the minimum standard of the ACS set in motion?
   - ☐ a. Licensure
   - ☐ b. Regulation
   - ☐ c. Audits
   - ☒ d. Accreditation

5. For which of the following processes have many states adopted the Joint Commission's accreditation requirements?
   - ☐ a. Licensure
   - ☐ b. Regulation

☐ c. Certification
☐ d. Registration

6. The purpose of incorporating standards for hospitals such as licensure, accreditation, and Medicare approval is to reduce the number of what?
    ☐ a. Beds
    ☐ b. Hospitals
    ☐ c. Surveys
    ☐ d. Audits

7. What is the accrediting organization for osteopathic hospitals?
    ☐ a. American Osteopathic Agency
    ☐ b. Healthcare Facilities Accreditation Program
    ☐ c. Osteopathic Accreditation Agency
    ☐ d. American Association for Accreditation of Osteopathic Healthcare

8. What is the most frequently used accrediting body for managed care organizations?
    ☐ a. American Managed Care Association
    ☐ b. National Managed Care Association
    ☐ c. National Committee for Quality Assurance
    ☐ d. National Association of Managed Care

9. Which organization accredits utilization review and worker's compensation programs?
    ☐ a. National Committee for Quality Assurance
    ☐ b. URAC
    ☐ c. American Osteopathic Association
    ☐ d. The Joint Commission

10. Which of the following organizations does *not* accredit ambulatory healthcare facilities?
    ☐ a. American Association for Accreditation of Ambulatory Surgery Facilities
    ☐ b. American Association for Ambulatory Health Care
    ☐ c. The Joint Commission
    ☐ d. URAC

Quiz 3

Chapter 3: The Medical Staff Organization

1. To which body is the medical staff organization ultimately accountable?
   - ☐ a. Medical executive committee
   - ☐ b. Joint conference committee
   - ☐ c. Governing body
   - ☐ d. Credentials committee

2. Which of the following is *not* a function of the organized medical staff?
   - ☐ a. Establishing professional standards
   - ☐ b. Providing continuous surveillance to see that standards are met
   - ☐ c. Taking final action on medical staff appointments and privileges
   - ☐ d. Taking disciplinary action when necessary

3. Which of the following is *not* a usual working component of a medical staff organization structure?
   - ☐ a. Medical staff officers
   - ☐ b. Clinical departments
   - ☐ c. Medical staff committees
   - ☐ d. Medical staff membership categories

4. What does a medical staff membership category usually signify?
   - ☐ a. Level of clinical privileges
   - ☐ b. Committee appointment status
   - ☐ c. Tenure as a medical staff member
   - ☐ d. Activity level of the member

5. Medical staff members can be appointed to more than one clinical department.
   - ☐ a. True
   - ☐ b. False

6. Which of the following medical staff committees does the Joint Commission require?
   - ☐ a. Infection control
   - ☐ b. Utilization review

☐ c. Medical executive
☐ d. Credentials

7. Which of the following documents is considered to be the blueprint for the medical staff organization?
   ☐ a. Job description
   ☐ b. Rules and regulations
   ☐ c. Bylaws
   ☐ d. Policy manual

8. Which of the following documents should exist to assist a medical staff leader in his or her role?
   ☐ a. Rules and regulations
   ☐ b. Policy manual
   ☐ c. Governing body bylaws
   ☐ d. Job description

9. Which of the following are barriers to a successful medical staff organization? (Choose all that apply.)
   ☐ a. Physicians have less time than they had in the past for medical staff organization work.
   ☐ b. Physicians are not as loyal to hospitals as they once were.
   ☐ c. Serving as a medical staff leader does not hold the same honor and respect as it did in the past.
   ☐ d. Physicians have privileges at several hospitals due to current reimbursement systems.

10. What are steps the medical staff services professional can take to make the medical staff organization more effective and efficient?
    ☐ a. Schedule a meeting when there are no substantive agenda items.
    ☐ b. Wait until the last minute to do a meeting agenda to determine whether there are additional agenda items.
    ☐ c. Resist changing the medical staff organization structure for fear of upsetting long-standing medical staff members.
    ☐ d. Do as much work outside committee meetings as possible.

Quiz 4

Chapter 4: Medical Staff Bylaws and Related Documents

1. Medical staff bylaws provide: (Choose all that apply.)
    a. A system of rights and responsibilities between the medical staff and governing body
    b. Protection of the patient, medical staff, and governing body
    c. A contract between the organized medical staff and the hospital, according to the AMA
    d. Confidential, protected information relevant to the medical staff

2. According to the Joint Commission standards, which of the following are considered functions of a medical staff's self-governance and, therefore, should be included in the bylaws? (Choose all that apply.)
    a. Approving/disapproving amendments to the bylaws
    b. Selecting and removing medical staff officers
    c. Establishing a nominating committee
    d. Engaging in performance improvement activities

3. The hospital bylaws are the same document as the medical staff bylaws.
    a. True
    b. False

4. Who are key stakeholders in revising a set of bylaws? (Choose all that apply.)
    a. Hospital legal counsel
    b. Medical staff legal counsel
    c. Hospital administration
    d. External accrediting agencies

5. Which of the following are indications of an organization's culture? (Choose all that apply.)
    a. The number of specialists on the medical staff
    b. The degree of governing body control
    c. Level of medical staff authority and representation on board committees
    d. The way in which medical staff dues money is spent

6. A bylaws revision project is an opportunity to restructure the medical staff.
   a. True
   b. False

7. A successful bylaws revision project requires which of the following? (Choose all that apply.)
   a. At least seven interested medical staff members
   b. Hospital administrative support
   c. Access to current regulatory and accreditation requirements
   d. At least one "respected" medical staff leader

8. Why is it important to maintain a chronological history of bylaws documents?

9. List two alternatives to distribution of bylaws to medical staff members besides making paper copies.

10. Any member of the medical staff is allowed to submit recommendations for bylaws amendments.
    a. True
    b. False

Quiz 5

Chapter 5: Physician Executives

1. Hospital trustees (governing boards) rely on the medical staff not only to deliver an acceptable level of care, but also to document and report information about which of the following?
   - ☐ a. Financial status of the hospital
   - ☐ b. Quality and appropriateness of care
   - ☐ c. Staffing levels
   - ☐ d. Long-range planning

2. With decreasing reimbursement due to implementation of the prospective payment system (DRGs), hospitals must be managed efficiently or risk losing money on patients who are insured by which of the following payers?
   - ☐ a. Blue Cross
   - ☐ b. Blue Shield
   - ☐ c. Medicare
   - ☐ d. HMOs

3. Elected medical staff leaders rarely have significant training or expertise in which of the following functions?
   - ☐ a. Medical
   - ☐ b. Surgical
   - ☐ c. Political
   - ☐ d. Managerial

4. What built-in barriers to effective medical staff leadership do practitioners potentially have?
   - ☐ a. Conflict of interest
   - ☐ b. Communication
   - ☐ c. Motivation
   - ☐ d. Ambition

5. In some hospitals, the demands of leading the medical staff organization have led to the emergence of which position?
   - ☐ a. Chief of staff
   - ☐ b. Medical director or physician executive

☐ c. Vice chief of staff
☐ d. Secretary/treasurer of staff

6. As a result of changes in health care, physician executives now play a greater role in which of the following areas?
   ☐ a. Financial accountability
   ☐ b. Staffing
   ☐ c. Overall management of the organization
   ☐ d. Public relations

7. The American College of Physician Executives recommends that prospective physician executives become board-certified physicians and practice medicine for what period of time?
   ☐ a. 10 years
   ☐ b. 15 years
   ☐ c. 1 year
   ☐ d. 3–5 years

8. Which concerns must the physician executive always place over concerns regarding the organization or the individual physician?
   ☐ a. Quality and safety of patient care
   ☐ b. Personal concerns
   ☐ c. Financial concerns
   ☐ d. Public relations concerns

9. Knowing how to manage which of the following may be a determinant of the physician executive's success or failure?
   ☐ a. Conflicting interests
   ☐ b. Competing interests
   ☐ c. Financial interests
   ☐ d. Personal interests

10. Healthcare organizations increasingly want their physician executives to hold a degree in which of the following fields?
    ☐ a. Finance
    ☐ b. Philosophy
    ☐ c. Finance
    ☐ d. Management

Quiz 6

Chapter 6: The Hospital Credentials Process

1. Hospitals and their governing bodies have a duty to the public to ensure that only qualified, competent practitioners are allowed to provide care in healthcare organizations.
    a. True
    b. False

2. The license of a physician identifies which procedures he or she is qualified to perform.
    a. True
    b. False

3. Licensed independent practitioners (LIPs) may be granted which of the following?
    a. Membership only
    b. Privileges only
    c. Membership and privileges
    d. All of the above

4. It is the responsibility of the medical staff services professional to review application materials to assure that they are complete prior to beginning the verification process.
    a. True
    b. False

5. Which of the following is an important role played by the medical staff services professional in the credentialing process?
    a. Identification of "red flags"
    b. Telling the department chairs which privileges to approve
    c. Making the decision about which applications should be denied
    d. Determining the number of peer references to obtain

6. A credentials committee is required by:
    a. The Joint Commission
    b. Medicare Conditions of Participation

c. None of the above

d. Both of the above

7. A credentials committee can play an important role in credentialing by:
    a. Doing the work of the department chairs because they are usually too busy to handle this task
    b. Making sure that medical staff bylaws and credentialing policies and procedures are appropriately implemented
    c. Making a recommendation directly to the governing board because the medical executive committee's agenda is usually too full to consider credentialing
    d. Granting temporary privileges

8. Medical staff bylaws should describe which of the following?
    a. The type of licensed independent practitioners eligible for medical staff membership and clinical privileges
    b. Medical staff membership categories
    c. Elements of a complete application
    d. All of the above

9. Which of the following requires that healthcare organizations establish a pre-application process?
    a. The Joint Committee
    b. Medicare Conditions of Participation
    c. American Health Lawyers Association
    d. None of the above

10. New applicants to the medical staff must always be interviewed by the credentials committee.
    a. True
    b. False

11. A manual checklist attached to the front of a credentials file is the preferred method of tracking the status of the file.
    a. True
    b. False

12. The Joint Committee requires that all state licenses that a practitioner has ever had be verified at the time of initial appointment.
    a. True
    b. False

13. Under which conditions should the term "board eligible" be used in regard to a credentialing application?
    a. It should never be used.
    b. It should be used to describe a practitioner's board status.
    c. It should be used only to describe the board status of a practitioner with ABMS board status.
    d. It should be used if a practitioner states that he or she intends to become board certified.

14. A healthcare organization may seek peer recommendations only from names submitted by the applicant.
    a. True
    b. False

15. What does a "red flag" signify?
    a. The applicant should be denied.
    b. There is something that must be further investigated or resolved prior to making a recommendation about membership or privileges.
    c. The applicant is probably incompetent.
    d. The applicant should be instructed to withdraw his or her application.

16. According to the Joint Commission, how often must reappointment occur?
    a. One year after the initial appointment
    b. At least every 24 months
    c. When the medical staff office gets around to it
    d. On the birthday of each practitioner

QUIZ 7

Chapter 7: Hospital Privileging

1. List two different formats for delineation of privileges that have been used.
   a. _____
   b. _____

2. What is a major disadvantage of the laundry list format?
   a. It is too short.
   b. It is too long.
   c. It is too cumbersome and difficult to maintain.
   d. It is too simple.

3. Privileges to care for a patient on a ventilator would most likely be granted to all internists.
   a. True
   b. False

4. If you were a recent graduate from a residency training program and were applying for privileges at a hospital but the privilege form did not include two procedures you were trained to perform and wanted to perform, should you add those privileges to your request form? Why or why not?
   a. Yes
   b. No

   Explanation: _____

5. What is the goal of privileging?
   a. To limit a practitioner's practice
   b. To provide the practitioner with as many privileges as possible
   c. To identify the practitioner's competency level and recommend and authorize him or her to practice within that competency level
   d. To control the practitioner so as to keep him or her from competing for patients

6. The November 2004 CMS statement concerning privileges requires which of the following? (Choose all that apply.)
   a. The privilege criteria are authorized by the governing body.

b. The individual practitioner's ability to perform each privilege must be assessed.

c. The medical staff bylaws must describe the privileging process.

d. Privileges can be recommended by only one department.

7. Each hospital's privilege forms should be in place for at least three years before being revised.

    a. True

    b. False

8. If an applicant is not granted a privilege because he or she did not fulfill the basic criteria, should withholding the privilege be reported to the NPDB? Why or why not?

    a. No

    b. Yes

    Explanation: _____

9. What is proctoring?

    a. A mechanism for competing physicians to show who is best

    b. A requirement established by NCQA

    c. A means to observe and assess new appointees or someone with new privileges

    d. Always an objective process

10. It is not necessary to query the NPDB when someone requests temporary privileges.

    a. True

    b. False

QUIZ 8

Chapter 8: Credentialing Allied Health Professionals

1. Which of the following types of employment status may be held by an allied health professional? (Choose all that apply.)
   a. Physician employed
   b. Hospital employed
   c. Contract with organization
   d. Independent practitioner

2. The hospital board and medical staff organization should determine which categories of allied health professionals are permitted to work in the hospital.
   a. True
   b. False

3. The source of an allied health professional's employment has a bearing on the person's need to be authorized to provide services in the hospital.
   a. True
   b. False

4. Which of the following are credentials that an allied health professional may hold? (Choose all that apply.)
   a. Licensure
   b. Certification
   c. Registration
   d. Narcotics prescribing permit

5. In what manner should a licensed independent allied health professional exercising independent medical judgment be authorized to provide services?
   a. Authorized by human resources
   b. Credentialed in the same manner as a physician
   c. No credentialing is necessary
   d. Functions under a job description

6. In which of the following manners is it permissible to authorize a physician-employed surgical assistant to provide services in a healthcare organization? (Choose all that apply.)

a. The medical staff organization's credentialing process
   b. May function under a job description
   c. A mechanism provided by human resources
   d. Should function with delineated clinical privileges

7. For allied health professional disciplines other than physician assistants and advanced practice registered nurses, the authorization process can include which of the following? (Choose all that apply.)
   a. Primary source verification of licensure, certification, or registration
   b. Education and experience
   c. Peer recommendations
   d. Criminal background check
   e. Other verifications that human resources may perform

8. Dependent allied health professionals may have a performance evaluation at the same frequency as a hospital employee.
   a. True
   b. False

9. Physician assistants and advanced practice registered nurses must have delineated clinical privileges and are subject to the ongoing professional practice evaluation and the focused professional practice evaluation processes.
   a. True
   b. False

10. All allied health professionals should have due process rights identical to those of medical staff members.
    a. True
    b. False

QUIZ 9

Chapter 9: The Managed Care Credentials Process

1. Which of the following words describes credentialing in managed care organizations prior to the early 1990s?
   a. Impossible
   b. Invisible
   c. Impractical
   d. Inefficient

2. Before National Committee for Quality Assurance (NCQA) standards were issued in 1991, on which entity or entities did managed care organizations rely for credentialing?
   a. State licensing boards
   b. National Practitioner Data Bank
   c. Contracted hospitals
   d. Credentials verification organizations

3. Which of the following factors led to the need for managed care organizations to credential providers? (Choose all that apply.)
   a. Case law
   b. Reporting requirements of the Health Care Quality Improvement Act
   c. Issuance of provider directories
   d. Restriction of member access to providers

4. Which of the following are minimum qualifications criteria required by NCQA for providers? (Choose all that apply.)
   a. Board certification
   b. Current licensure
   c. Relevant training and experience
   d. Disclosure of health issues affecting a provider's ability to practice

5. According to NCQA standards, it is possible to separate criteria used to evaluate professional competence from criteria used to make a business decision as to need for specific categories of provider.
   a. True
   b. False

6. Which of the following are elements required by NCQA for primary source verification? (Choose all that apply.)
   a. A valid license to practice
   b. A valid DEA or CDS certificate
   c. Highest level of education
   d. Hospital affiliations

7. NCQA does not require the managed care organization to credential practitioners who have which of the following characteristics? (Choose all that apply.)
   a. Practice exclusively in an inpatient hospital setting
   b. Are hospital-based practitioners
   c. Are dentists who provide primary dental care
   d. Do not provide care for health plan members in a treatment setting

8. If a healthcare organization chooses to use a credential verification organization to verify the credentials of healthcare practitioners, it should confirm that the CVO selected understands how to perform verifications on all the types of healthcare professionals that the organization must credential.
   a. True
   b. False

9. NCQA standards do not require that a managed care organization designate a credentialing committee.
   a. True
   b. False

10. According to NCQA standards, which of the following methods are appropriate for credentials verification? (Choose all that apply.)
    a. Electronic
    b. Written
    c. Verbal
    d. None of the above

QUIZ 10

Chapter 10: Health System Credentialing and Credentials Verification Organizations

1. A healthcare system is an integrated delivery system and always has a single governing body.
   a. True
   b. False

2. The staff working in a centralized credentialing department must be skilled in:
   a. Data management
   b. Verification procedures
   c. Using technology effectively
   d. All of the above

3. For what primary purpose are centralized credentialing departments established by healthcare systems?
   a. Eliminate jobs
   b. Eliminate duplication of credentialing
   c. Satisfy NCQA requirements
   d. Save money

4. If it is determined to be feasible to establish a centralized credentialing department in a healthcare system, it is critical to determine which of the following? (Choose all that apply.)
   a. Which services will be provided by the centralized credentialing department
   b. Which credentialing software will be used
   c. Where the centralized credentialing department will be located
   d. All of the above

5. If a centralized credentialing department ensures that the credentialing work product it provides meets the Joint Commission requirements, all other regulatory requirements will automatically be met.
   a. True
   b. False

6. Data from the credentialing database in a healthcare system should never be shared with contracting personnel.
   a. True
   b. False

7. When establishing a centralized credentialing department, the most preferable location would be the largest medical staff office in the healthcare system.
   a. True
   b. False

8. The centralized credentialing department must be located:
   a. In an office close to its customer organizations
   b. At one of the customer organizations
   c. At corporate headquarters
   d. Anywhere, if the service is electronic

9. Each entity in a healthcare system should select the credentialing software that best meets its needs.
   a. True
   b. False

10. A users group made up of representatives of customers of the centralized credentialing department should be made responsible for supervising the staff of the centralized credentialing department.
    a. True
    b. False

11. Which of the following established the first credentials verification organization?
    a. Physician professional associations
    b. Hospitals
    c. Proprietary groups
    d. Local and state medical societies

12. Which event caused an explosive need for centralized credentialing services?
    a. When the Joint Commission standards began requiring it
    b. When managed care organizations that sought NCQA accreditation began to credential their practitioners

c. When URAC began accrediting credentials verification organizations

d. When networks were first established by hospitals

13. Which of the following is *not* a service provided by credentials verification organizations?

    a. Primary source verification

    b. Application management services

    c. Management of information subject to expiration

    d. Approval of delineation of privileges

14. Application management services refers to initial application distribution, collection, and tracking prior to verification.

    a. True

    b. False

15. Which of the following is a benefit of outsourcing credentials verification to a credentials verification organization?

    a. Justifying hiring of additional staff

    b. Additional time for completing applications

    c. Efficiencies of scale

    d. Loss of control over the process

16. What does NCQA survey credentials verification organizations for with regard to verification, frequency of reporting, and data management of credentials? (Choose all that apply.)

    a. Hospital reference verification

    b. Sources used for primary source verification

    c. Peer reference verification

    d. Time frame within which verifications are completed

17. Within what time frame does NCQA require a credentials verification organization to complete the credentials verification process?

    a. 100 days

    b. 110 days

c. 180 days

d. 200 days

18. NCQA does not require managed care organizations to credential practitioners who practice exclusively in the inpatient hospital setting or ambulatory free-standing facilities and who provide care for organization members only as a result of the members being directed to the hospital or facility.

    a. True
    b. False

19. For which of the following does NCQA *not* require office site visits?

    a. Primary care practitioners
    b. Obstetrician/gynecologists
    c. High-volume behavioral health providers
    d. Orthopedic surgeons

20. Which of the following queries/statements does NCQA *not* require for a credentials verification organization–developed application form?

    a. Mother's maiden name
    b. ADA requirements regarding accommodation for disabilities
    c. Attestation for completeness and accuracy
    d. Felony convictions

QUIZ 11

Chapter 11: The Role of the Medical Staff in Quality Improvement

1. Information regarding certain aspects of hospital quality of care is available on the Internet.
   a. True
   b. False

2. The quality improvement program and performance with key performance metrics is now vital to the organization because it is compared against data for other organizations by which of the following? (Choose all that apply.)
   a. Accrediting agencies
   b. Insurance payers
   c. Healthcare consumers
   d. Licensing agencies

3. With increasing emphasis on interdisciplinary quality improvement, which of the following have emerged in hospitals? (Choose all that apply.)
   a. Medical staff committees
   b. Quality improvement teams
   c. Quality councils
   d. Hospital quality improvement committees

4. In which of the following quality functions does the Joint Commission require the medical staff to be involved? (Choose all that apply.)
   a. Use of medications
   b. Medical assessment and treatment of patients
   c. Nursing staffing levels
   d. Operative and other procedures

5. Reasons for evaluating use of medications include which of the following? (Choose all that apply.)
   a. Virtually all hospital patients receive medications.
   b. Many new drugs are being introduced.
   c. Untoward drug reactions may occur.
   d. The cost of drugs is drawing attention.

6. Reasons for evaluating blood and blood products usage include which of the following?
   a. Blood and blood products are a precious commodity.
   b. Blood and blood products are always readily available.
   c. Blood and blood products can cause harm.
   d. Blood and blood products can be life saving.

7. Many hospitals have eliminated their use of a blood usage committee and a pathologist performs that function.
   a. True
   b. False

8. Review of operative procedures is required only for those procedures performed in operating rooms.
   a. True
   b. False

9. The medical staff services professional must be aware of the practitioner-specific information produced by quality committees and must facilitate the availability of this information for use in which of the following? (Choose all that apply.)
   a. The evaluation of practitioner performance at reappointment
   b. The medical staff's ongoing professional practice evaluation
   c. Selection of peer review panels
   d. The medical staff's focused professional practice evaluation process

10. Reasons for using external peer review include which of the following? (Choose all that apply.)
    a. Adequate expertise in the specialty under review
    b. Internal peer review has not been effective in improving performance
    c. Conflicting or ambiguous recommendations from peer reviewers
    d. Conflict of interest with internal peer review

QUIZ 12

Chapter 12: Program-Specific Accreditation

1. Hospital institutional review boards (IRBs) are required to oversee which of the following with regard to human subjects involved in clinical investigations?
   a. Medication dosage
   b. Clinical trials
   c. Protection of rights and welfare
   d. Clinical investigations

2. Products under investigation that must be evaluated by the Food and Drug Administration (FDA) include which of the following? (Choose all that apply.)
   a. Medical devices
   b. Durable medical equipment
   c. Drugs
   d. Oxygen tents

3. In addition to review and approval of protocols for study, what is the institutional review board required to do with regard to investigations?
   a. Grade them
   b. Summarize them
   c. Monitor them
   d. Disregard them

4. Which of the following persons must be included in the membership of an institutional review board? (Choose all that apply.)
   a. All members of the same gender
   b. One member who has a nonscientific background
   c. One member whose only affiliation with the institution is institutional review board membership
   d. One member who has a scientific background

5. The FDA specifies that in addition to minutes and protocols, which records and reports must the institutional review board maintain?
   a. Positive results
   b. Cure rates
   c. Patient noncompliance with the study protocol
   d. Adverse reactions

6. Which organization sponsors a voluntary approval program for hospital cancer programs?

    a. American Cancer Society

    b. American College of Surgeons

    c. American Medical Association

    d. American Hospital Association

7. Which of the following are American College of Surgeons requirements for a committee that oversees the cancer program? (Choose all that apply.)

    a. Must be a standing committee

    b. Must have scheduled meetings

    c. Must be multidisciplinary

    d. Must have defined authority

8. Which of the following are American College of Surgeons–required functions of the cancer committee? (Choose all that apply.)

    a. Development of treatment plans

    b. Development and evaluation of goals for patient care

    c. Development of critical pathways

    d. Development and implementation of plans to evaluate the quality of cancer registry data and activity

9. Match the description below with the trauma center level. Note the matching letter in the space provided.

    a. Level I   _____ Provides advanced trauma life support

    b. Level II   _____ Provides initial definitive trauma care

    c. Level III   _____ Is usually a university-based teaching hospital

    d. Level IV   _____ Provides prompt assessment, resuscitation, and patient stabilization

10. According to the American College of Surgeons' trauma guidelines, which of the following is required for Level I and Level II trauma centers?

    a. Emergency room call list

    b. Emergency services committee

    c. Medical specialty roster

    d. Multidisciplinary trauma committee

QUIZ 13

Chapter 13: Practitioner Health and Behavior Issues

1. What percentage of physicians is estimated by the literature, to be impaired by drug or alcohol abuse?

    a. 50–60%

    b. 14–20%

    c. 8–10%

    d. 35–45%

2. The Joint Commission standards require hospitals to have a process to address physician well-being that is separate from the disciplinary action process.

    a. True

    b. False

3. Which of the following is a word that would describe a successful "impaired physician" program?

    a. Retaliatory

    b. Accusatory

    c. Judgmental

    d. Nonpunitive

4. Prospective members of a committee that deals with practitioner well-being could include which of the following?

    a. Partners or associates

    b. Family members

    c. Staff members or administrators recovering from impairment

    d. The individual who reported the practitioner

5. Which of the following is the term associated with the activity of discussing issues with an impaired practitioner and supporting his or her removal from active practice to find formal assistance?

    a. Interception

    b. Intemperance

    c. Intervention

    d. Summary suspension

6. Which of the following could be a possible symptom that would alert to a physician having problems with alcohol or drugs?
   a. High performance with increased productivity
   b. Consistent promptness
   c. Developing large numbers of friends
   d. Inappropriate orders and treatment

7. Wording in a contract between an impaired physician and a practitioner well-being committee would include which of the following?
   a. Agreement to continue the practice of medicine while receiving treatment
   b. Agreement to identify a primary care physician who will consult with the well-being committee
   c. Agreement to notify his or her patients of the outcome of the therapy
   d. Agreement to have six months of treatment

8. The monitoring process is the gathering and evaluation of information concerning an impaired physician and his or her treatment. This information should come from which of the following?
   a. Friends of the physician
   b. Office colleagues
   c. Ongoing therapist
   d. Department chair

9. A monitoring plan for a practitioner recovering from alcohol or drug addiction should incorporate which of the following elements?
   a. Release of information
   b. List of symptoms noted
   c. Reasons given by physician as to why he or she became impaired
   d. Length of time of impairment

10. Respect and long-standing service often prevent a medical staff from addressing the aging physician who no longer has the skills to provide high-quality care. Which of the following could be included in a policy for addressing the aging physician?
    a. Automatic honorary staff status after age 65
    b. Automatic replacement in practice with a younger physician at age 65
    c. Annual reappointments
    d. Automatic review of 100% of medical records after age 65

QUIZ 14

Chapter 14: Effective Meeting Management

1. To efficiently and effectively schedule medical staff meetings, what should the medical staff services department prepare?

    a. List of committees

    b. Annual calendar

    c. Biennial calendar

    d. Master calendar

2. Well-prepared meeting agendas can be powerful tools.

    a. True

    b. False

3. How does a well-prepared agenda assist with the conduct of meetings? (Choose all that apply.)

    a. It can influence the outcome of agenda items.

    b. It helps the chair maintain control during the meeting.

    c. It assists with preparation of meeting minutes.

    d. It allows committee members to prepare for discussion.

4. If there is potential for negotiation or deliberation of important issues in a meeting, it may be helpful for the chair of the meeting to sit on one side of a rectangular table.

    a. True

    b. False

5. Establishing a paper or electronic agenda hold file is not an effective means for keeping track of agenda items.

    a. True

    b. False

6. What is the purpose of parliamentary procedure? (Choose all that apply.)

    a. Assists with orderly consideration of issues

    b. Guarantees the minority a voice

    c. Assures that the majority rules

    d. Assures that the minority rules

7. Strict adherence to parliamentary procedure can be a hindrance in some meetings.
   a. True
   b. False

8. According to *Robert's Rules of Order*, in which order do these agenda items appear? List them in order from 1 to 4.
   _____ a. New business
   _____ b. Committee reports
   _____ c. Unfinished business
   _____ d. Reading of minutes

9. According to *Robert's Rules of Order*, when a motion is made, which action is required prior to further discussion of the matter?
   a. The item is tabled
   b. The motion is amended
   c. The chair calls for a vote
   d. The motion is seconded

10. According to *Robert's Rules of Order*, when a motion has been made, seconded, and discussed, what is the next step?
    a. The item is deferred
    b. The motion is amended
    c. The item is tabled
    d. The chair calls for a vote

QUIZ 15

Chapter 15: Introduction to the Law

1. Which of the following is highest in the hierarchy of law?
   a. U.S. Constitution
   b. U.S. Supreme Court decisions
   c. Common law decisions
   d. State decisions

2. Where did the common law used in the United States have its origins?
   a. Greece
   b. Roman Empire
   c. England
   d. France

3. Which of the following is known as the common law principle that provides that the courts apply previous decisions to subsequent cases involving similar facts and questions?
   a. Respondeat superior
   b. Stare decisis
   c. Res gestae
   d. Res judicata

4. Which of the following are branches of government? (Choose all that apply.)
   a. Executive
   b. Legislative
   c. Judicial
   d. Constitutional

5. Which of the following is a civil wrong committed by one person against the person or property of another?
   a. Crime
   b. Misdemeanor
   c. Tort
   d. Trespass

6. What is the commission or omission of an act that a reasonably prudent person would or would not do?
   a. Negligence
   b. Retribution
   c. Tort
   d. Vengeance

7. What, in negligence, is the failure to act when there is a duty to act?
   a. Nonfeasance
   b. Malfeasance
   c. Malpractice
   d. Misfeasance

8. In a malpractice case, which of the following individuals could be accused of negligence? (Choose all that apply.)
   a. Physician
   b. Pharmacist
   c. Licensed registered nurse
   d. Dietary aide

9. Which of the following describes the conduct expected of an individual in a given situation?
   a. Duty to use due care
   b. Standard of care
   c. Breach of duty
   d. Proximate cause

10. Which of the following is an element of negligence that must be present to establish negligence? (Choose all that apply.)
    a. Proximate cause
    b. Duty to use due care
    c. Breach of duty
    d. Injury

QUIZ 16

Chapter 16: Medical Staff Law and Important Legal Cases

1. The relationship between a hospital and its medical staff, as well as the relationship between the medical staff and practitioners seeking access to the medical staff, is the subject of which of the following? (Choose all that apply.)
   a. State legislation
   b. Case law
   c. Federal legislation
   d. Local legislation

2. Which of the following mandate a hospital to credential practitioners seeking to provide services in the hospital?
   a. Federal legislation
   b. Accreditation requirements
   c. Hospital licensure requirements
   d. Case law

3. Self-governance by the medical staff may support a finding by the courts that the medical staff is an entity separate from the hospital.
   a. True
   b. False

4. Whether the medical staff is a separate entity from the hospital has been addressed conclusively in the courts in all jurisdictions.
   a. True
   b. False

5. State statutes or regulations may address which of the following issues pertinent to the medical staff setting? (Choose all that apply.)
   a. Medical professionals can access the medical staff
   b. Procedures must be afforded if appointment is denied
   c. Membership criteria may be required as a condition of appointment or as a basis for denial
   d. Privileges of confidentiality and immunity are available for peer review actions and participants in peer review

6. Which of the following does case law in medical staff areas generally address?
   a. Reasons a hospital may use to exclude or terminate a practitioner
   b. Specifics as to which provisions are required for inclusion in the medical staff bylaws
   c. Procedures used to accomplish exclusion or termination of membership or privileges
   d. Whether the hospital may be liable for credentialing of practitioners

7. Which legal doctrines are used to hold a hospital liable for actions of a practitioner providing services in the hospital setting? (Choose all that apply.)
   a. Respondeat superior/vicarious liability
   b. Charitable immunity
   c. Ostensible agency
   d. Independent liability/corporate liability

8. A practitioner may seek to hold the hospital liable for denying membership or for terminating membership or privileges focusing on which of the following?
   a. Reasons for the hospital's action
   b. The manner in which the action was taken
   c. Both a and b
   d. Neither a nor b

9. Which of the following are standards established for taking professional review actions that would qualify for limited immunity under the Health Care Quality Improvement Act (HCQIA)? (Choose all that apply.)
   a. In the reasonable belief that the action was in the furtherance of quality health care
   b. After a reasonable effort to obtain the facts
   c. After adequate notice and fair hearing procedures are afforded
   d. In the reasonable belief that the action was warranted by the facts known

10. Which of the following are rights afforded by HCQIA to an adversely affected practitioner in a hearing situation?
    a. Notice of the proposed action
    b. A list of witnesses who will testify
    c. Representation by an attorney or other person of practitioner's choice
    d. A copy of the hearing transcript at the facility's expense